Emergency Radiology

Emergency Radiology

Edited by

Mayil S. Krishnam
UCI Medical Center, University of California, Irvine, USA

and

John Curtis
University Hospital Aintree, Liverpool, UK

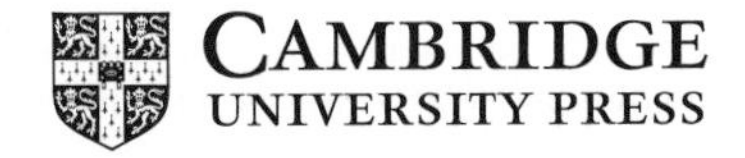

CAMBRIDGE UNIVERSITY PRESS
Cambridge, New York, Melbourne, Madrid, Cape Town, Singapore,
São Paulo, Delhi, Dubai, Tokyo

Cambridge University Press
The Edinburgh Building, Cambridge CB2 8RU, UK

Published in the United States of America by
Cambridge University Press, New York

www.cambridge.org
Information on this title: www.cambridge.org/9780521672474

First published 2010

Printed in the United Kingdom at the University Press, Cambridge

A catalogue record for this publication is available from the British Library

Library of Congress Cataloging-in-Publication Data

Emergency radiology / edited by Mayil S. Krishnam and John Curtis.
p. ; cm.
Includes bibliographical references and index.
ISBN 978-0-521-67247-4 (pbk.)
1. Radiography, Medical–Handbooks, manuals, etc. 2. Medical emergencies–Imaging–Handbooks, manuals, etc. I. Krishnam, Mayil S. II. Curtis, John (John Michael)
[DNLM: 1. Emergencies–Handbooks. 2. Radiography–Handbooks. WN 39 E53 2009]
RC78.E5823 2009
616.07′572–dc22

2009036358

ISBN 978-0-521-67247-4 Paperback

To my wife, Shafiqa and our beautiful kids, Neha and Kavin, you are my joy!
To my mother, father and brothers, for their endless love and support.

Mayil S. Krishnam

To Juliet and Matthew, for your constant love and encouragement, always – I dedicate my work to you both.
To my parents for their love.

John Curtis

Contents

Contributors

Shivarama Avula
Consultant Radiologist,
Department of Radiology,
Alder Hey Children's NHS Foundation Trust,
Liverpool, UK

Nick Barnes
Consultant Radiologist,
Clinical Director,
Department of Radiology,
Alder Hey Children's NHS Foundation Trust,
Liverpool, UK

John Curtis
Consultant Radiologist,
University Hospital Aintree,
Liverpool, UK

Swati P. Deshmane
Diagnostic Cardiovascular Imaging,
Department of Radiological Sciences,
University of California, Ronald Reagan Medical Center,
Los Angeles, CA, USA

Mayil S. Krishnam
Associate Clinical Professor of Radiology,
Division Director, Cardiovascular and Thoracic Imaging,
UCI Medical Center
University of California, Irvine
California, USA

Michael Murphy
Consultant Interventional Radiologist,
South Infirmary-Victoria University Hospital,
Cork, Ireland

Sacha Niven
Consultant Neuroradiologist,
The Walton Centre for Neurology and Neurosurgery, Liverpool, UK

Jolanta Webb
Consultant Radiologist,
Ultrasound Specialist,
University Hospital Aintree,
Liverpool, UK

Advisory contributors

Amin Matin
Resident,
Department of Radiological Sciences,
University of California at Los Angeles,
Los Angeles, CA, USA

Anderanik Tomasian
Resident,
Mallinckrodt Institute of Radiology,
Washington University School of Medicine,
St. Louis, Missouri, USA

Special acknowledgments

Barbara Kadell
(GI Radiology Chief, UCLA)

Noriko Salamon
(Neuroradiologist, UCLA)

Ines Boechat
(Pediatric Radiologist, UCLA)

Antoinette Gomes
(Interventional Radiologist, UCLA)

Nagesh Ragavendra
(Ultrasound Specialist, UCLA)

Allen Cohen
(Body CT Radiologist, UCI)

Foreword

This is a highly informative radiology pocket book dealing with general principles, instructions and techniques for procedures, use of contrast, analgesia, monitoring, interventional equipment and 'pearls' that summarize the essence of each chapter. Radiology, anatomy and pathology, pediatrics and adult radiology; they are all in one book. This is clearly written and a great bench book to have at hand for clinicians and radiologists to help decide on best practice for requesting imaging in and out of hours. It will be useful for registrars and consultants in all specialities. The pocket book is easy to read and is well worth owning.

Professor Philip Gishen
MB, B.ch., DMRD, FRCR

Director of Imaging
Imperial College Healthcare NHS Trust, UK

Preface

The principal aim of this pocket book is to provide a quick radiological reference in the vast array of medical and surgical emergencies encountered on-call. It aims to assist radiology residents and specialist registrars throughout the globe in accurately interpreting the various diagnostic images and investigations during emergency situations. It will also serve to improve the understanding of performing therapeutic and diagnostic interventional procedures that are commonly encountered during emergencies.

This book is intended to be a quick reference handbook in every radiology and A&E department globally. It covers a wide range of emergencies and specifically targets on-call radiologists and trainees who deal with these emergencies. We feel that this guide in emergency radiology will be very useful for all radiologists who want to regain or retain their skills and confidence in acute care imaging.

This book is primarily intended for radiology residents, registrars, junior attending physicians and consultants across the world. Radiologists in private practice may find this book useful to maintain their skills in a wide range of emergencies. The intended readership is not limited to radiologists but also includes medical students, radiology assistants, physicians, surgeons, ER doctors and radiographers who work closely with radiologists.

This book has numerous high-quality images of various radiological emergencies involving head, cardiovascular, chest, abdomen, pelvis and extremities. It also covers radiological emergencies in pediatrics and musculoskeletal imaging and in modalities such as fluoroscopy, ultrasound and MRI with depiction of corresponding high-resolution images. Under each diagnosis/topic in this book, there are technical notes which will assist on-call radiologists to provide a protocol for the study specific to the need of patients. In addition to salient radiological features, each topic in the book briefly mentions some useful tips and pitfalls under "pearls" and some helpful information on signs and symptoms under "clinical features," which would assist the on-call radiologist especially when receiving calls out-of-hours.

This book will be very useful to trainees in the preparation of international radiology exams including FRCR, DMRD, ABR, MD (Radiodiagnosis) and also in the preparation of medical and surgical exams such as MRCP and MRCS.

We are grateful to various authors and contributors of this book for their excellent work to make a practical and useful survival guide for on-call radiologists. We also express our gratitude to Drs Barbara Kadell, Ines Boechat, Noriko Salamon, Antoinette Gomes, Nagesh Ragavendra, and Allen Cohen and Allison Louie (Research Assistant at UCI) for their excellent contributions to the book. Finally, we are greatly indebted to our families for their constant support and love throughout this process to complete this book successfully.

Mayil S. Krishnam, USA
John Curtis, UK

CT emergencies

Head

Mayil S. Krishnam

1.1 General principles

A CT scan of the brain is the most commonly performed cross-sectional imaging during out-of-hours periods. See Fig. 1.1.

Indications

Altered Glasgow Coma Scale (GCS), acute confusional state, sudden onset severe headache, head injury, drowsiness, status epilepticus, post-epileptic with decreasing consciousness level or with focal neurology, anoxic–hypoxic injury to brain (post-cardiac arrest).

Technique

Axial CT brain.

Contrast

Intravenous (IV) contrast is usually not needed except in cases of suspected intracranial or meningeal infection, arteriovenous malformations (AVMs) and suspected tumors. Following a road traffic accident (RTA), an initial non-contrast head scan should be carried out to exclude extra-axial or intracranial hemorrhage before a dynamic contrast scan of chest or abdomen. A contrast-enhanced CT scan of the brain may be helpful in suspected isodense subdural hematoma.

Review areas in a "near normal" CT head scan:

1. Foramen magnum: High density blood around the brainstem - sub-arachnoid hemorrhage (SAH), tight foramen magnum–tonsillar herniation suggests raised intracranial pressure.

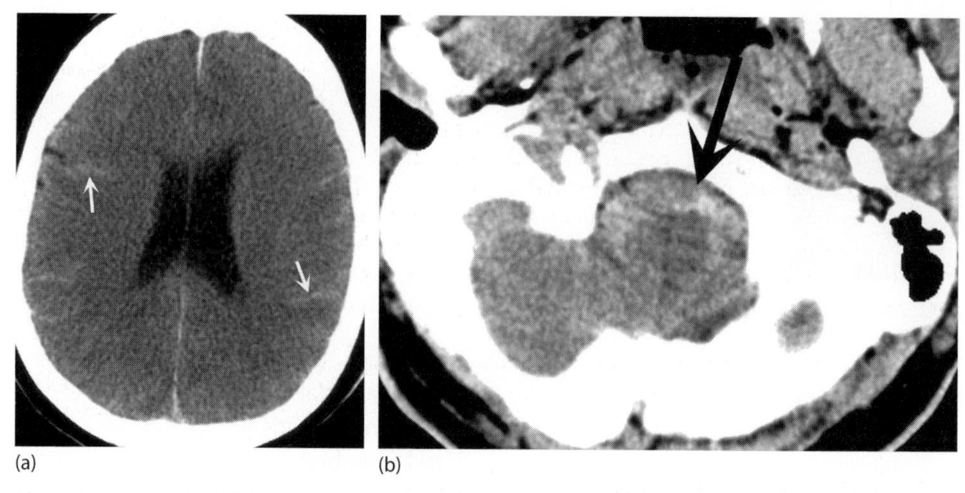

Fig. 1.1. (a) Traumatic SAH. Axial non-contrast CT shows linear hyperdensities within the cerebral sulci (arrows), consistent with blood in the subarachnoid space. (b) Spontaneous SAH. Axial non-contrast CT shows hyperdensity anterior to the brainstem at the level of the foramen magnum (arrow), where only hypodense CSF should normally be present. Note the tight foramen magnum without free CSF space.

2. Cerebello-pontine (CP) angle and pituitary fossa: Isodense soft tissue mass – give IV contrast. High density in the pituitary on a non-contrast brain scan may indicate hemorrhage.
3. Brainstem: Hemorrhage, infarct, central pontine myelinolysis (low attenuation).
4. Gyri recti: Hidden area for contusions, mass.
5. Vessels: Dense middle cerebral (MCA) and basilar arteries may represent early thrombus – look for infarct.

   Hyperdense venous sinuses on unenhanced CT in venous sinus thrombosis.
6. Cisterns: High density in the ambient, quadrigeminal and pre-pontine cisterns – (SAH).
7. Ventricles: High-density blood/CSF level in the dependent posterior horn ventricle – a sign of SAH, extending into the ventricle.

   Temporal horn dilatation is an early sign of obstructive hydrocephalus. This temporal horn dilatation is disproportionate to the sulci.

   Inter- and intraventricular regions for abnormal soft tissue mass (colloid cyst of the third ventricle).
8. Interhemispheric fissure: High density in SAH, non-accidental injury (NAI).

   Low density suggests subdural empyema in appropriate clinical context – give IV contrast to demonstrate peripheral rim enhancement.

   Very low density equal to CSF density implies cerebral atrophy.
9. Sulci and gyri: Asymmetry, mass effect, isolated high density within the sulci (traumatic SAH), effacement insular ribbon – sign of early infarction.
10. Temporal lobe: Unilateral hypodensity may be due to herpes simplex encephalitis. Can be bilateral (often difficult to differentiate from artefact). Suggests lumbar puncture and MRI.
11. Superior slices of the scan: Always ensure that the uppermost slices of the brain are obtained to look for hidden pathologies like parafalcine meningioma, traumatic SAH or a small subdural bleed.
12. Bones: Review mandibular condyles, mastoid bones, skull base, inferior orbits, posterior occipital bone, foramen magnum as well as C1 and C2 on bone windows.

Pearls

- A doubtful abnormality noticed on thick section can be resolved by a thin section through the apparent lesion.
- Know and understand the Glasgow Coma Scale.
- Go through the above review areas of the brain before calling a normal study.
- The sulci should be visible as hypodense clefts in the peripheral cortex. Note: In young patients, higher brain volume relative to intracranial space may render sulci more difficult to see, although sulci in the vertex will usually still be clearly identifiable. While sulci may sometimes be hard to visualize, hyperdensity within sulcal spaces is always abnormal.
- High-density beam-hardening artefact can simulate SAH but the foramen magnum is usually not squashed.
- The anteroinferior temporal and frontal lobes are common locations for brain contusions following deceleration trauma.

1.2 Acute subarachnoid hemorrhage

Blood in the subarachnoid spaces. See Fig. 1.2.

Clinical

Sudden onset of severe headache associated with nausea, vomiting or altered level of consciousness. Altered conscious level and/or focal neurological deficit warrants an urgent CT brain to identify hydrocephalus and/or hematoma, which may need urgent neurosurgical treatment. 75–80% of SAH is due to spontaneous rupture of cerebral aneurysms. The site of hematoma is not considered as a reliable indicator of the site of aneurysm.

Technique

Non-contrast CT brain. Computerized tomographic angiography (CTA) of the brain can be performed to look for ruptured intracranial aneurysm as the cause of SAH.

CT brain findings

1. High attenuation (blood) in the cisterns and sulci. Typically blood is present in the suprasellar cistern near the circle of Willis.
   Sylvian fissure/temporal lobe hematoma – in middle cerebral artery aneurysm rupture.
   Frontal horn and frontal lobe blood – anterior communicating artery aneurysm rupture.
   Blood in the interpeduncular and CP cistern and extending to brainstem – basilar artery aneurysm rupture.
   Blood in the 4th ventricle, foramen magnum and around the brainstem – internal carotid artery (ICA) rupture.
2. Blood–fluid levels in the posterior horn of the lateral ventricle suggest intraventricular extension of SAH.
3. Subtle signs of SAH: Blood in the interpeduncular cistern, foramen magnum and ventricle. High-density asymmetrical tentorium cerebelli, and high-density sulci in traumatic SAH.

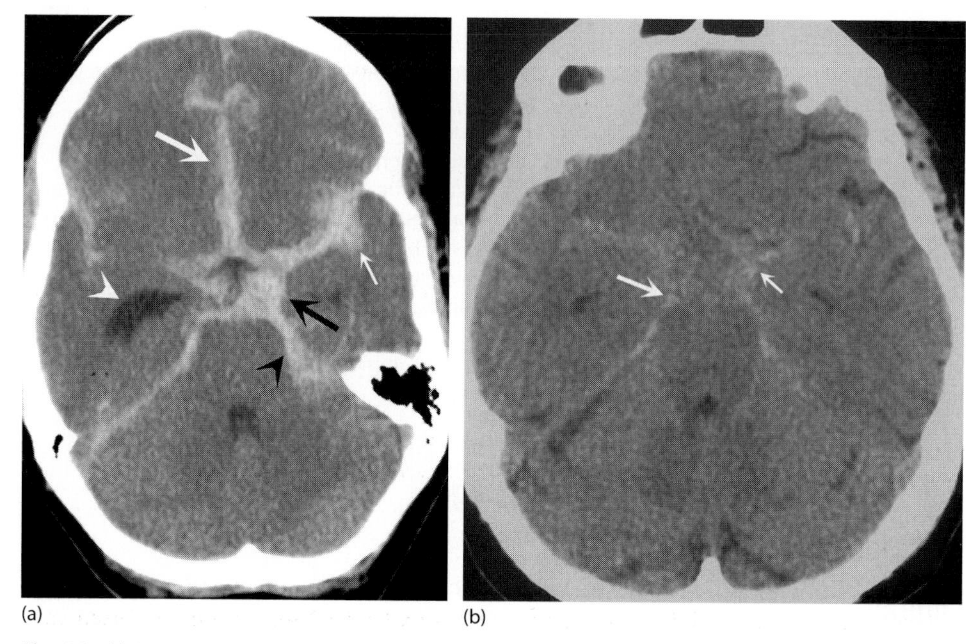

Fig. 1.2. (a) Acute spontaneous SAH. Axial non-contrast CT shows marked hyperdensity in the suprasellar cistern (black arrow), interhemispheric fissure (white large arrow), cerebellopontine cistern (black arrowhead), and sylvian fissure (thin white arrow) indicative of acute subarachnoid blood. Note secondary hydrocephalus of the lateral ventricles (white arrowhead). (b) Subtle SAH. Axial non-contrast CT shows mild hyperdensity in the subarachnoid spaces of the suprasellar (thin arrow) and perimesencephalic (thick arrow) cisterns.

4. Mass effect: Subfalcine/tentorial herniation. Hydrocephalus – earliest sign is temporal horn dilatation – results from decreased CSF resorption by the arachnoid granulations in the presence of blood. Tight foramen magnum and/or basal cistern effacement are signs of impending coning.
5. An aneurysm may be visible as a rounded soft tissue mass with or without rim calcification which enhances intensely following intravenous contrast.

Pearls

- Suggest urgent neurosurgical opinion and make sure images are available to the neurosurgeon.
- CT of the brain is very sensitive in the first 48 hours and thereafter its sensitivity falls to 50%. Chronic anemia patients can have low-density blood. A negative CT brain requires lumbar puncture to exclude SAH.
- CT cerebral angiography with or without more invasive digital subtraction angiography is often required at a later stage to identify aneurysms.
- Perimesencephalic bleeding is due to venous hemorrhage with no aneurysm and usually carries a good prognosis.
- Normal cerebellar tentorium reflection is symmetrical and uniformly of high density with well-defined anterior concave margin towards the ventricles.

Suggested reading

Besenski N. Traumatic injuries: imaging of head injuries. *Eur Radiol* 2002;**12**(6):1237–1252.

Lenhart M *et al.* Cerebral CT angiography in the diagnosis of acute subarachnoid hemorrhage. *Acta Radiol* 1997;**38**(5):791–796.

Zee CS, Go JL. CT of head trauma. *Neuroimaging Clin N Am* 1998;**8**:525–539.

1.3 Acute subdural hematoma

Extra-axial collection of blood between the dura mater and cortical surface of the brain is due to venous hemorrhage. See Fig. 1.3.

Clinical

Headache, drowsiness, focal neurology and unequal pupils.
Etiology: Trauma, surgery, shunts, anticoagulant therapy.

Technique

Unenhanced CT brain is the first procedure of choice. Intravenous contrast may be helpful to identify an isodense subdural hematoma. MR is particularly sensitive in its detection.

Findings

1. Concavo-convex high-density extra-axial collection of blood seen along the surface of the brain with concavity towards the midline.
2. Fluid level due to different stages of hematoma. High density in acute ($<$ 1 week), intermediate/isodensity recent (1–2 weeks) and low density/CSF density represents 2–3 weeks old. High-density acute blood is seen in the dependent posterior subdural space in a supine position.
3. Mass effect: Effacement of ipsilateral sulci and ventricles, sub-falcine or sub-tentorial herniation with contralateral ventricular hydrocephalus.
4. *Contre coup* parenchymal contusions or hematoma.
5. Associated skull vault and basal skull fractures and soft tissue hematoma.

Pearls

- Subdural hematoma (SDH) is crescent shaped (concavo-convex) with the concavity towards midline of the brain. Extradural hematoma (EDH) is biconvex or lens shaped with the convexity towards the midline. EDH is usually smaller in volume compared with SDH. EDH does not cross the suture line. Subdural hematomas cross the suture line of the skull vault but do not cross the interhemisphere fissure.
- Small SDH: can be easily missed. Look for apparent asymmetrical "thickening" of the skull vault, effacement of cortical sulci and lateral ventricle, and dilated temporal horns. You should always widen the window width to better evaluate for subtle bleeds along the calvarium (WL 40 WW 150).
- Isodense SDH is associated with a subacute presentation and has similar density to the adjacent brain tissue. Look for sulci buckling, and absence of sulci at the peripheries.

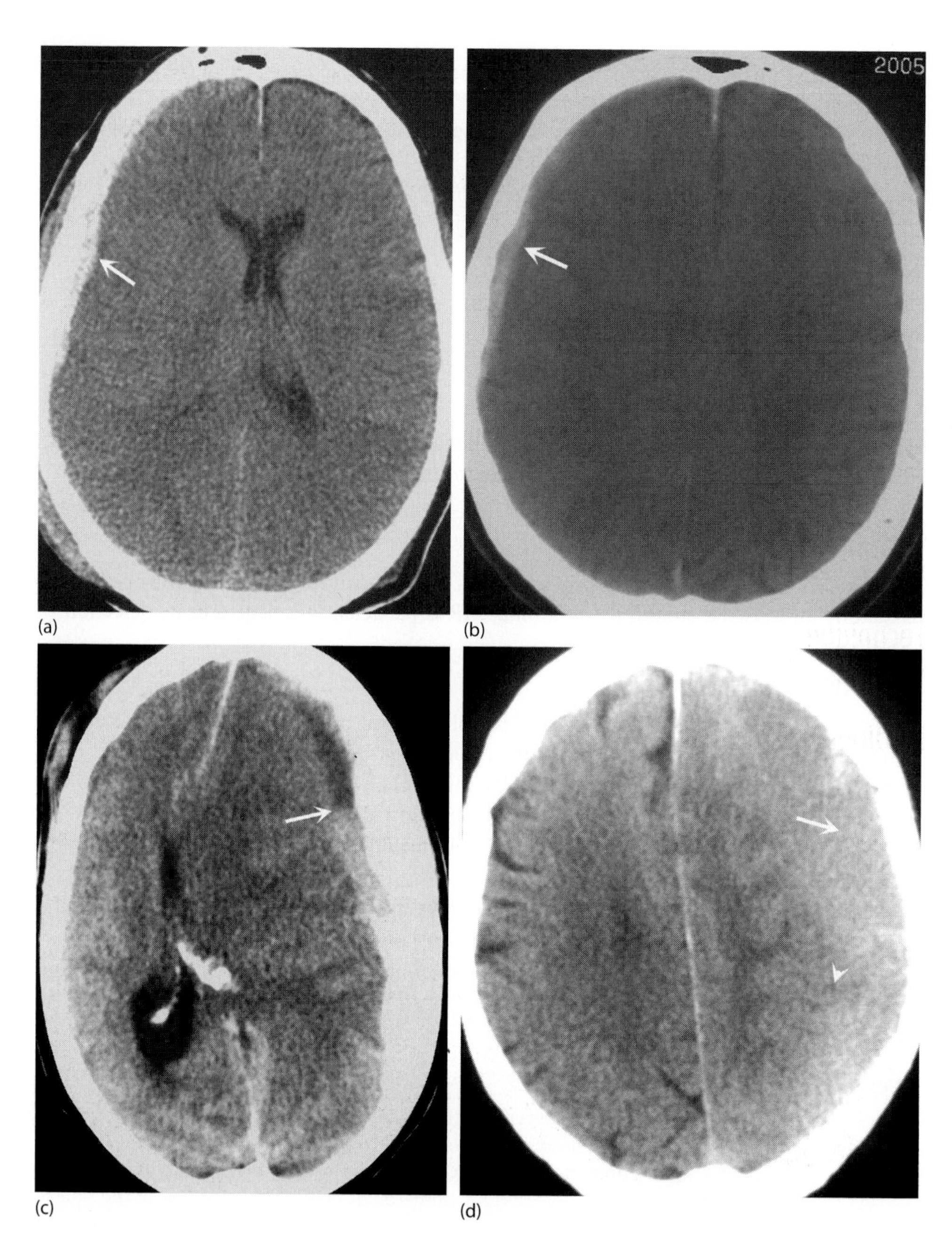

(a) (b) (c) (d)

Fig. 1.3. (a, b) Acute SDH. (a) Non-contrast CT shows a subtle thin rim of hyperdensity (arrow) along the right inner table of the skull, with mild sulcal effacement. (b) The same patient's study with "hematoma windows" (L40, W150) more easily demonstrates the hematoma (arrow). (c) Acute on chronic SDH. Non-contrast axial CT image shows fluid–fluid level (arrow), with higher-density acute blood layering dependently. Note the marked mass effect with effacement of the left lateral ventricle and midline shift to the right. (d) Isodense SDH. Non-contrast CT shows effacement of sulci on the left side (arrowhead) and a large subdural collection (arrow) that is isodense to cortical parenchyma.

Enhancement of the cortical interface but not the hematoma following IV contrast is helpful in identifying an isodense SDH.
- Blood within the sulci and ventricle suggests extension into subarachnoid space. Slit-like ventricles may be seen in bilateral SDH.
- Over time, a hyperdense acute bleed will evolve through isodense and ultimately hypodense phases with the breakdown of blood products.

Suggested reading

Refer to Section 1.2.

1.4 Extradural hematoma

Extra-axial collection of blood between the dura mater and inner table of the skull is usually due to arterial injury as a result of head trauma. See Fig. 1.4.

Clinical

Refer to Section 1.3.

Technique

Unenhanced CT brain scan.

Findings

1. Biconvex shape of high-density blood located in the periphery of the cranial cavity.
2. Unlike SDH it crosses the dural reflection but not the vault sutures.
3. Mass effect: Subfalcine, tentorial, brainstem herniations and diffuse or localized cerebral edema.
4. Associated vault or base of skull fractures, pneumocephalus and soft tissue hematoma.

Pearls

- EDH represents arterial hemorrhage and it needs immediate neurosurgical attention. Hypodensity within the hematoma represents unclotted active extravasation of blood (the "swirl sign").
- Alter the window to look for associated skull fractures, subdural hematoma.
- Look for associated signs of traumatic subarachnoid hemorrhage, *coup* and *contre coup* parenchymal contusions.

Suggested reading

Refer to Section 1.2.

1.5 Traumatic parenchymal brain injury

Brain parenchymal injury can occur with or without evidence of subdural or extradural hematoma, and is most likely due to traumatic acceleration and deceleration injury. See Fig. 1.5.

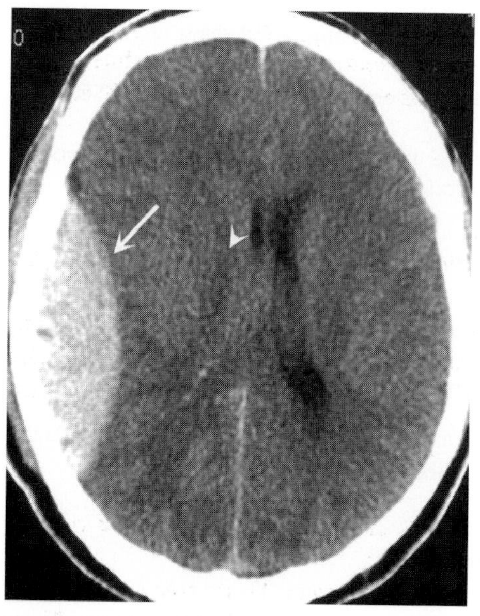

Fig. 1.4. Acute extradural (epidural) hematoma. Non-contrast CT shows a biconvex or lens-shaped hyperdense extradural hematoma (arrow). Note effacement of the right lateral ventricle (arrowhead) and midline shift to the left indicative of subfalcine herniation. Posteriorly it is limited by the lambdoid suture.

Clinical

Headache, altered level of consciousness, falling GCS level.

Technique

Unenhanced CT scan is sufficient.

Findings

Can be classified as contusions, diffuse axonal brain injury, diffuse cerebral edema and brainstem herniations.

Contusions

Focal small hemorrhagic foci are seen usually within the frontal and temporal lobes.

Focal hypodensity areas seen due to associated cerebral edema.

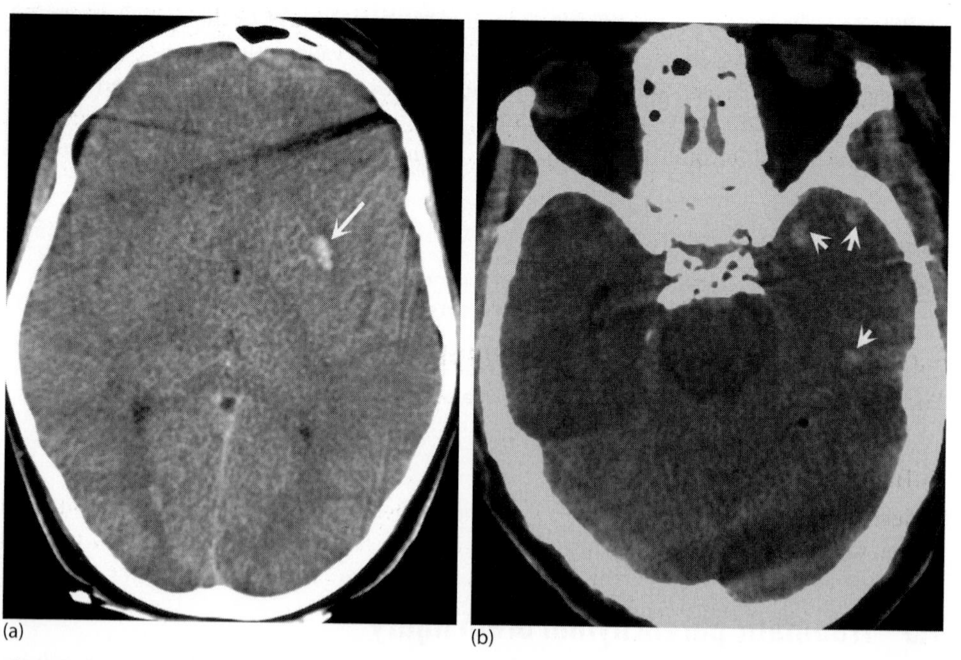

Fig. 1.5. (a) Axonal brain injury. Axial non-contrast CT shows gray–white matter interface focal hyperdensity (arrow) in the left frontal lobe. (b) Brain contusions. Axial non-contrast CT shows several hyperdense foci (arrows) along the anteroinferior left temporal lobe, consistent with small intraparenchymal foci of blood.

Diffuse axonal brain injury (DAI)

Small foci of hemorrhage are present at the gray–white matter junction, deep white matter, corpus callosum and brainstem. DAI may be associated with herniations and cerebral edema.

Diffuse cerebral edema

Either due to hyperemia or increased interstitial edema.

Seen as mass effect causing effacement of cortical sulci, ventricles with associated dilated temporal horns.

Diffuse low-density cerebral parenchyma due to cerebral edema causes an apparently high attenuation of cerebellum (white sign) relative to the rest of the brain. There is also increased attenuation of the arterial vessels and meninges and effacement of the cisterns (pseudo-SAH).

Brainstem herniations

Subfalcine: Common type with cingular gyri herniations. Distortion of anterior cerebral artery can cause secondary ischemia and infarction in the frontal lobe.

Tentorial: Due to herniations of temporal lobe and brainstem. This is seen as effacement of basal cisterns, dilatation of temporal horns and midline shift of brain parenchyma. These are all signs of raised intracranial pressure.

Tonsillar: herniation of the cerebellar tonsils causes a tight and effaced foramen magnum. This is a sign of imminent coning.

Pearls

- Contusions and DAI are seen well on a MR of the brain.
- DAI is associated with high morbidity and mortality.
- Always look for associated extra-axial hematoma, soft tissue injury and skull fracture.
- *Coup* injuries are smaller than *contre coup*.

Suggested reading

Refer to Section 1.2.

1.6 Intracerebral/cerebellar hemorrhage

Focal collection of blood in the cerebellum or cerebral hemispheres. See Fig. 1.6.

Clinical

Sudden onset headache, unexplained confusion, altered level of consciousness and focal motor weakness. Risk factors: Hypertension, blood disorders, anticoagulants and amyloid microangiopathy. The most common locations of hypertensive bleeds are the putamen, subcortical white matter, cerebellum, thalamus and pons.

Technique

Non-contrast CT brain.

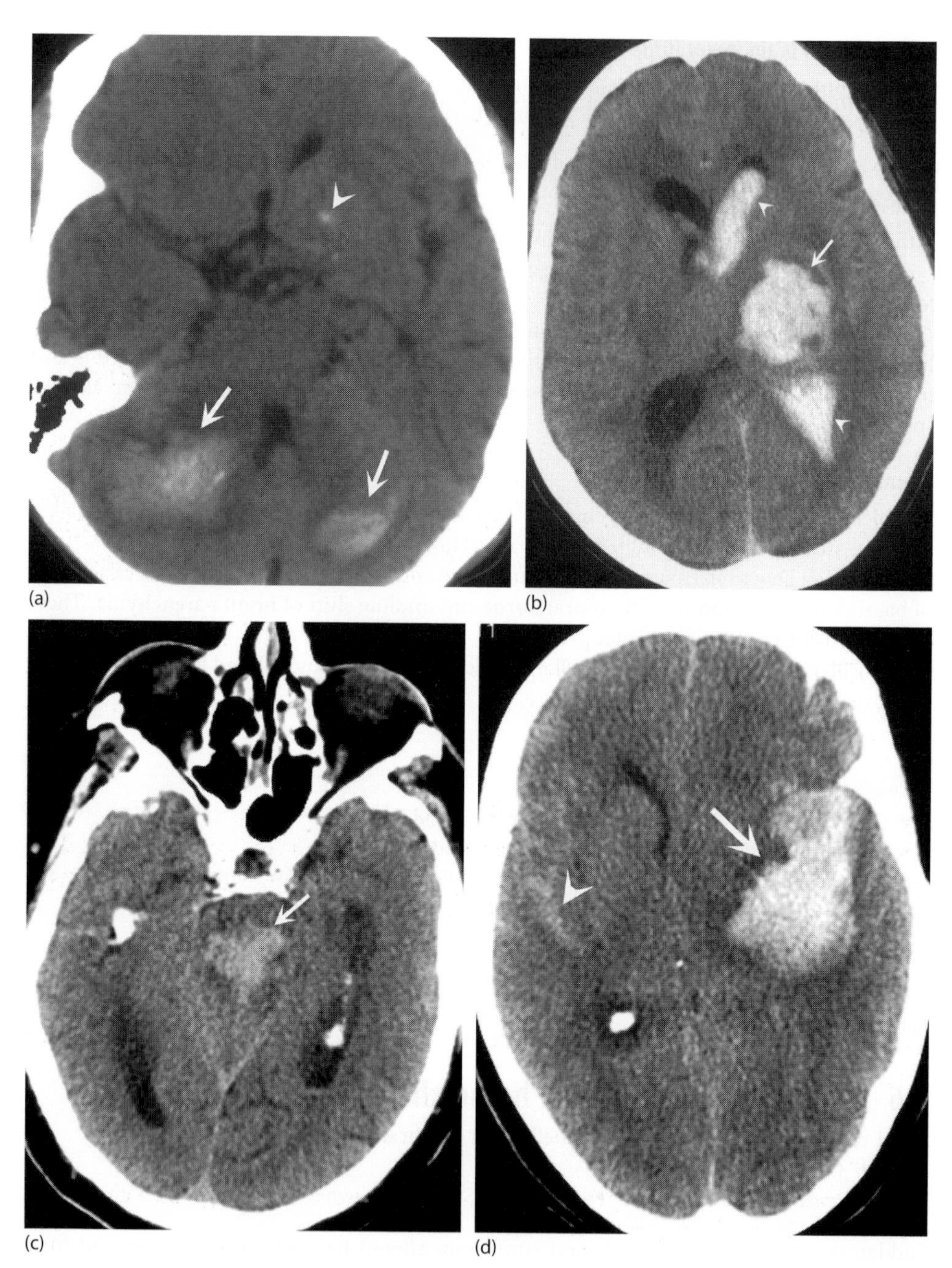

Fig. 1.6. (a) Cerebellar hematomas. Axial non-contrast CT shows large regions of hyperdense hematomas with surrounding hypodensities (arrows) in bilateral cerebellar hemispheres. Note the age-related calcification in the region of the left globus pallidus (arrowhead). (b) Intracerebral hemorrhage. Axial non-contrast CT shows a large hyperdense hematoma in the left basal ganglia and thalamus (arrow) with surrounding hypodensity as well as hyperdensity (blood) within the left lateral ventricle (arrowheads). (c) Pontine hemorrhage. Axial non-contrast CT with abnormal hyperdensity in the pons (arrow) is consistent with hemorrhage into the pons. (d) Sylvian fissure hematoma. Axial non-contrast CT shows a large Sylvian fissure hematoma (arrow) with extension into the cerebral parenchyma, with effacement of the left lateral ventricle and midline shift to the right. There is subarachnoid blood in the right Sylvian fissure (arrowhead).

Findings

1. Homogeneous and high density intraparenchymal hematoma with well-defined margins. Clot retraction may result in perihematoma low-density rim.
2. Extension of blood into dependent occipital horns seen as blood/CSF level or as complete opacification.
3. Look for hydrocephalus and features of tentorial herniation.

Pearls

- A cerebellar hematoma needs urgent neurosurgical intervention as the raised pressure in the posterior fossa predisposes to tentorial herniation. Be sure to evaluate for tonsillar herniation (downward through the foramen magnum) and upward transtentorial herniation in these patients.
- Exclude underlying aneurysm or vascular malformation in a young patient.
- Thalamic hemorrhage is most likely due to systemic hypertension.
- Hemorrhagic infarction (HI) is due to development of hemorrhage within the focal low density infarct. A focal low-density area is usually evident on the initial CT brain scan prior to hemorrhagic transformation. The larger infarcts are more prone to undergo secondary hemorrhage.

Suggested reading

Smith EE, Rosand J, Greenberg SM. Hemorrhagic stroke. *Neuroimaging Clin N Am* 2005;**15**(2):259–272.

Young RJ, Destian S. Imaging of traumatic intracranial hemorrhage. *Neuroimaging Clin N Am* 2002;**12**:189–204.

1.7 Cerebral venous sinus thrombosis

Cerebral venous sinus thrombosis represents clot formation in the superficial and deep venous sinus with or without extension into the cortical veins. The superior sagittal sinus, transverse sinus and vein of Galen are usually involved. See Fig. 1.7.

Clinical

Risk factors include infection (especially mastoid or middle ear), hypercoagulable states (pregnancy, puerperium etc.), oral contraceptive pill, dehydration. It can be idiopathic in 25% of cases.

It may present with thunderclap headache, drowsiness and sepsis.

Technique

Non-contrast CT brain and if there is a suspicion of hyperdense cord sign then a contrast-enhanced study should be performed.

Non-contrast CT brain findings

1. Hyperdense cord sign, due to acute thrombus within the vein. This may be seen along the transverse sinus, sagittal sinus or vein of Galen.
2. Ovoid bulging dense sagittal sinus.
3. Small focal cortical hemorrhage or infarct due to cortical vein infarction (suggests severity).
4. Small ventricular size.

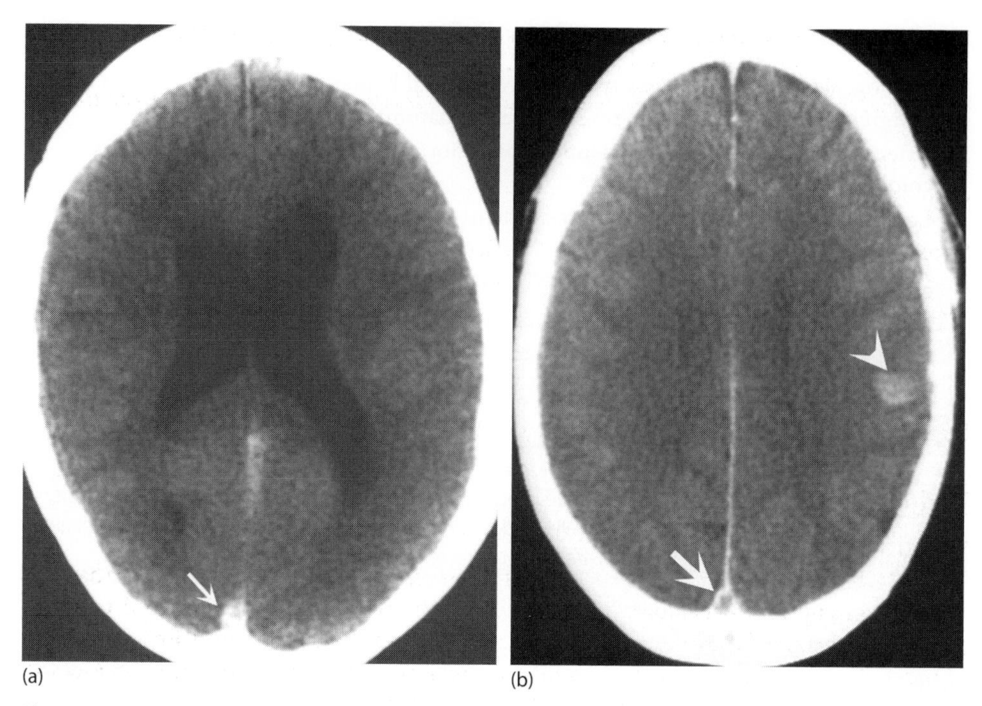

Fig. 1.7. (a, b) Venous sinus thrombosis. (a) Axial non-contrast CT shows subtle ovoid bulging of the sagittal sinus to the right (arrow). (b) CECT shows the "empty delta sign" (arrow) and a small focal cortical hyperdensity due to hemorrhage from a focal cortical venous infarction (arrowhead) in the left cerebrum.

Contrast-enhanced CT brain findings

1. "Empty delta sign"; in transverse section, the sagittal sinus exhibits rim enhancement with a low-attenuation filling defect (thrombus) within the lumen.
2. Infarcts may show "luxury perfusion" with some gyral enhancement adjacent to the infarct.
3. Look for a potential source of infection such as mastoiditis and sinusitis. Look for any associated complication such as cavernous sinus thrombosis.

Pearls

- Always remember to look at the venous sinuses. Give an IV contrast medium if the sagittal sinus or vein of Galen are hyperdense on the unenhanced study.
- Bilateral thalamic or basal ganglion hemorrhage should raise the suspicion of deep cerebral venous thrombosis.
- MR brain and MRV are helpful if CT findings are equivocal.

Suggested reading

Connor SE, Jarosz JM. Magnetic resonance imaging of cerebral venous sinus thrombosis. *Clin Radiol* 2002;57(6):449–461.

Leach JL, Fortuna RB, Jones BV, Gaskill-Shipley MF. Imaging of cerebral venous thrombosis: current techniques, spectrum of findings, and diagnostic pitfalls. *RadioGraphics* 2006;**26**:S19–S41.

Poon CS, Chang JK, Swarnkar A, Johnson MH, Wasenko J. Radiologic diagnosis of cerebral venous thrombosis: pictorial review. *Am J Radiol* 2007;**189**:S64–S75.

Rodallec MH *et al.* Cerebral venous thrombosis and multidetector CT angiography: tips and tricks. *RadioGraphics* 2006;**26**:S5–S18.

1.8 Ischemic brain injury

Stroke is defined as a focal neurological deficit which persists for more than 24 hours. In a transient ischemic attack, focal neurological deficit will recover within 24 hours. See Fig. 1.8.

Clinical

Stroke classically presents with sudden onset of focal neurology.

Technique

Unenhanced CT brain scan.

A CT brain scan is indicated in the acute stage to exclude intracranial hemorrhage so that aspirin and anticoagulation, if indicated, can be commenced. CT is useful to triage patients for thrombolysis in the correct clinical settings (if patient presents within 3–6 hours of onset of stroke). In some centers where thrombolysis is being used routinely, CTA of the carotid circulation and CT perfusion of the brain can be performed.

Findings

Early infarction

1. May be normal within first 3–6 hours.
2. Loss of insular ribbon sign: Effacement of lateral insular cortex.
3. Hypodensity and effacement of lentiform nucleus. Effacement of gray and white matter and mild sulcal effacement.
4. Hyperdense middle cerebral artery due to acute intraluminal clot.
5. MCA or insular dot sign represents a focal high-density acute clot distal to the M1 segment of MCA.

Subacute ischemic infarction

CT is usually positive for infarction after 3–6 hours.

1. Peripheral wedge-shaped hypoattentuation involving gray and white matter in the vascular territory.
2. Luxury perfusion of the infarction after intravenous contrast due to hypervascularity.
3. Rarely, fogging effect causes near-normal density of the infarct due to decreasing edema and hypervascularity.

Chronic infarction

1. Encephalolamacia: Very low density with HU similar to CSF.
2. Ipsilateral ex-vacuo ventricular enlargement due to atrophy.
3. No mass effect.

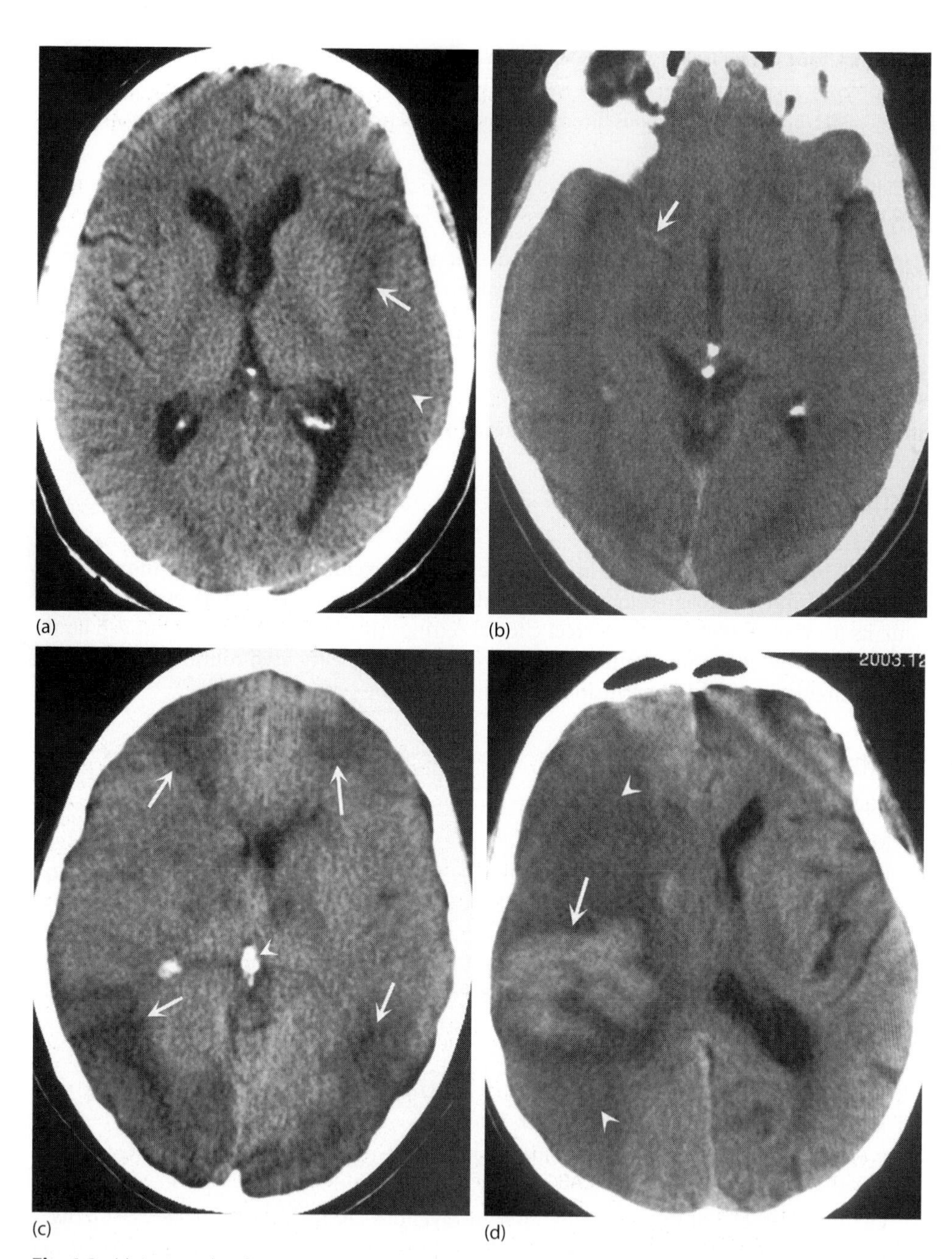

Fig. 1.8. (a) Acute early infarction. Axial non-contrast CT shows hypodensity in the left MCA territory, with loss of the insular ribbon (arrow) and loss of gray–white matter differentiation in the left cerebral hemisphere (arrowhead). Note the hypodense left external capsule. (b) Dense middle cerebral artery. Axial non-contrast CT shows linear hyperdensity in the region of the M1 branch of the right MCA (arrow), concerning for a clot within this vessel – an early sign of acute infarction. (c) Watershed infarcts. Axial non-contrast CT shows large areas of hypodensity (large arrows) bilaterally in the "watershed" areas. Note a calcified pineal gland (arrowhead) and calcified arachnoid granulations in the lateral ventricle. (d) Hemorrhagic infarction. Axial non-contrast CT shows a large irregular area of hyperdensity (hemorrhage) (arrow) within the markedly hypodense right MCA infarct (arrowheads). There is mass effect with effacement of the right lateral ventricle and midline shift to the left.

Watershed infarction

Border-zone infarcts occur between the vascular territories (between ACA/MCA and MCA/PCA) in the superficial cortex and in the deep white matter and are associated with poor prognosis.

Usually they are multiple and bilateral and are associated with hypotension from hemodynamic compromise or due to multiple emboli within the small peripheral arteries.

Hemorrhagic infarction (HI)

HI is due to development of hemorrhage within the focal low-density infarct. A focal low-density area is usually evident on the initial CT brain scan prior to hemorrhagic transformation. The larger infarcts are more prone to later HI, which can occur with or without anticoagulant therapy. Hemorrhagic infarction does not necessarily indicate discontinuation of anticoagulant therapy (e.g. in AF, LV thrombus).

Venous infarction

Refer to Section 1.7.

Lacunar infarction

Very small low-density lesions in the deep gray matter, usually involve the basal ganglion, thalamus, pons and internal capsule. Commonly associated with hypertension. Cytotoxic edema is usually absent. Lacunar infarcts are easily overlooked or missed on CT.

Pearls

- Presence of a large infarct (more than one-third size of the MCA territory) and hemorrhage are contraindications to thrombolysis. T1-weighted GRE MRI imaging may be useful to identify small intracerebral hemorrhage, which is an absolute contraindication to thrombolysis.
- The "insular ribbon", is normally seen as a thin hyperdense line (gray matter) marginating the Sylvian fissure.
- CT brain perfusion (quantifies relative areas of infarction to penumbra) and CT carotid angiography (identifies occlusion) are useful techniques to further triage patients for initiation of stroke thrombolysis.
- Multiple bilateral low-density areas in the watershed region typically occur in post-CABG or carotid artery surgery patients.
- MRI is more sensitive in the detection of lacunar infarction and also helps in the triage of patients for thrombolysis.
- Multiple cerebral infarctions; consider carotid artery dissection with embolism, cardiac pathology, Moyamoya, post-CABG or carotid artery surgery, and reversible posterior leukoencephalopathy.
- Also refer to Section 6.3.

Suggested reading

Beauchamp NJ, Barker PB, Wang PY, vanZijl PCM. Imaging of acute cerebral ischemia. *Radiology* 1999;**212**:307–324.

Tomandl BF *et al.* Comprehensive imaging of ischemic stroke with multisection CT. *RadioGraphics* 2003;**23**(3):565–592.

1.9 Bacterial meningitis

Infectious or inflammatory process involving the meningeal layer of the brain. See Fig. 1.9.

Clinical

Headache, vomiting, fever, drowsiness, confusion, cloudy conciousness, seizures and focal neurological deficit. Complications include focal abscess, hydrocephalus, venous thrombosis and subdural empyema. CT of the brain is indicated in the presence of deteriorating consciousness and/or focal neurological deficit prior to lumbar puncture. Empirical parenteral antibiotics can be given immediately in suspected meningitis, prior to CT scan or LP.

Technique

Unenhanced and contrast-enhanced scan. If an unenhanced scan is completely normal then a contrast-enhanced scan may not be essential. The normal unenhanced CT scan serves to significantly lower the likelihood of raised intracranial pressure.

Findings

1. Normal study in early phase.
2. Unenhanced scan may demonstrate dense meningeal layers especially along the cisterns. Intense meningeal enhancement after the intravenous contrast.
3. Temporal horn dilatation is an early sign of hydrocephalus.
4. Focal low-density lesions representing ischemia due to vasculitis.

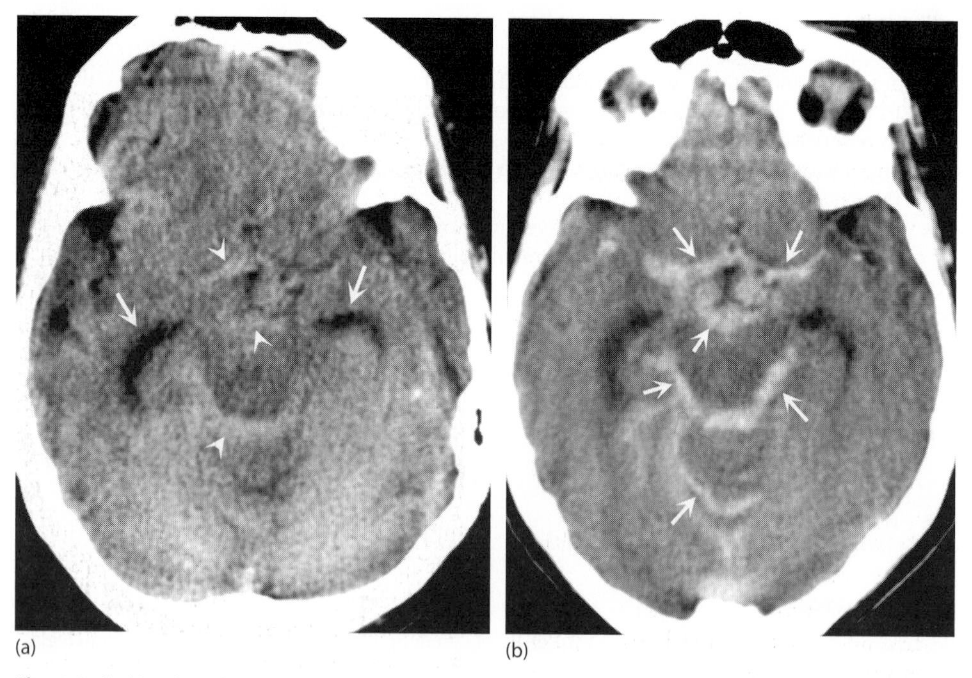

Fig. 1.9. (a, b) Tuberculous meningitis. (a) Axial non-contrast CT shows dilated temporal horns of the lateral ventricles (arrows) and increased density in the suprasellar, interpeduncular and ambient cisterns (arrowheads). (b) Post-contrast CT shows marked meningeal enhancement along the basal cisterns (arrows).

5. Look for signs of venous thrombosis.
6. Source of infections like mastoiditis, skull base fracture, sinusitis.

Pearls

- A normal scan does not exclude raised intracranial pressure; therefore, herniation rarely occurs following lumbar puncture after a completely normal CT brain.
- Hydrocephalus may be the only presenting feature of bacterial meningitis, especially in tuberculous meningitis.
- Persistent meningeal signs and drowsiness, despite treatment, requires a repeat CT scan of the brain to evaluate for complications such as focal abscess, resorptive hydrocephalus, venous sinus thrombosis. CT venography may be useful to evaluate for venous sinus thrombosis.
- MRI is a superior technique to CT in evaluating complications like focal abscess, venous thrombosis, ischemia.
- Meningeal metastases and neurosarcoidosis can demonstrate meningeal enhancement but typically do not have hyperdense meninges on non-contrast CT.

Suggested reading

Anslow P. Cranial bacterial infection. *Eur Radiol* 2004;**14** Suppl. 3:E145–E154.

Karampekios S, Hesselink J. Cerebral infections. *Eur Radiol* 2005;**15**(3):485–493.

1.10 Encephalitis

Inflammation of the brain secondary to infectious or non-infectious causes. See Fig. 1.10.

Clinical

Herpes simplex encephalitis is a clinical emergency. Symptoms are headache, nausea, fever, drowsiness, reduced GCS and seizures.

Technique

Unenhanced and enhanced CT scan of the brain.

Findings

1. Normal brain scan in the early phase (3–5 days).
2. Temporal lobe hypodensity. Usually unilateral but can be bilateral.
3. Effacement of cortical sulci and the ipsilateral lateral ventricle are suggestive of brain swelling.
4. Contrast-enhanced scan may demonstrate gyriform enhancement,

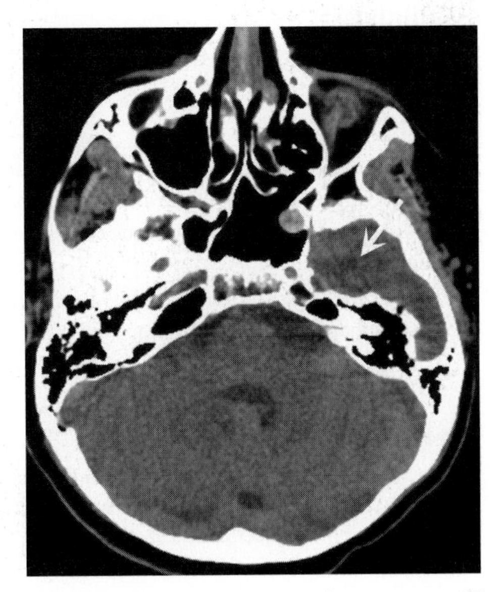

Fig. 1.10. HSV encephalitis. Axial non-contrast CT shows subtle hypodensity of the left temporal lobe (arrow), suggestive of herpes encephalitis in the proper clinical setting.

usually in the temporal and parietal lobes. Temporal lobe hypodensity becomes more conspicuous after contrast enhancement.

Pearls

- Have a high degree of suspicion in the appropriate clinical settings. Streak artefacts in the skull base can resemble a temporal lobe hypodensity.
- Lumbar puncture is mandatory in the absence of a contraindication.
- MRI is the choice of imaging modality.
- Differential diagnoses include glioma and lymphoma.

Suggested reading

Foerster BR, Sundgren PC. Intracranial infections: clinical and imaging characteristics. *Acta Radiol* 2007;**48**(8):875–893. [Review.]

Karampekios S, Hesselink J. Cerebral infections. *Eur Radiol* 2005;**15**(3):485–493.

1.11 Cerebral abscess

Focal parenchymal necrosis/pus formation in the brain. See Fig. 1.11.

Clinical

Headache, nausea and vomiting, cloudy consciousness, sepsis, seizures and focal neurological deficit. Causes include pyogenic, tuberculous, opportunistic (toxoplamosis), fungal, general septicemia and sarcoidosis.

Technique

Unenhanced and enhanced CT brain.

Findings

1. Unenhanced scan: Focal low-density lesion with a less-dense surrounding rim and perifocal low-density white matter edema. It is helpful to identify calcification and hemorrhage. In most cases only white matter edema (finger-in-glove white-matter edema) is seen.
2. Post-contrast scan demonstrates typical peripheral ring enhancing lesion with central necrosis and perifocal edema.
3. If an unenhanced brain scan is completely normal then a post-contrast scan can be foregone.

Pearls

- Differential considerations include glioma, lymphoma and metastasis. Knowledge of the clinical presentation is therefore vital. Abscess is usually located in the peripheral brain parenchyma adjacent to calvarium.

Suggested reading

Refer to Section 1.10.

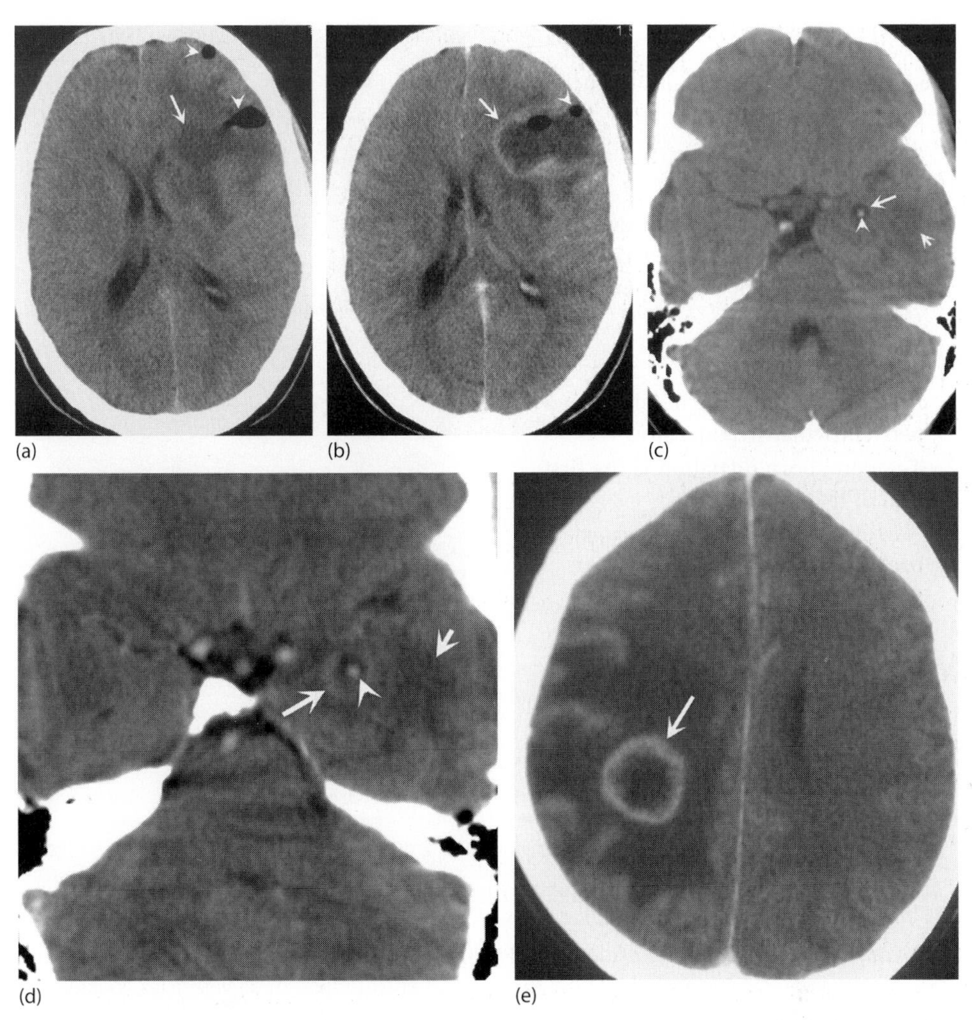

Fig. 1.11. (a, b) Frontal lobe abscess. (a) Axial unenhanced CT shows a large area of decreased attenuation (arrow) due to vasogenic edema in the anterior left frontal lobe, gas pockets (arrowheads) and rightward midline shift. (b) Post-contrast image shows peripheral enhancement (arrow) with central low density and gas bubbles (arrowhead). (c, d) Tuberculoma. (c) Axial unenhanced CT shows a calcification (arrowhead) within the left temporal lobe with surrounding low-density halo (large arrow). Note subtle edema (small arrow) in the adjacent temporal lobe. (d) Post-contrast CT shows peripheral rim-enhancement (arrow). Note calcification (arrowhead) and perilesional edema (small arrow). (e) Ring-enhancing lesion. CECT shows peripheral rim-enhancing lesion (arrow) in the right parietal lobe with central necrosis and significant vasogenic edema. This may represent a solitary necrotic mass versus abscess.

1.12 Hydrocephalus

Dilatation of the ventricular system of the brain is due to increased production of, or decreased absorption of, cerebrospinal fluid. See Fig. 1.12.

It can be classified as obstructive and non-obstructive. The former is subdivided into communicating and non-communicating hydrocephalus.

Clinical

Headache, vomiting and signs of meningitis such as a stiff neck.

Technique

Unenhanced CT brain. Intravenous contrast is useful to assess for underlying meningitis, ventriculitis or occult tumor.

Findings

1. Round frontal and occipital horns with periventricular hypodensity.
2. Temporal horn dilatation is the first sign of hydrocephalus.
3. Narrowing of the angle anteriorly between the frontal horns at the midline.
4. Effacement of the cortical sulci.
5. Look for an important underlying cause – tumors along the CSF pathway, intracranial hemorrhage, meningitis (dense thick meninges) etc.

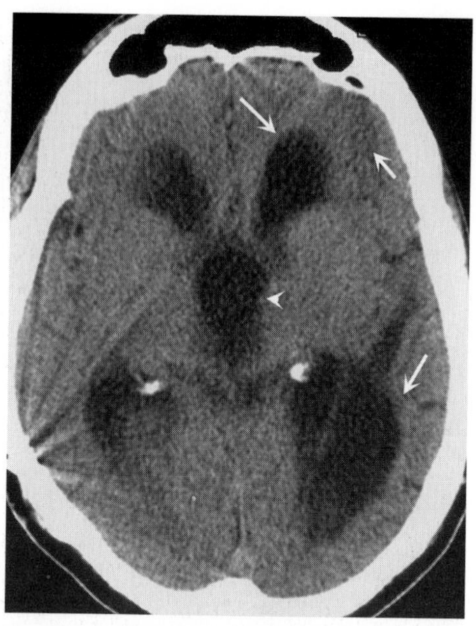

Fig. 1.12. Acute hydrocephalus. Axial unenhanced CT shows marked dilatation of bilateral frontal and occipital horns of the lateral ventricles (large arrows), third ventricle (arrowhead) (midline) and effacement (small arrow) of the cerebral sulci. Bilateral periventricular hypodensities (small arrow) favor acute hydrocephalus.

Pearls

- Periventricular hypodensity (anterior to the frontal and posterior to the occipital horns) can imply recent-onset hydrocephalus.
- Communicating types of obstructive hydrocephalus are due to obstruction of CSF distal to the 4th ventricle and present with a symmetrical enlargement of all ventricles, including the 4th ventricle (e.g. SAH, meningeal disease).
- Asymmetric enlargement of ventricles occurs in the non-communicating type of obstructive hydrocephalus due to obstruction of CSF within the ventricles (tumors).
- Normal-pressure hydrocephalus is a communicating type of obstructive hydrocephalus. Disproportionate dilatation of the ventricles to cortical sulci. Flat gyri.
- In cerebral atrophy there is a proportionate dilatation of the ventricles and cortical sulci with symmetrical periventricular hypodensities. Round gyri.

Suggested reading

Refer to Section 1.2.

Goeser CD, McLeary MS, Young LW. Diagnostic imaging of ventriculoperitoneal shunt malfunctions and complications. *RadioGraphics* 1998;**18**:635–651.

1.13 Intracranial aneurysm

Abnormal dilatation of the intracranial cerebral arteries. See Fig. 1.13.

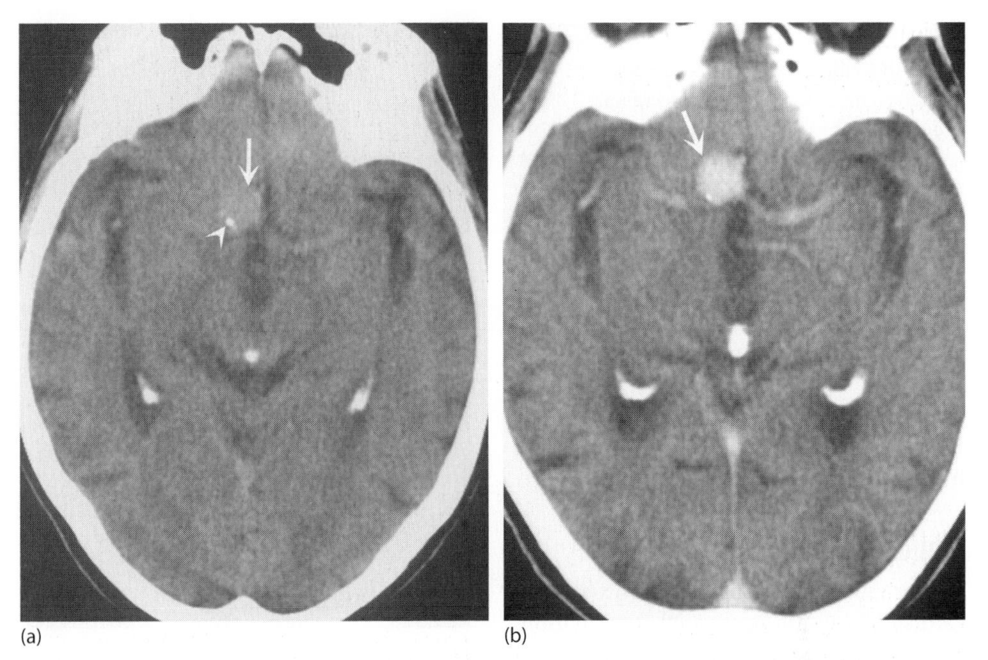

Fig. 1.13. (a, b) Intracranial aneurysm. (a) Axial unenhanced CT shows subtle round high attenuation (arrow) structure with peripheral calcifications (arrowhead) in the suprasellar cistern. (b) Post-contrast CT shows intense rounded enhancement of this lesion (arrow), consistent with a right A-commissure aneurysm.

Clinical

Cerebral aneurysms can present with headache, painful ophthalmoplegia, seizures and stroke. Posterior communicating artery aneurysms may cause an ipsilateral third nerve palsy.

Multiple aneurysms can occur in 20–25%.

Technique

Pre- and post-contrast scan and CT angiography.

Findings

1. On the pre-contrast images, there may be curvilinear peripheral calcification with central intermediate density of the aneurysm, which is slightly higher than the surrounding brain tissue.
2. Post-contrast images demonstrate well-defined intense homogeneous enhancement of the spherical aneurysm. Partially thrombosed aneurysms may lack uniform enhancement.

Pearls

- Look for location, size and number of aneurysms and for SAH.
- Understand the anatomy of carotid and vertebro-basilar artery circulation.
- CTA may be needed to further characterize the aneurysm in symptomatic patients.
- Always look for the source and post-processing datasets to identify and characterize the aneurysm.

Suggested reading

Cloft HJ, Kallmes DF. Detection and characterization of very small cerebral aneurysms by using 2D and 3D helical CT angiography. *Am J Neuroradiol* 2003;**24**(1):154.

Tomandl BF *et al.* CT angiography of intracranial aneurysms: a focus on postprocessing. *RadioGraphics* 2004;**24**: 637–655.

1.14 Hypoxic–anoxic brain injury

Ischemic injury to brain due to prolonged hypoxia. See Fig. 1.14.

Clinical

Causes include prenatal asphyxia, and cardiac arrest with prolonged resuscitation. Usually the patient is in a pre-terminal condition.

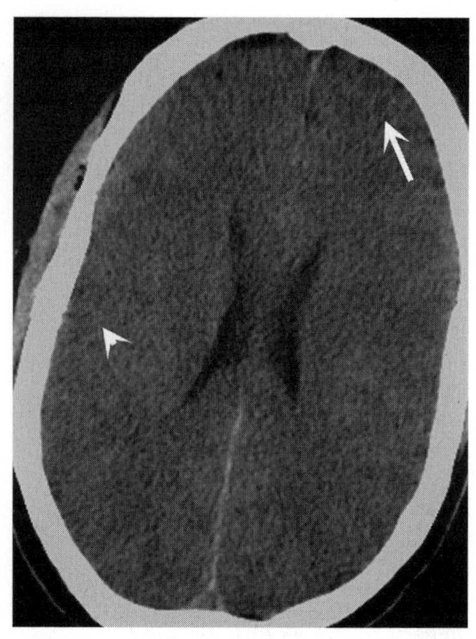

Fig. 1.14. Hypoxic–anoxic brain injury. Axial unenhanced CT brain of a patient who had recovered from cardiac arrest shows effacement of bilateral cerebral sulci (arrowhead) and diffuse loss of gray–white differentiation (arrow).

Findings

1. Non-contrast CT scan may demonstrate diffuse cerebral edema, bilateral loss of gray and white matter differentiation, reversal of gray and white matter density, low-density deep gray matter involving the thalamus and lentiform nucleus and typical watershed infarcts.

Pearls

- MRI is helpful in demonstrating high signal on T1-weighted imaging of hemorrhage in the basal ganglion and cortical areas.
- Cerebral atrophy is a late complication.

Suggested reading

Kjos BO, Brant-Zawadzki M, Young RG. Early CT findings of global central nervous system hypoperfusion. *Am J Roentgenol* 1983;**141**(6):1227–1232.

1.15 Carotid/vertebral artery dissection

Intimal tear or intramural hematoma of carotid and vertebral arteries. See Fig. 1.15.

Clinical

It is a common cause of stroke in young individuals.

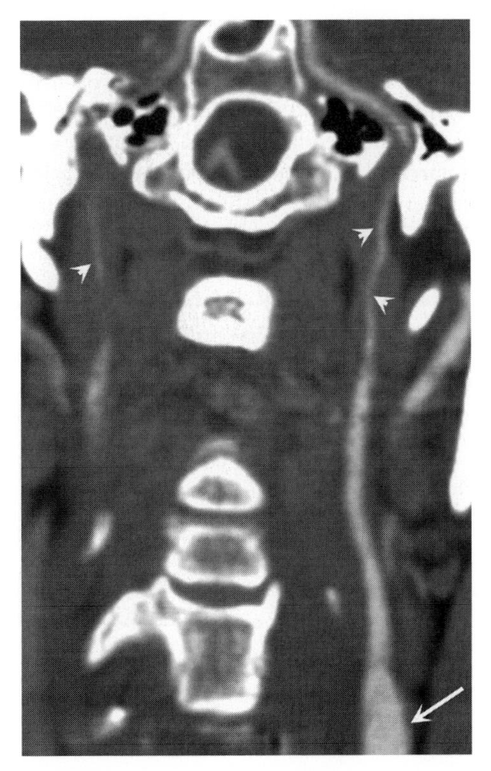

Fig. 1.15. Traumatic carotid artery dissection. Coronal CTA of the neck in a trauma patient shows normal left common carotid artery (arrow), and irregularity and marked attenuation of bilateral ICAs (string sign, arrowheads) with mural hematoma.

Causes include spontaneous, neck trauma, vasculitis, connective tissue disease and hypertension. Involvement of the anterior circulation is suggested by features such as transient visual loss and hemiparesis, vertigo, dizziness, light-headedness; cerebellar signs such as ataxia and incordination suggest vertebral artery involvement.

Technique

Multislice CTA of the neck and brain following 120 ml of IV contrast at 3 ml/s, with automatic bolus tracking with ROI at the aortic arch.

In addition to axial reconstruction, sagittal and coronal reformatted images should be obtained.

Findings

1. Dilatation and irregularity of vessel.
2. Intraluminal flap.
3. True and false lumen.
4. String sign.
5. Occlusion.
6. Soft-tissue brain parenchyma may show evidence of scattered foci of low-density areas of infarction.

Pearls

- Neck ultrasound is useful to diagnose dissection of cervical carotid and vertebral arteries.
- Liaise with neuroradiologist and neurologist. Immediate anticoagulation treatment may be needed.
- Refer to Section 6.9.

Suggested reading

Flis CM, Jager HR, Sidhu PS. Carotid and vertebral artery dissections: clinical aspects, imaging features and endovascular treatment. *Eur Radiol* 2007;**17**(3):820–834.

LeBlang SD, Nunez DB, Jr. Non-invasive imaging of cervical vascular injuries. *Am J Roentgenol* 2000;**174**:1269–1278.

Núñez DB, Torres-Leon M, Munera F. Vascular injuries of the neck and thoracic inlet: helical CT–angiographic correlation. *RadioGraphics* 2004;**24**:1087–1098.

1.16 Miscellaneous

Spontaneous intracranial hypotension: Presents with acute onset headache. Non-contrast CT scan may not be useful, however contrast CT may show subdural collections, cerebellar tonsillar herniation and meningeal thickening. Gadolinium-enhanced MRI is helpful.

Moyamoya: Presents with multiple cerebral infarcts due to stenoses of bilateral internal carotid, proximal anterior and middle cerebral arteries. There is intimal thickening and proliferation at the terminal portions of the bilateral internal carotid arteries. Etiology is unknown, but it is associated with various diseases.

Reversible posterior leukoencephalopathy: Reversible multiple and bilateral areas of ischemia in the territory of the posterior circulation are associated with hypertension, eclampsia, renal disease and chemotherapy.

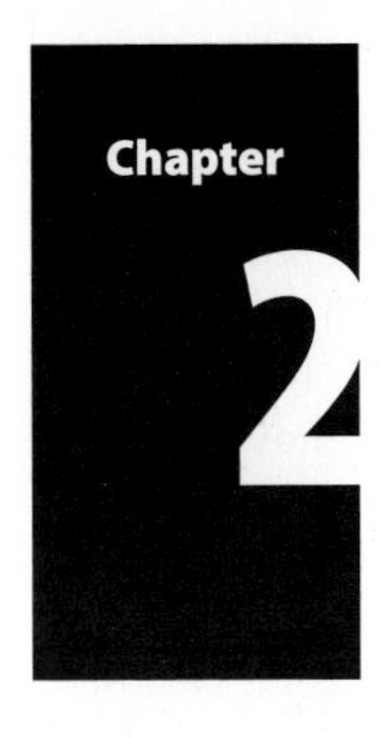

Cardiovascular and chest

Mayil S. Krishnam

2.1 General principles

Worldwide, chest pain is the most common reason for admission to the emergency department. Life-threatening emergencies such as aortic dissection, pulmonary embolism, aortic aneurysm or rupture and myocardial ischemia/infarction all present with chest pain. In upper or lower extremity trauma, rapid non-invasive assessment of peripheral arteries for vascular injury is important to plan for appropriate management. In certain clinical circumstances, non-invasive assessment of the deep veins is required. With 16- and 64-slice multi-detector CT, high-quality images of the coronary arteries, aorta, pulmonary vessels and peripheral vessels including deep veins can be obtained to reliably evaluate acute pathologies. See Fig. 2.1.

Indications

Acute pulmonary embolism (PE).
Aortic dissection.
Aortic aneurysm – to evaluate for imminent rupture.
Coronary artery occlusion.
Traumatic aortic injury.

Technical considerations

Bolus tracking of the aorta or pulmonary artery as per the clinical indication is a preferred rapid technique in the emergency setting.

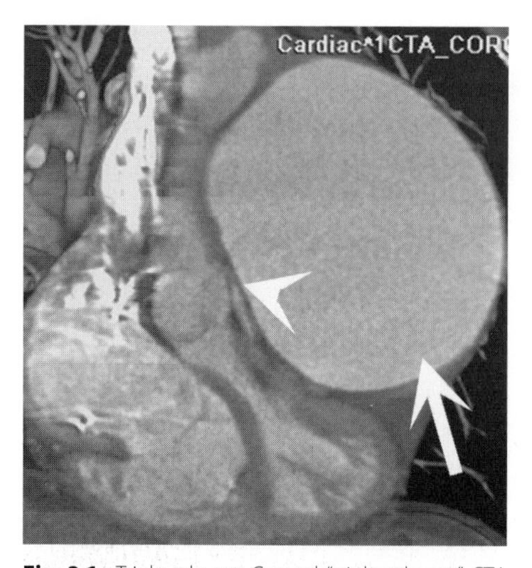

Fig. 2.1. Triple rule-out. Coronal "triple rule out" CTA image shows a main pulmonary artery aneurysm (arrow) with resultant significant compression of the left main stem coronary artery (arrowhead).

However in "double rule out" protocol for aortic dissection and PE, bolus tracking of the ascending aorta with contrast continuously filling the right heart (3 ml/s) throughout the scan time should be considered supplemented by 30 ml of 0.9% saline to flush the contrast stasis in the veins on the side of injection and to keep a tight contrast bolus. Total contrast dose = scan time × contrast injection rate + additional 20 ml. If the scan time is 20 s, then the total contrast dose is approximately 80 ml (20 × 3 + 20). This is readily achievable using the latest multi-detector CT. The study should be gated if the primary clinical indication is to rule out aortic dissection.

It is more challenging to carry out a "triple rule out" protocol for aortic dissection/aneurysm, pulmonary embolism, and coronary artery disease, especially in the ER setting. The contrast injection rate should be 4–5 ml/s to opacify the coronary arteries and the study should always be gated. Bolus tracking, with use of a region of interest (ROI) is placed in the ascending or descending aorta to trigger the start of scanning when an optimal attenuation value (usually 150 HU) has been reached.

A non-contrast scan can be useful in the assessment of intramural hematoma. In all other emergencies, the arterial phase scan is sufficient. Oral contrast is not routinely needed but can be useful in patients with suspected esophageal dissection or rupture, where non-ionic iodinated contrast media such as iopamidol or iohexol, or 2% diluted barium should be used just before the study. Coronal and sagittal reformats are useful and are readily viewed on PACS.

Important review areas in a "near-normal thoracic CTA chest"

Transverse aortic arch for pseudoaneurysm in trauma.

Aortic root for dissection or rupture (aortic valve is a trileaflet and in root dissection the intimal flap usually starts just above the valve annulus and extends into the ascending aorta).

Intramural hematoma.

Segmental pulmonary embolism.

Pneumomediastinum.

Anomalous coronary arteries.

Acute osseous fracture.

Pericardial hematoma.

Pneumoperitoneum.

Intracardiac thrombus or mass.

2.2 Chest trauma

Blunt injury to the chest is the second most common cause of death in chest trauma, due to shearing aortic injury. In addition, compression and/or direct impact injuries to lung parenchyma, pleura, diaphragm, appendicular and axial skeletons can occur. See Fig. 2.2.

Clinical

Chest pain, breathlessness, tachycardia, hypotension and hypoxia. Widening of the mediastinum on CXR.

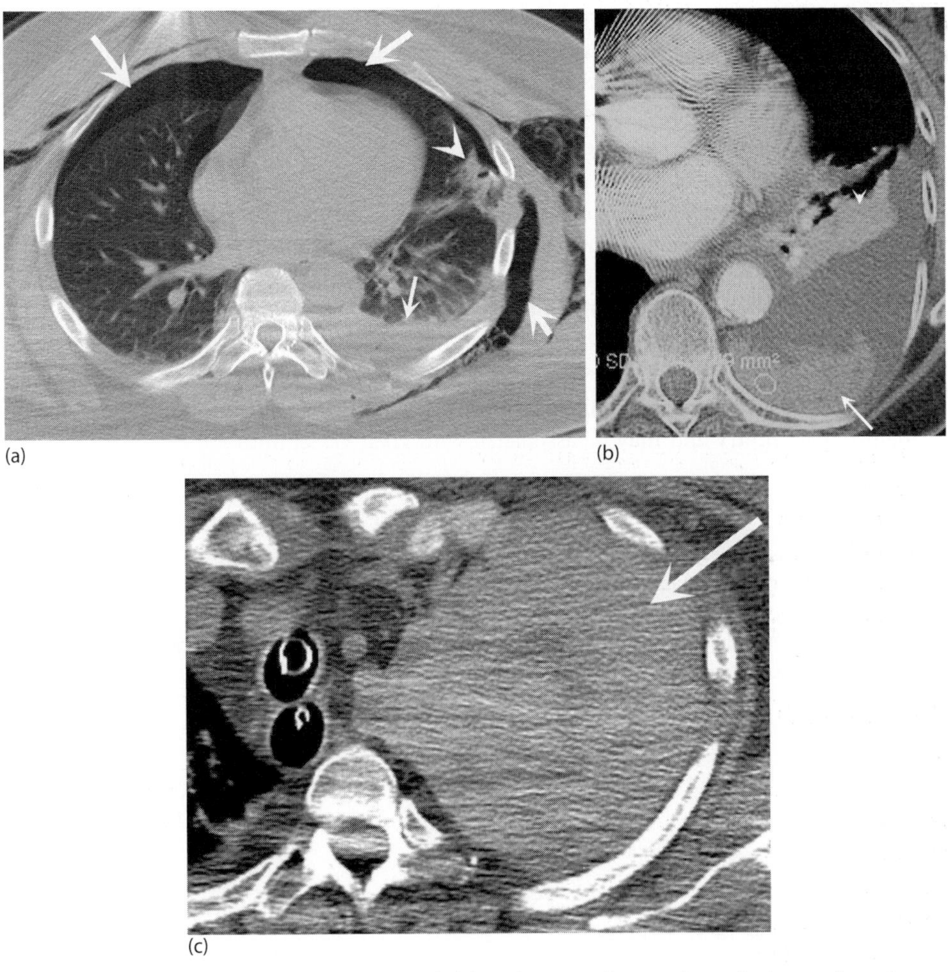

Fig. 2.2. (a) Lung contusion. Axial CT shows with bilateral pneumothoraces (arrows), chest wall emphysema (small arrow), left hemothorax (thin arrow) and non-segmental pulmonary parenchymal opacities (arrowhead). (b) Hemothorax. CECT of the chest shows a large left pleural collection with a high-density material posteriorly that represents blood (Hematocrit sign, arrow). Note atelectatic lung (arrowhead), which enhances on post-contrast scans. (c) Traumatic pleural hematoma. Axial non-contrast chest CT in a patient with failed left jugular vein instrumentation demonstrates a large high-attenuation well-defined hematoma in the left upper hemi-thorax (arrow).

Technique

Contrast-enhanced CT chest. Oral contrast can be given if there is a suspected esophageal injury or pneumomediastinum.
Sagittal and coronal reformations.

Findings

1. Lung contusion: Non-segmental, discrete or ill-defined groundglass, alveolar and interstitial opacities.
2. Lung laceration: Parenchymal cyst containing air or air and fluid. The cyst is due to a tear in the lung parenchyma. A cyst which contains high-density fluid is called a pulmonary hematoma. There may be adjacent atelectasis or contusion.
3. Hemothorax: Look for any extravasation of intravenous contrast from the intercostal arteries. Hematocrit sign-posterior layering of high-density blood beneath low-attenuation plasma.
4. Pneumothorax and pneumomediastinum.
5. Tracheobronchial laceration: Fallen lung (lung is cut off from the hilum and abuts the postero-lateral chest wall or the hemidiaphragm), pneumomediastinum, hydropneumothorax, subcutaneous emphysema (cervical), fistula between airway and the mediastinum, abnormal location and balloon distension of the ET tube. A focal or complete tear in the trachea or bronchus.
6. Diaphragmatic injury: A focal diaphragmatic defect with herniation of abdominal fat or organs into the chest.
7. Bone injury: Fractures of scapula, sternum and upper ribs (1–3) are associated with high-impact injury and may be associated with great vessel injury.

Pearls

- Contusions can occur immediately and usually subside within 7 days.
- Lacerations are commonly associated with rib fracture.
- Suspect tracheobronchial or esophageal injury in the presence of pneumothorax or pneumomediastinum, especially if the pneumothorax persists in spite of intercostal chest drain placement.
- Focal disruption of the diaphragm is usually well depicted on the sagittal and coronal reformatted images.

Suggested reading

Van Hise ML, Primack SL, Israel RS, Muller NL. CT in blunt chest trauma: indications and limitations. *RadioGraphics* 1998;**18**(5):1071–1084.

Zinck SE, Primack SL. Radiographic and CT findings in acute chest trauma. *J Thoracic Imaging* 2000;**15**(2):87–96.

2.3 Acute aortic dissection/intramural hematoma

Spontaneous intimal tear in the aortic wall. See Fig. 2.3.

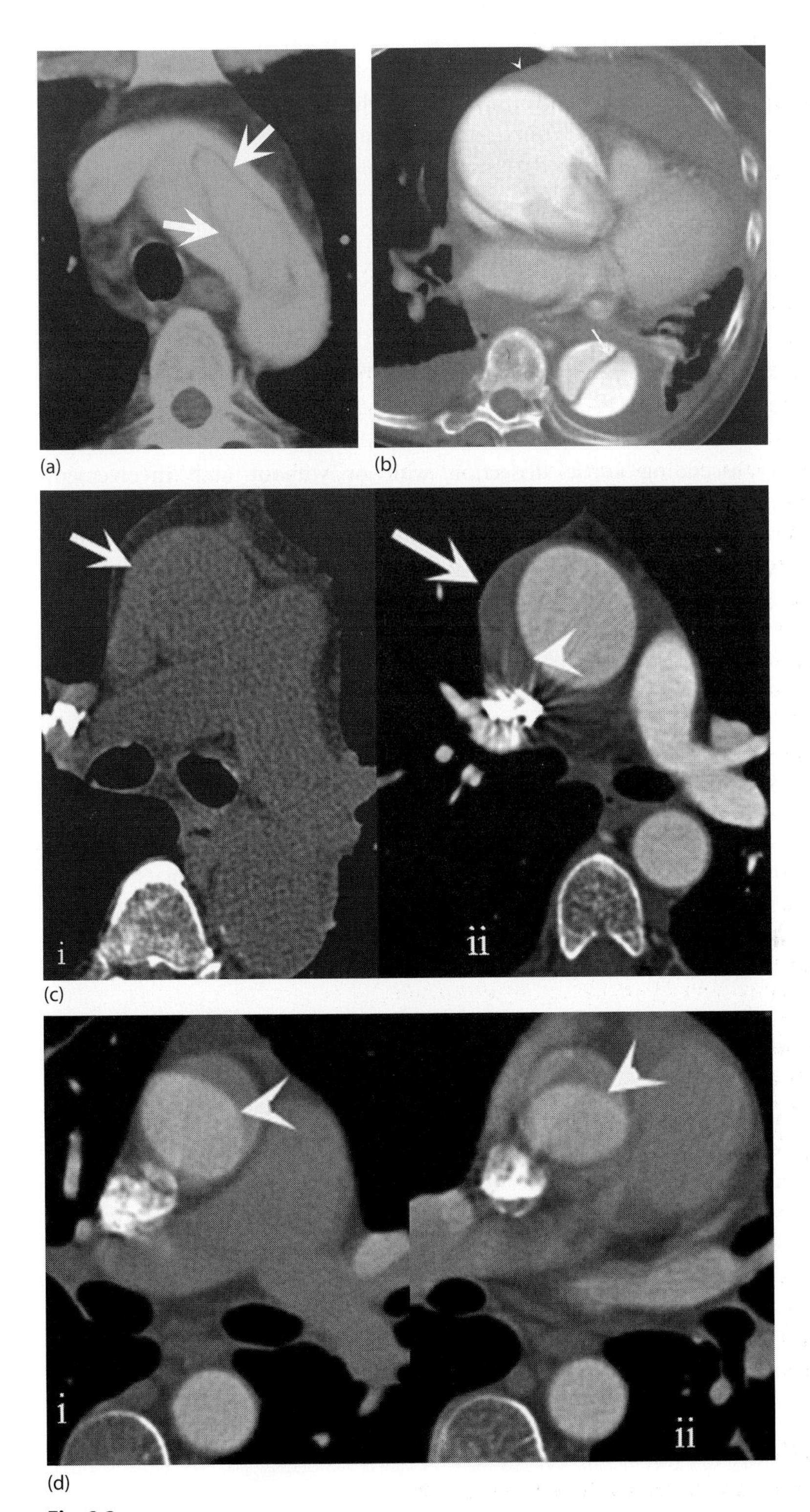

Fig. 2.3.

Clinical

Sudden onset of constant chest pain radiating between the shoulder blades. May mimic a myocardial infarction. Blood pressure difference in the upper limbs.

Chest X-ray may show a widened mediastinum, pleural effusion, left apical pleural cap, displacement of calcium.

Thin section spiral CECT of the aorta has sensitivity and specificity of 100%. The negative predictive value (NPV) is almost 100%.

Causes

Trauma, hypertension, idiopathic, connective tissue diseases, aortic aneurysm etc.

Types

Stanford: Type A = ascending aortic dissection with or without arch involvement. Rx Surgical intervention to prevent rupture and progressive aortic valve insufficiency

Type B = descending aortic dissection distal to the origin of left subclavian artery. Rx Conservative, consisting mainly of hypotensive therapy. Intervention is needed if there is end organ damage, progressive aneurysmal dilatation and uncontrollable chest pain.

A and B dissections = Dissections from the aortic root to a point distal to the origin of the left subclavian artery.

Technique

Limited non-contrast (depends upon the local hospital policy) and whole aorta contrast-enhanced scan. Consider cardiac gating for chest to avoid motion artefacts.

Scan from thoracic inlet to femoral vessels. Scan delay approximately 23 s.

Thin overlapping contiguous slices (1.5–2.5 mm) are obtained with reformats.

Bolus tracking injection method to trigger the start of scanning when an optimal attenuation value has been reached (usually 150 HU) with region of interest (ROI) placed in the ascending or descending aorta or abdominal aorta as indicated.

CECT aorta findings

1. Intimal flap: A thin curvilinear low density structure separates the true and false lumen of the aorta. The intimal flap can be either flat or curved and occasionally complex and highly mobile, especially in the arch.
2. Entry and re-entry point: The communication or entry point between the false and true lumen indicates the origin of the dissection. Usually lies just above the aortic root in the right antero-lateral wall or just after the origin of the left subclavian artery. Not always

Caption for Fig. 2.3 (a) Aortic dissection. Axial CT angiogram shows linear low density areas (intimal flap) within the aortic lumen (arrows), consistent with aortic dissection. (b) Leaking type A dissection. CTA shows an intimal flap in the descending aorta (arrow) and in the dilated aortic root, periaortic soft tissue, pericardial collection (arrowhead), and right pleural space hematoma. (c) Type A intramural hematoma. Axial non-contrast CT (i) shows a subtle crescentic area of relatively increased density in the ascending aorta (arrow). Axial CECT (ii) shows low-density ascending aortic wall thickening (arrow) and smooth inner aortic wall margin (arrowhead). (d) Pseudo intimal flap. Axial non-gated CTA shows multiple short segment curvilinear low-density areas (arrowheads) which are changing in positions.

visible on the scan. There may be further communication between the false and true lumen distally (re-entry point).

3. Extent of dissection: Can extend from aortic root to any point along the aorta to the bifurcation of vessels.
4. Branch vessel involvement (Great vessels, mesenteric, renal and iliac arteries): Extension of dissection flap into the branch vessels narrows the diameter of the true lumen. Identification of luminal origin of the branch vessels from the true or false lumen is important for planning management.
5. Fluid in the pericardial recess and pericardial space: Fluid could be due to leakage of blood through the dissection, however, presence of significant blood suggests rupture of dissection and urgent surgical advice is needed.
6. Identification of false and true lumen:

   True lumen: Usually opacifies first on bolus tracking.

   Smaller in size compared to false lumen. Continues as the normal aorta distal to the dissection flap.

   False lumen: Lentiform shape.

   Beak sign (acute angle between the dissection flap and aortic wall). Rarely (10%) cobwebs (thin linear filling defects due to debris of the media) are seen within the false lumen.

   Usually located in the right lateral position within the ascending aorta, anteriorly in the arch and then takes a left lateral course in the descending aorta. Look for low-density thrombus in the false lumen.

7. Size of aorta (aortic root, ascending, proximal arch, distal arch, descending, upper abdomen, below renal arteries, iliac and femoral arteries): Look for associated aortic aneurysm. Femoral artery size and the neck of the aorta between the left subclavian artery and start of the dissection in type B are important for planning endovascular stent graft.
8. Renal and bowel ischemia: Reduced or absent cortical enhancement of the kidney. Bowel wall thickening, intra-mural lucency (gas) with narrowing of the true lumen of the superior mesenteric artery (SMA) suggests bowel ischemia.
9. Secondary signs: In the absence of an intimal flap, true luminal narrowing, aortic wall thickening and widening of the aorta are less specific signs of dissection.

Pearls

- Pseudo intimal flap: Aortic wall motion and post-surgical graft infolding may simulate an intimal flap especially in the aortic root and ascending aorta. However, the curvilinear interface changes position from one image to another. This artefact is less likely to occur in ECG-gated multi-slice CT.
- Pseudo false lumen: The left superior intercostal and left superior pulmonary vein, superior pericardial recess, pleural thickening, lung atelectasis adjacent to the aortic wall may simulate a false lumen.
- Differentiation of the true from false lumen may be challenging on CTA images due to multiple fenestrations (communications through the intima) resulting in equal or mildly asymmetrical opacification of both lumens.

- Intramural hematoma (IMH): 3–13% of acute aortic dissections. Non-communicating aortic dissection. Hematoma in the media forms the false lumen. No visible intimal tear. Typical unenhanced CT features are smooth high-density rim with regular inner aortic wall margin (cf. atherosclerosis – patchy and irregular aortic inner margin). Displacement of intimal calcification into the aortic lumen (better seen on narrow window settings). In the absence of non-contrast images, presence of a smooth aortic margin (irregular in mural thrombus) with surrounding homogeneous low density has a high index of suspicion for acute IMH.

Suggested reading

Bonomo L *et al.* Non-traumatic thoracic emergencies: acute chest pain: diagnostic strategies: *Eur Radiol* 2002;**12**(8):1869–1871.

Katarzyna JM, Corl FM, Fishman EK, Bluemke DA. Pathogenesis in acute aortic syndromes: aortic dissection, intramural hematoma, and penetrating atherosclerotic aortic ulcer. *Am J Roentgenol* 2003;**181**:309–316.

2.4 Traumatic aortic injury

Traumatic aortic transection or rupture is rare but it is a major cause of mortality if untreated. There is an aortic tear (intima or media) due to a rapid acceleration/deceleration injury to chest. See Fig. 2.4.

Clinical

Causes: Blunt chest trauma due to motor vehicle accidents and falls. Clinical features include chest pain, hypotension, tachycardia and diaphoresis.

In suspected aortic injury CT angiogram of the aorta is the modality of imaging if the patient is hemodynamically stable. In a hemodynamically unstable patient with suspected aortic injury, resuscitation followed by surgical intervention is the better option. In chest injury or polytrauma, presence of hypotension and tachycardia with or without abnormal widening of mediastinum on CXR, should raise the suspicion of aortic injury.

Indication: Polytrauma, high-speed injury to chest, chest pain and radiographic evidence of abnormal widening of mediastinum with or without pleural effusion and displacement of intimal aortic calcification. An apical pleural cap is due to extravasation of blood from the mediastinum into the extrapleural space.

Technique

Limited non-contrast chest CT and contrast-enhanced CT of the whole aorta including supra aortic branch vessels and femoral arteries. In low pretest probability patients, CT of the thoracic aorta alone would be sufficient. Bolus tracking can be employed with ROI in the proximal descending aorta for whole aorta imaging. Contrast: 100–120 ml, rate 3 ml/s. Non-ECG gating study is sufficient but gated study would alleviate motion artifact at aortic root.

Findings

1. Displacement of intima with mural curvilinear high density.
2. Intimal tear evident by linear hypodensity at the level of isthmus just distal to the origin of the left subclavian artery (LSA).

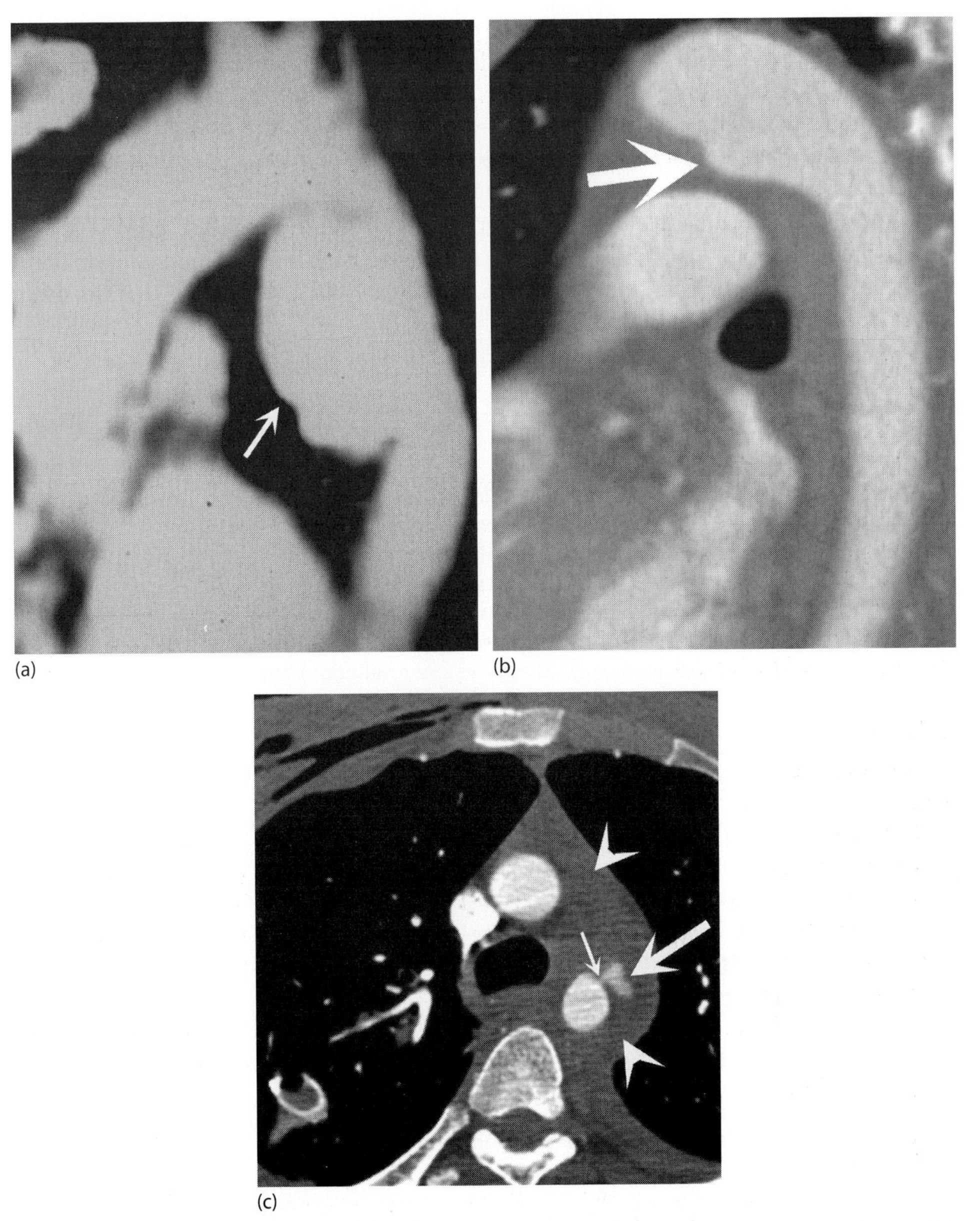

Fig. 2.4. (a) Traumatic aortic pseudoaneurysm. Sagittal CTA shows irregular anterior outpouching (arrow) at the junction of the aortic arch and descending aorta, with abrupt change in contour of the aorta at the ends of the abnormal segment. (b) Ductus diverticulum. Sagittal CECT shows a focal bulge forming smooth obtuse angles with the aortic wall along the anteromedial aspect of the proximal descending aorta (arrow). (c) Traumatic aortic transection. Axial CECT shows an irregular area of contrast pooling (arrow) antero-lateral to the transverse arch with an apparent small communication (thin arrow) to the aortic arch surrounded by periaortic and mediastinal hematoma (arrowheads), features are consistent with acute aortic pseudoaneurysm.

3. Pseudoaneurysm: This is due to a tear in the media with resulting subadventitial and surrounding peri-aortic hematoma. This is seen as an irregular small contrast-filled out-pouching/sac which is attached to the inferior wall of the distal aortic arch/proximal descending aorta via a small channel. It is commonly surrounded by an intermediate to high-density hematoma. It makes an acute angle with the aorta.
4. Extravasation of contrast indicates rupture.
5. Mediastinal hematoma, pleural and/or pericardial effusion.
6. Focal aortic luminal thrombus, periaortic fluid, irregular aortic contour, abnormally small calibre aortic lumen, small size aorta, focal linear filling defects due to intimal flap are other signs of aortic injury.

Pearls

- Negative CTA scan rules out aortic injury.
- Mediastinal hematoma alone may be related due to venous injury. Traumatic aortic transection is the cause of mediastinal hematoma in fewer than 15%.
- Traumatic pseudoaneurysm is consistent with acute injury to the aorta. Always look at the sagittal reformatted images for pseudoaneurysm.
- Mention the size of pseudoaneurysm, its distance from the LSA, extension of tear, patency and measurement of iliac and femoral arteries, for planning endovascular intervention.
- Remnant ductus diverticulum (DD), along the antero-inferior transverse arch distal to the take off of the left subclavian artery, usually has a smooth margin, and an obtuse angle to the aorta. It is not associated with mediastinal hematoma.
- Virtual angioscopy of the aorta at workstation may demonstrate intimal flap and irregular intima in traumatic aortic pseudoaneurysm, but not in DD.
- Penetrating ulcer is commonly located in descending aorta of elderly patients and it appears as a small irregular area of contrast out-pouching with adjacent calcification and mural thrombus. The aorta is generally atherosclerotic.
- DD is a normal variant seen in approximately 10–20% of adults.
- An aortic tear usually seen along the anterior-lateral aortic arch at the isthmus. It classically has an acute margin, is irregularly shaped, and almost always has associated mediastinal hematoma.

Suggested reading

Cleverley JR *et al.* Direct findings of aortic injury on contrast-enhanced CT in surgically proven traumatic aortic injury. *Clin Radiol* 2002;**57**:281–286.

Mirvis SE, Kostrubiak I, Whitley NO, Goldstein LD, Rodriguez A. Use of spiral computed tomography for the assessment of blunt trauma patients with potential aortic injury. *J Trauma* 2004;**56**:243–250.

Scaglione M *et al.* Role of contrast enhanced helical CT in evaluation of acute thoracic aortic injuries after blunt chest trauma. *Eur Radiol* 2001;**11**(12):2444–2448.

2.5 Traumatic peripheral vascular injury

In trauma, vascular compromise due to dissection, rupture and vasospasm can occur in peripheral arteries due to lower or upper limb fractures. It represents a vascular emergency. See Fig. 2.5.

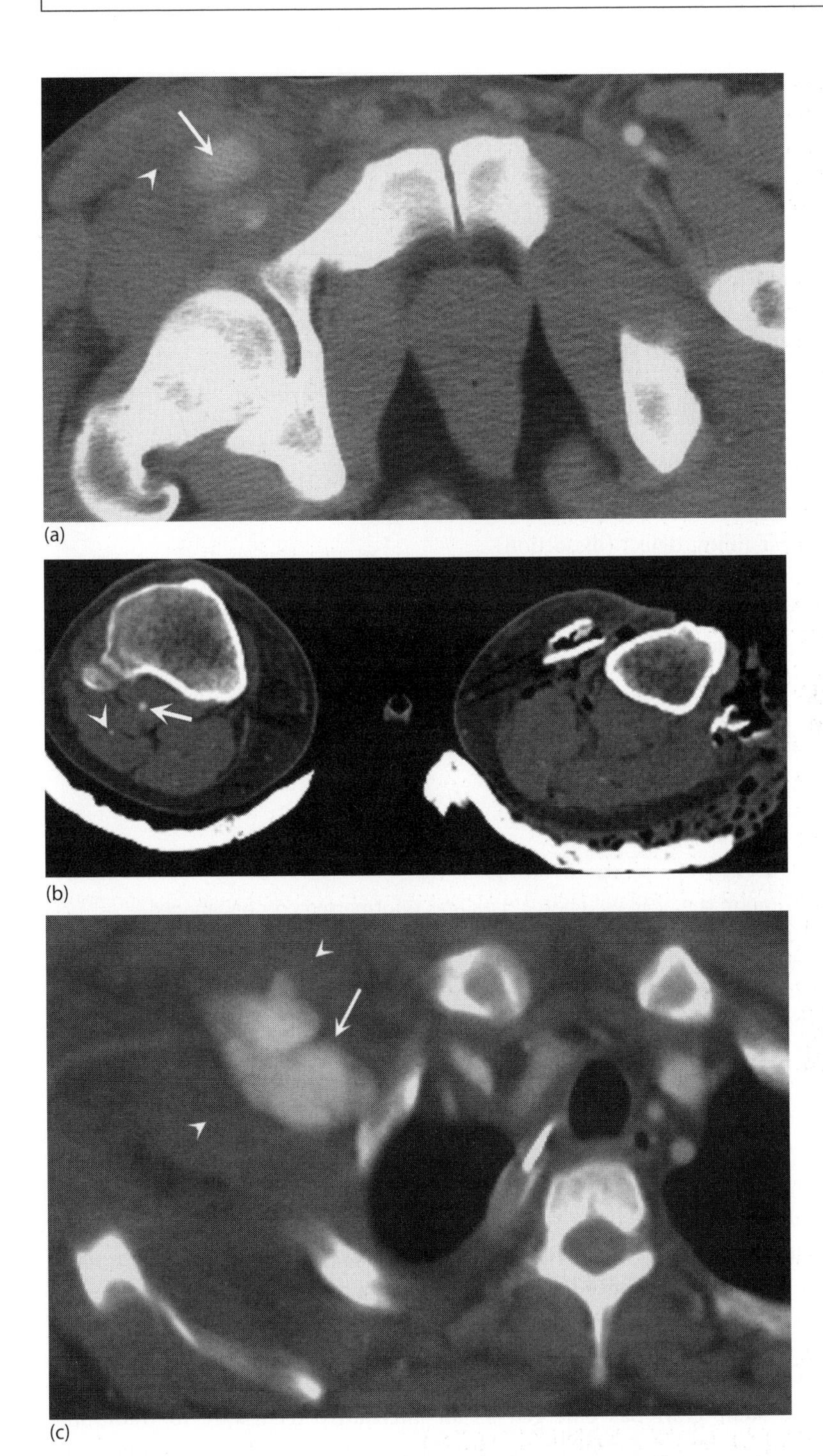

Fig. 2.5. (a) Femoral artery pseudoaneurysm. Axial CTA in a patient with trauma shows an ill-defined saccular contrast filled outpouching (arrow) of right femoral artery with adjacent thrombus (arrowhead) and hematoma due to a leaking femoral artery pseudoaneurysm. (b) Lower extremity arterial injury. Axial CTA in a trauma patient shows normal popliteal artery (arrow) and trifurcation arteries (arrowhead) on the right side, with no arterial enhancement on the left side due to severe vasospasm or dissection. (c) Right subclavian artery injury. Axial CTA shows a contrast filled outpouching extending from the proximal subclavian artery (arrow) and adjacent soft tissue hematoma (arrowheads), consistent with traumatic pseudoaneurysm.

Clinical

Cold peripheries, decreased or absent pulse, pain, purple skin all suggest peripheral vascular compromise. Indication includes traumatic bone injury with suspected vascular compromise to peripheral arteries.

Technique

Lower limb: CT angiogram: 120–140 ml of contrast at 3–4 ml/s. Bolus tracking with ROI at distal abdominal aorta (120–150 HU). Field of view includes from pelvis to feet.
Upper limb: Target to relevant arm. Contrast 100–120 ml at 3–4 ml/s with ROI placed at aortic arch. Cover from aortic arch to R or L distal forearm.

Findings

1. Intimal flap/linear filling defect (dissection).
2. Extravasation of contrast (in rupture).
3. Enhancement of veins during arterial phase scan (traumatic arteriovenous fistula).
4. Pseudoaneurysm (dissection).
5. Markedly attenuated or sudden disappearance of arteries (intimal dissection or intense vasospasm).
6. Look for associated osseous fractures and soft tissue hematoma, foreign body and gas pockets.

Pearls

- Always scroll through the axial volumetric data and reformatted coronal images.
- Careful evaluation of vascular anatomy is recommended.
- Sudden disappearance of peripheral arteries suggests occlusion due to peripheral thrombo-embolism, dissection and/or intense vasospasm in trauma. Consider vasculitis in the absence of trauma.

Suggested reading

Rieger M, Mallouhi A, Tauscher T, Lutz M, Jaschke WR. Traumatic arterial injuries of the extremities: initial evaluation with MDCT. *Am J Roentgenol* 2006;**186**:656–664.

Soto JA *et al.* Focal arterial injuries of the proximal extremities: helical CT arteriography as the initial method of diagnosis. *Radiology* 2001;**218**:188–194.

2.6 Endovascular aortic stent graft

Endovascular aortic stent graft has emerged as an alternative technique to traditional surgical repair of thoracic and abdominal aortic pathologies. Post-treatment complications are common including endoleaks. Normally there should not be any blood within the excluded thrombosed aneurysmal sac or false lumen of dissection. Presence of blood within the excluded aneurysmal sac is called endoleak. See Fig. 2.6.

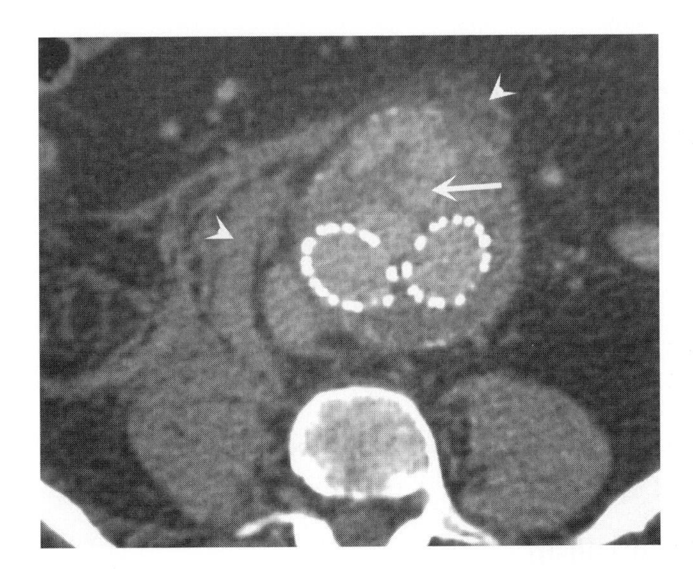

Fig. 2.6. Ruptured endoleak. Axial CTA shows an infrarenal abdominal aortic aneurysm, endovascular stent grafting, and endoleak (arrow) and retroperitoneal/para-aortic hematoma (arrowheads).

Clinical

Usually patients are asymptomatic but endoleaks may present with abdominal pain. Hypotension and tachycardia may indicate infection, rupture or severe endoleak.

Technique

Contrast-enhanced CTA of the aorta. Single arterial phase is sufficient. In doubtful versus suspected endoleaks, arterial and 90–120 s late phase scan may be useful to identify endoleaks.

Complications

1. Leakage of contrast into the aneurysm sac or near the proximal or distal segment of the graft.
2. Extravasation of contrast into abdomen or chest due to graft or aortic rupture.
3. Enlarging aneurysmal sac with apparent high-density thrombus (Endotension-type V).
4. Perigraft collection or hematoma. Air-fluid level and air pockets suggest infection.
5. Occlusion of mesenteric vessels or renal arteries.
6. Occlusion of the stent or in-stent thrombosis.
7. Graft struts fracture (type IV).
8. Retraction of grafts causing inadequate anchoring.

Pearls

- Endoleak is a complication in over 20% of patients.
- Type I leaks are due to an inadequate landing zone at the proximal and distal attachment site of the stent graft and type II leaks are due to collateral filling of the residual aneurysmal sac. The latter is usually due to patent inferior mesenteric artery at the origin

(high-density blood is seen anteriorly in the aneurysmal sac) but also due to lumbar arteries, in which blood is seen posteriorly within the sac. Type 3 endoleak is due to graft porosity.

- In the immediate post-stent check scan, look for retroperitoneal hemorrhage due to iliac or femoral arterial injury.
- Important complications should be discussed with an interventional vascular radiologist or surgeon.

Suggested reading

Garzon G *et al.* Endovascular stent-graft treatment of thoracic aortic disease. *Radiographics* 2005;**25** Suppl. 1:S229–S244.

Katzen BT, Dake MD, MacLean AA, Wang DS. Endovascular repair of abdominal and thoracic aortic aneurysms. *Circulation* 2005;**13**:1663–1675.

2.7 Acute pulmonary embolism

Presence of clot in the pulmonary arteries. See Fig. 2.7.

Clinical

Acute onset of chest pain, breathlessness and tachycardia. Other presentations include atrial fibrillation, collapse, cardiac arrest. Hypotension, tachycardia and respiratory failure are suggestive of severe PE. Chest radiography is usually unremarkable but may show peripheral wedge-shaped consolidation, pleural effusion, enlarged pulmonary arteries and focal oligemia (Westermark's sign).

Indications

Suspected pulmonary embolism in an unstable patient.
Equivocal ventilation/perfusion (V/Q) imaging.
Acute presentation.
Coexisting cardiorespiratory disease or abnormalities on the chest radiograph (V/Q scan is not helpful here).
CT pulmonary angiogram (CTPA): Sensitivity and specificity are approximately 95–100% for thin (1–2 mm) collimation spiral CT technique. Negative predictive value (NPV) for PE is almost 100% with good quality spiral CTPA.

Technique

Contrast-enhanced scans only. Precaution in renal failure patients (make the clinician aware of contrast-induced nephropathy).

Scan delay 15–25 s (1 mm–2.5 mm), but bolus tracking is preferable.

Thin collimation spiral CT of the entire thorax (can identify subsegmental pulmonary arteries). 1.5 mm collimation scan of entire thorax will probably give sufficient information on the central and segmental arteries in a sick and uncooperative patient.

Prior hyperventilation increases the patient breath-hold time and improves the scan quality.

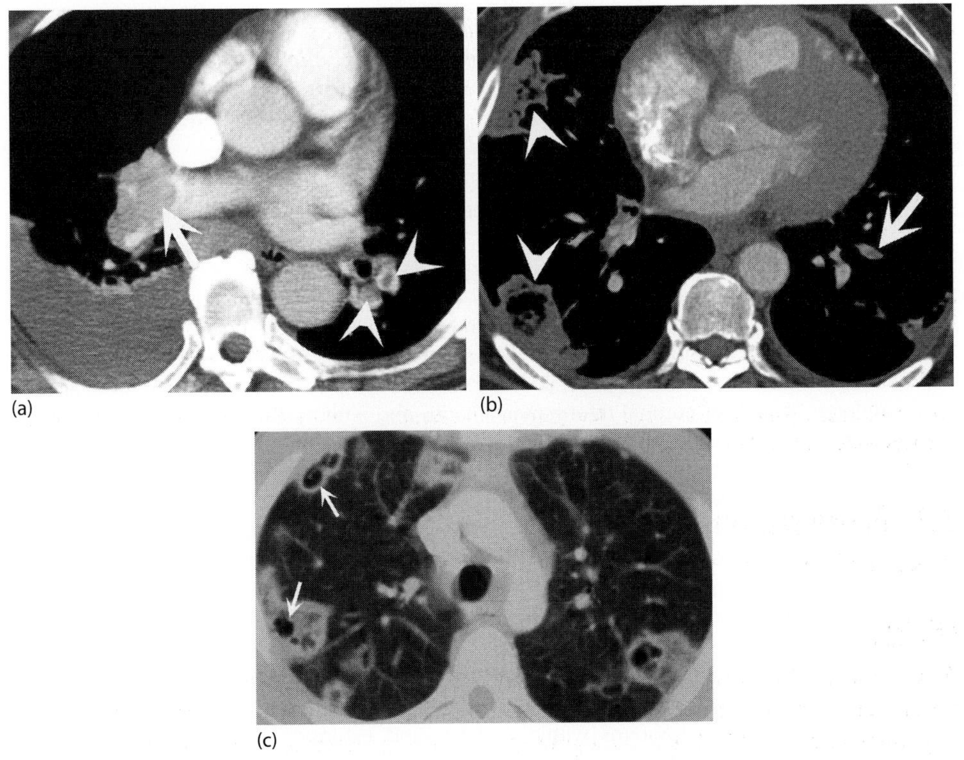

Fig. 2.7. (a) Acute PE. CTA chest shows large globular filling defects within the distal right main pulmonary artery (arrow) and filling defects within segmental pulmonary arteries in the left lower lobe (arrowheads) and a large right-sided pleural effusion. (b) Chronic PE. CTA chest shows non-occlusive intraluminal filling defects (arrows) adherent to the wall and multiple peripheral cavitary infarcts (arrowhead). (c) Septic emboli. Axial CT chest of an intravenous drug abuse patient shows multiple peripheral cavitary nodules (arrows) due to septic emboli. Echocardiography demonstrated tricuspid valve vegetations.

Data acquisition in deep inspiration: For intubated and ventilated patients, the ventilator is manually suspended in deep inspiration while obtaining the scan.

Findings

Examine the lobar, segmental and subsegmental pulmonary arteries at the workstation in axial, sagittal and coronal reformatted images.

1. Endoluminal clot: This is seen as a partial intravascular central or marginal filling defect surrounded by contrast forming an acute angle with the vessel wall ("polo mint" or "tram line" sign). A complete intravascular filling defect occupies the entire vessel, without rim enhancement.
2. Dilated pulmonary artery proximal to the clot.
3. Other non-specific signs: Peripheral wedge-shaped consolidation represents a pulmonary infarction especially if it is non-enhancing and displays a thick vessel running towards the bubbly consolidation (vascular sign).
4. Pleural effusion and right-heart dilation. The central pulmonary arteries may be dilated in subacute PE.

Pearls

- Pseudo-filling defects; apparent filling defects seen on only one or two images are likely due to artefact.
  Causes:
  Vertically oriented vessels. Unlikely to occur in thin collimation MSCT.
  Breathing artefact.
  Laminar blood flow-inadequate contrast opacification at either the beginning or the end of the scan.
  Beam hardening artefacts from SVC contrast – saline flush after bolus, caudo-cranial scanning helps to avoid these.
  Cardiac failure causes prominent intersegmental lymph nodes, peri broncho-vascular tissue thickening and slow flow in pulmonary veins. Also dilated bronchial artery in the peri broncho-vascular space, partially calcified lymph nodes mimic vascular filling defects. Sagittal or coronal reformatted images and altering the window level may be useful to overcome some of these problems.
  "Stair-step" artefact: On axial images there is low density in the vessel lumen simulating PE, however, on MPR images horizontal band-like low-density areas alternate with high-density areas due to Z axis artefact. True endoluminal clot in PE extends cranio-caudally.
  Extensive air space consolidation and reactive pulmonary vasoconstriction can lead to false positive diagnosis of PE.
- Look for an alternative diagnosis: pneumomediastinum, pneumothorax, pneumonia, neoplasia.
- Septic emboli: Findings include multiple peripheral cavitary lung nodules (common), feeding vessel leading to the nodules, wedge-shaped peripheral lesions abutting the pleura, air bronchograms within nodules, and extension into the pleural space, sometimes complicated by empyema formation. Intravenous drug users with right-heart endocarditis and patients with central venous line are at high risk of developing septic emboli.
- Chronic PE: Non-occlusive intraluminal filling defects adherent to the wall, multiple peripheral cavitary lesions, pulmonary artery webs, luminal irregularities, calcification, areas of abrupt vessel narrowing and/or obstruction, and dilated central pulmonary arteries (i.e. main pulmonary artery > 2.9 cm in diameter), RV strain. Pulmonary findings are usually bilateral.

Suggested reading

Wittram C *et al.* Acute and chronic pulmonary emboli: angiography-CT correlation. *Am J Roentgenol* 2006;**186**:S421–S429.

Wittram C *et al.* CT angiography of pulmonary embolism: diagnostic criteria and causes of misdiagnosis. *Radiographics* 2004;**24**:1219–1238.

2.8 Aortic aneurysm/rupture

A focal irreversible dilatation of the aorta. See Fig. 2.8.

True aneurysm involves dilatation of all three layers (intima, media and adventitia) of the aortic wall. At least one of these layers is not involved in false aneurysm or pseudoaneurysm.

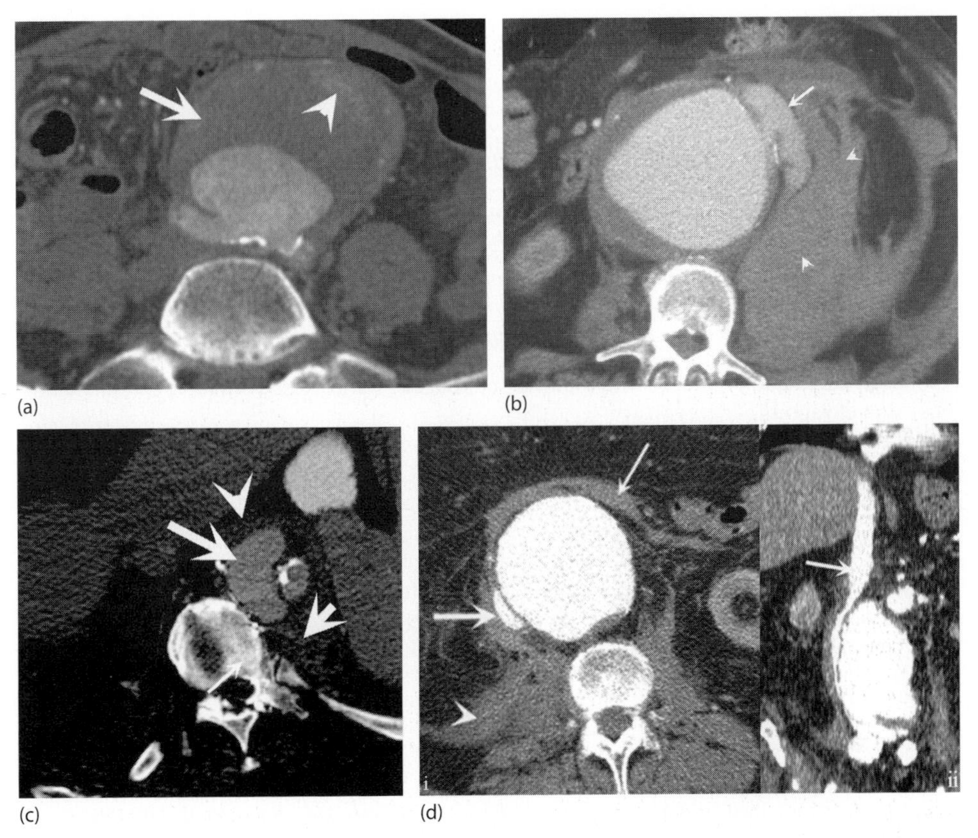

Fig. 2.8. (a) Imminent rupture of AAA. Axial CTA shows a large outpouching (arrow) near the bifurcation of the abdominal aorta into the iliac arteries. Note the small crescent-shaped area of hyperdensity (arrowhead) within the large thrombus anteriorly. (b) Ruptured AAA. Axial CTA shows a large infrarenal AAA with extravasation of contrast (arrow) and a large left retroperitoneal hematoma (arrowheads). (c) Septic aortic pseudoaneurysm. Axial CTA image shows a saccular outpouching (arrow) from the descending thoracic aorta, increased peri-aortic thickening (arrowhead), left paravertebral soft tissue enhancement, right pleural effusion and chronic osteomyelitis of vertebral body (note increased bone sclerosis – thin arrow). (d) Aorto-caval fistula CTA images show a large abdominal aortic aneurysm with simultaneous enhancement of the entire inferior vena cava (arrows), consistent with aorto-caval fistula. Enlarged right psoas muscle (arrowhead) and soft tissue stranding (thin arrow) represents hematoma due to leaking AAA. (Fig. 2.8d courtesy of Dr. A. Camenzuli, Radiologist, Liverpool, UK.)

Focal dilatation of ascending or descending thoracic aorta greater than 4 cm and focal dilatation of the abdominal aorta greater than 3 cm are considered as aortic aneurysm.

Clinical

Abdominal pain, and palpable pulsatile mass. Aortic rupture can present with shock, and rarely with hemoptysis or GI bleeding.

Technique

Non-contrast and contrast-enhanced scan.

Limited non-contrast images are useful to clearly demonstrate a high attenuation crescent with the sac.

Findings

1. Dilatation of the aorta.
2. Contained rupture: High-density sac.
3. Imminent sign of rupture: High-attenuation crescent within the sac but outside the perfused lumen.
4. Rupture: Extravasation of contrast, discontinuity of circumferential mural calcification of aorta, discontinuity of aortic wall, para aortic and retroperitoneal hematoma, pleural and pericardial hematoma.

Pearls

- High-attenuation crescent within the sac but outside the perfused lumen is an imminent sign of rupture.
- Complications include aortocaval fistula and aorto-enteric fistula which are recognized by demonstrating high-density contrast within the IVC and bowel loops.
- Luminal diameter of iliac and femoral arteries (especially stenosis) will help in planning the endovascular stent graft placement.
- Measurements: Transverse and AP diameter of the aneurysm, proximal neck length of the aneurysm – this is measured from the level of left subclavian artery to the descending aortic aneurysm and from the level of renal artery to infrarenal abdominal aortic aneurysm. Diameter of iliac and femoral arteries should be mentioned.

Suggested reading

Schwartz SA, Taljanovic MS, Smyth S, O'Brien MJ, Rogers LF. CT findings of rupture, impending rupture, and contained rupture of abdominal aortic aneurysms. *Am J Roentgenol* 2007;**188**: W57–W62.

Siegel CL *et al.* Abdominal aortic aneurysm morphology: CT features in patients with ruptured and nonruptured aneurysms. *Am J Roentgenol* 1994;**163**:1123–1129.

2.9 Coronary artery imaging

Ischemic heart disease is one of the most common causes of medical emergency. MDCT coronary artery imaging is emerging as an alternative attractive technique compared with catheter angiography excluding significant coronary artery stenosis. See Fig. 2.9.

Clinical

Typical ischemic-related chest pain with ECG changes needs conventional angiography and intervention if necessary. In patients with chest pain and non-specific ECG changes and equivocal cardiac enzymes, coronary CTA can be performed to exclude significant stenosis.

Indications include atypical chest pain, pre-operative evaluation of the coronary artery, coronary artery graft patency, coronary artery aneurysm, anomalous origin or course, coronary sinus fistula.

Technique

16-slice MDCT: 0.75 mm collimation, bolus tracking at ascending aorta, 120 ml of contrast at 5 ml/s followed by 40 ml of saline at 5 ml/s, scan coverage from pulmonary trunk to base

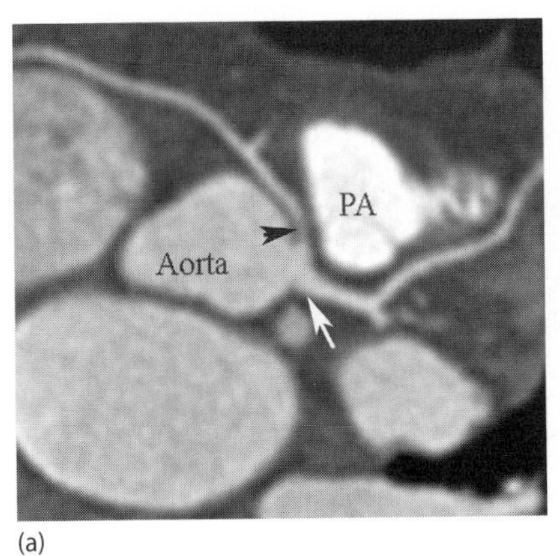

(a)

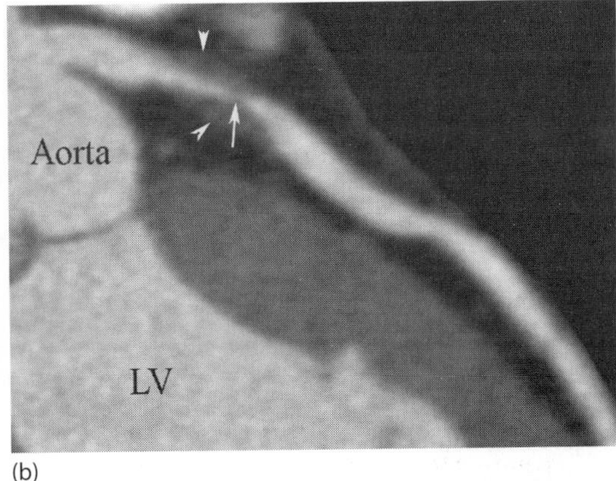

(b)

Fig. 2.9. (a) Anomalous right coronary artery. Coronary CTA shows anomalous origin of the right coronary artery from the left coronary cusp (arrow) with an inter-arterial course (arrowhead) between aorta and right ventricular outflow tract/pulmonary trunk. (b) Coronary artery stenosis. Coronary CTA shows a high-grade stenosis (arrow) due to non-calcified plaque (arrowheads) in the proximal LAD.

of heart (in LIMA or RIMA, include lung apices and supra aortic branch vessels). ECG gated scan during breath hold.

64-slice MDCT: 0.6 mm collimation, 80–100 ml of contrast at 5 ml/s followed by 40 ml of 0.9% saline. Reformat images at 0.75 mm slice thickness with 0.4 mm overlap using smooth kernel B26. For evaluation of in-stent restenosis, it is important to use an edge-enhancing kernel such as B46.

Pre-medication: Intravenous metoprolol 5 mg every 5 minutes to a maximum dose of 15 mg (some centers advocate up to 40 mg) to reduce the heart rate to less than 65/min on inspiration. Single dose of sublingual nitroglycerin spray of 400 mcg may be administered 2–4 minutes before the image acquisition. Continuous monitoring of pulse, blood pressure until 10 minutes after the scan is recommended if beta-blockers are given. Check for postural drop in blood pressure if sublingual nitroglycerin has been given. An oral beta blocker such as metoprolol 50–100 mg can be given ideally an hour before the scan. If the heart rate is still over 70/min at the time of scan, intravenous metoprolol can be administered just before the data acquisition while the patient is on the scanner. See Chapter 10.6.

Contraindication for beta-blocker: Asthma, heart block, severe aortic stenosis and cardiac failure. Alternatively a calcium channel blocker may be used as a rate-controlling drug.

Post-processing: Should be done at a special workstation for vessel tracking and to grade the stenosis.

Findings

1. Right coronary artery arises from anterior coronary cusp and left main stem artery from left coronary sinus. Normally, no artery arises from the posterior non-coronary cusp.
2. Look for an anomalous course of coronary artery between the aortic root and RVOT or pulmonary trunk. Check for posterior descending artery running along the posterior interventricular septum to determine the dominance (RCA: 85–90% and LCX: 10–15%).
3. Calcified and low-density non-calcified plaques.
4. Luminal stenosis – considered significant if the diameter stenosis is greater than 50%.
5. Abnormally large tortuous coronary arteries and veins suggest arteriovenous fistula.
6. Look for coronary artery aneurysms.

Pearls

- Evaluate LMS, left anterior descending coronary artery and its first and second diagonal branches, circumflex and its obtuse marginal branches, and right coronary and posterior descending arteries.
- Grading of luminal stenosis: mild $<50\%$, moderate 50–70%, high grade >70 but $<99\%$, and occlusion 100%.
- Look at the aorta and main pulmonary arteries for focal abnormality.
- Dual tube 64-slice CT scanner may obviate the need for beta blockade in patients with tachycardia.

Suggested reading

Achenbach S *et al.* Detection of coronary artery stenoses by contrast-enhanced retrospectively electrocardiographically-gated multislice spiral computed tomography. *Circulation* 2001;**103**: 2535–2538.

Hoffman U *et al.* Cardiac CT in emergency department patients with acute chest pain. *Radiographics* 2006;**26**(4):963–978.

2.10 Pleural empyema

Focal infected fluid collection in the potential pleural space. See Fig. 2.10.

Clinical

Usually unwell with fever, dull chest pain and dyspnea. Common causes include secondary to pneumonia, and immunocompromised state due to intravenous drug abuse and HIV infection.

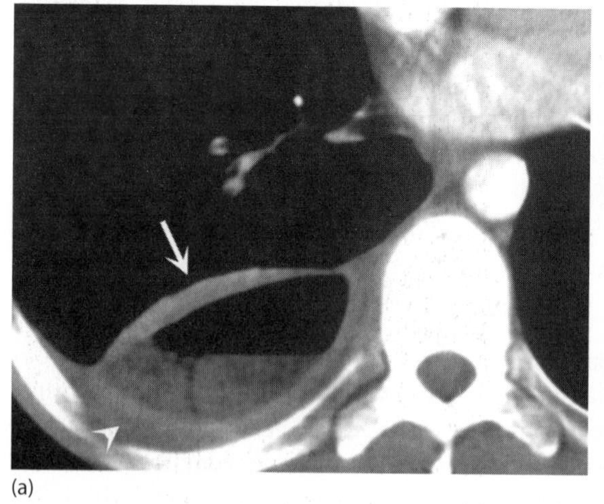

(a)

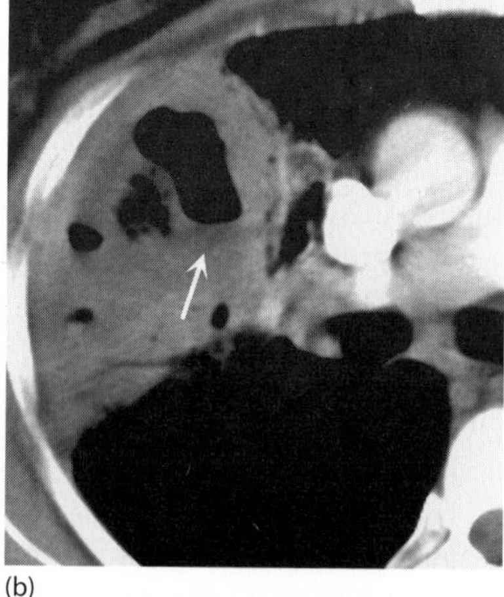

(b)

Fig. 2.10. (a) Empyema. Axial CECT shows a peripherally enhancing elliptical-shaped pleural collection with an air-fluid level (arrow). Note the thickening of the extrapleural subcostal fat (arrowhead), seen with chronic empyemas. (b) Lung abscess. Axial CECT shows an irregular non-elliptical intraparenchymal abscess cavity with an air-fluid level (arrow).

Technique

Contrast-enhanced chest CT.

Chest X-ray may show pleural opacification with or without air–fluid level.

CECT chest findings

1. Enhancing visceral and parietal pleura with fluid in between causing typical "split pleura" sign.
2. Elliptical shaped pleural collection.
3. Gas pockets, and an air–fluid level within the pleural collection.
4. Septations may be seen as linear intermediate density strands. Note that septations may be invisible on CT and only seen on US.
5. Extrapleural subcostal fat is of high attenuation in acute empyema. This fat layer becomes thickened with chronic empyemas.

Pearls

- US is more sensitive at identifying septations which appear as echogenic strands. This indicates a loculated collection.
- Lung abscess: Intra parenchymal, non-elliptical and has irregular wall. More spherical than elliptical. When close to the pleura, lung abscesses usually make an acute angle with the pleura whereas empyemas commonly result in an obtuse angle.

Suggested reading

Kuhlman JE, Singha NK. Complex disease of the pleural space: radiographic and CT evaluation. *Radiographics* 1997;17(1):63–79.

2.11 Acute mediastinitis

This is a rare but serious condition due to acute infection of the mediastinum. Chest CT is the best imaging modality of choice, which aids the diagnosis and guides percutaneous drainage of the mediastinal collection. See Fig. 2.11.

Causes include esophageal/pharyngeal perforation, post-sternotomy, extension of infection from elsewhere and may be associated with empyema.

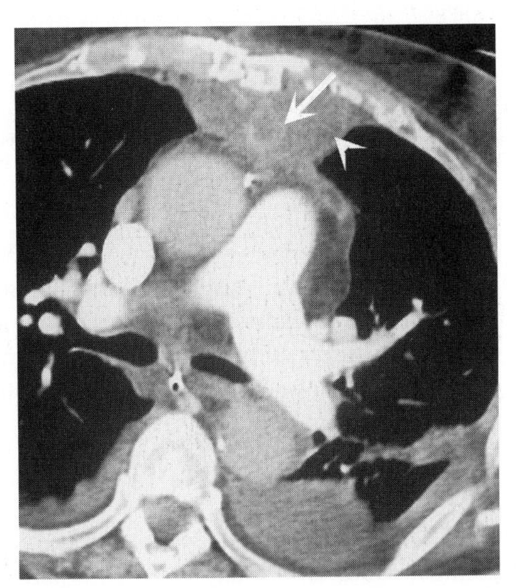

Fig. 2.11. Mediastinitis. Axial CECT shows a small pocket of enhancing loculated abscess (arrow) within the peripherally enhancing fluid collection (arrow head) in the anterior mediastinum. A small right pleural effusion and moderate left loculated pleural collection.

Clinical

Unwell, fever and chest pain.

Technique

CECT chest with oral contrast if indicated (lung and mediastinal settings, oral non-ionic contrast may be useful in suspected esophageal perforation).

Findings

1. Mediastinal enlargement.
2. Fluid collection with enhancing wall in the mediastinum (especially anterior and posterior).
3. Collection of air within the mediastinal fluid may be scattered (diffuse mediastinitis) or localized with air–fluid level (abscess).
4. Pneumomediastinum and/or effusion in esophageal perforation (in Boerhaave's syndrome there is a left pleural effusion and left lower lobe consolidation).
5. Look for associated empyema, pericardial effusion, jugular vein thrombosis. Contrast leak into the mediastinum or pleural space is associated with esophageal perforation.

Pearls

- Within 2 weeks after sternotomy, the above features are not specific of acute mediastinitis but are strongly suggestive of mediastinitis after the 14th post-operative day.
- Post-operative seroma or hematoma takes at least 2 weeks to resolve. Persistent and progressive air–fluid collection with an associated enhancing wall is highly suggestive of infection.
- In immediate post-sternotomy patients, evaluate for missing sternal wire, osteomyelitis (bone resorption indicates acute osteomyelitis; sclerosis and periostitis indicate chronic), bone fragmentation and widening of sternal fragments.

Suggested reading

Armstrong P. *Imaging of Diseases of the Chest, 2nd edition*. Mosby-Year Book, 1995.

Exarhos DN *et al.* Acute mediastinitis: spectrum of computed tomography findings. *Eur Radiol* 2005;**15**(8):1569–1574.

2.12 Esophageal perforation/dissection

Partial tear of the esophageal wall causes dissection. A complete tear through the wall results in perforation. See Fig. 2.12.

Clinical

Painful swallowing, dysphagia and chest pain. Causes include spontaneous, post-instrumentation, excessive retching, tumor necrosis, drugs, ulcers, retained foreign body, esophageal cancer and trauma. Iatrogenic injury is the most common cause of esophageal perforation, followed by spontaneous rupture (Boerhaave's syndrome) and blunt chest trauma.

Technique

MDCT of the chest and upper abdomen obtained following the administration of oral contrast which is typically given to a patient less than 30 minutes before the scan. 100–200 ml of non-ionic iodinated contrast medium should be utilized.

Oral gastrografin is contraindicated. This can result in pulmonary edema if the patient aspirates. Barium should be avoided to prevent barium mediastinitis and barium peritonitis if there is a communication with the peritoneum.

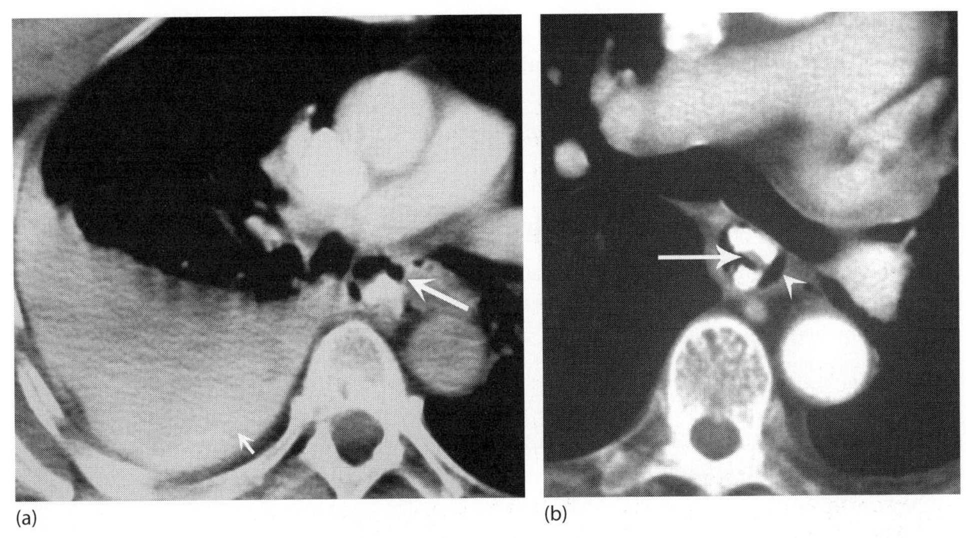

Fig. 2.12. (a) Esophageal perforation. Axial CECT shows a large amount of oral contrast layering posteriorly in the right hemithorax (small arrow), with some contrast and air seen within and adjacent to the esophagus (arrow). (b) Esophageal dissection. Chest CT shows a thin low-density mucosal dissection flap separating the false and true lumens (arrow). Note intramural air bubble in the esophagus (arrowhead).

Findings

1. Perforation
   Contrast can be seen passing through the complete tear.
   Extraluminal collection – mediastinal or pleural filled with high-density contrast.
   Pneumomediastinum.
   Pneumothorax.
   No double lumen.
2. Dissection
   Walled off double lumen (true and false lumen) which are filled with oral contrast. One of the lumina is blind-ending distally and the other is contiguous with the normal distal esophagus. Usually the false lumen is larger than the true lumen. Point of dissection is usually at the cervical esophagus (typically following instrumentation).
   "Mucosal stripe sign" – a thin radiolucent mucosal stripe separates the two lumina.
   Esophageal wall thickening.
   Intramural air.
   No pneumomediastinum.
   No extraluminal collection.

Pearls

- CT may also contribute to identify the cause of perforation, such as a tumor.
- Differentiation of dissection from perforation is important – the latter needs surgery, whereas the former is managed conservatively.
- Regular weekly fluoroscopy may be helpful in the follow up; the blind false lumen will gradually resolve in 4–6 weeks.

Suggested reading

Krishnam MS, Ramadan MF, Curtis J. Intramural esophageal dissection: CT imaging features. *Eur J Radiol Extra* 2005;**56**:17–19.

White CS, Templeton PA, Attar S. Esophageal perforation: CT findings. *Am J Roentgenol* 1994;**162** (4):767–770.

2.13 Superior vena cava syndrome

Progressive swelling and congestion of face and arms due to steno-occlusive disease of the superior vena cava. See Fig. 2.13.

Clinical

Intrinsic cause is due to thrombosis, and extrinsic causes include tumor.

SVC syndrome can be due to extrinsic or intrinsic causes and may need immediate treatment.

Technique

MDCT of the neck and chest covering from C3 through the heart using 1.5 mm collimation.

Scan delay 2–2.5 minutes after at least 120 ml of contrast administration with a 40 ml saline chaser. Rate of contrast injection is 2.5–3 ml/s.

Caudocranial acquisition.

Site of IV access depends on clinical information. Avoid side of pathology.

Images should be reformatted into coronal and sagittal planes.

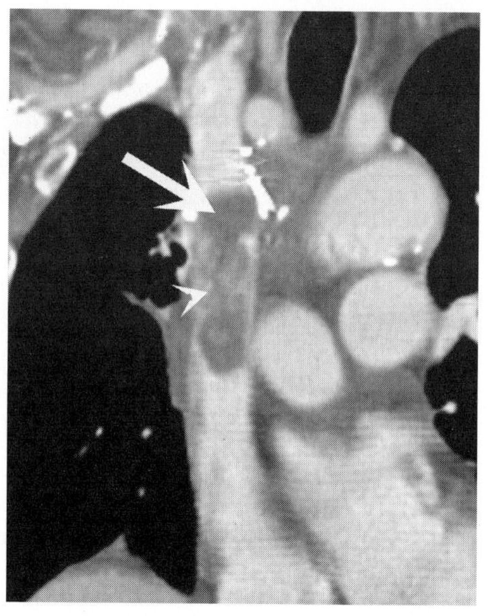

Fig. 2.13. SVC thrombosis. Venous phase CTA shows partial enhancement of (arrowhead) a large low-density thrombus (arrow) in the superior vena cava, representing tumor thrombus.

Findings

1. Clot is seen as a hypodensity within the lumen.
2. Occlusive – The clot is acute if the vessel lumen has been completely filled with clot and is dilated.
3. Non-occlusive; if there is a contrast around the intraluminal clot.
4. Collateral vessels – mediastinal and chest wall.
5. Look for pericatheter irregular low-density thrombus formation.
6. Look for extension of clot into the right atrium and IVC.

Pearls

- Evaluate bilateral internal jugular, bilateral subclavian, bilateral axillary and brachiocephalic veins.
- Coronal views are very helpful.

- Look for other causes such as stricture, post-thrombotic stenosis, and central tumor (tumor thrombi can demonstrate partial contrast enhancement).
- Normally thrombus does not enhance due to its avascularity, however tumor thrombus can show heterogeneous enhancement.

Suggested reading

Eren S, Karaman A, Okur A. The superior vena cava syndrome caused by malignant disease: imaging with multi-detector row CT. *Eur J Radiol* 2006;**59**(1):93–103.

2.14 Mesenteric vascular ischemia/occlusion

Steno-occlusive diseases of mesenteric artery or vein. Infection is one of the most common underlying causes of mesenteric vein thrombosis, with primary sources including diverticulitis, appendicitis and infected pancreatic necrosis. See Fig. 2.14.

Clinical

Recurrent abdominal pain, rectal bleeding or black stools. Risk factors for mesenteric vein thrombosis include cirrhosis, recent abdominal surgery or infection, and other hypercoagulable states (including clotting factor abnormalities, paroxysmal nocturnal hemoglobinuria, thrombocytosis, myeloproliferative disorders, sickle cell disease and homocystinemia).

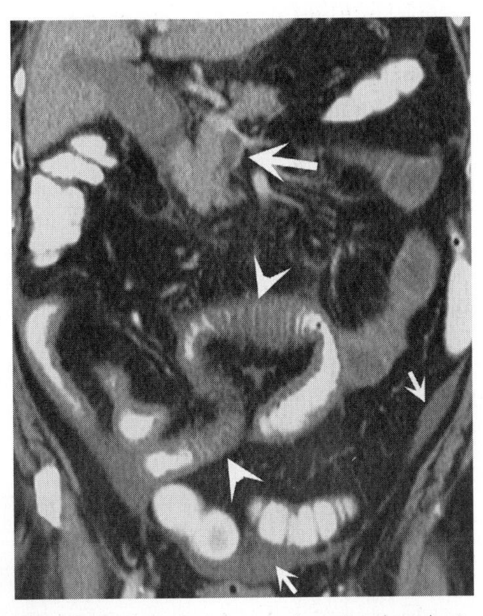

Fig. 2.14. Superior mesenteric vein thrombosis. CECT shows a low-density thrombus within the dilated SMV (arrow) and associated marked small bowel wall thickening (ischemia – likely secondary to edema from impaired venous drainage) (arrowheads), and ascites (small arrows).

Technique

Arterial phase alone is enough to evaluate the arteries but a venous phase scan is required to evaluate the SMV and end organs including the bowel.

Arterial phase scan: Bolus tracking of the suprarenal abdominal aorta following intravenous administration of 100–120 ml of contrast followed by 40 ml of saline chaser at a rate of 3 ml/s. A single portal venous phase scan is sufficient in an emergency setting.

Coronal and sagittal reformatted images are important.

Findings

1. Intraluminal clot within the superior mesenteric artery or vein.
2. Calcified and non-calcified plaque causing any significant stenosis.
3. Markedly diminished calibre of the SMA in shock.
4. Abnormal mural thickening of arteries in vasculitis.
5. Bowel wall thickening (refer to bowel ischemia).

Pearls

- Evaluate SMA/SMV, celiac axis and IMA.
- Evaluate end organs, including bowel.
- Evaluate aorta for atherosclerosis, dissection and vasculitis.

Suggested reading

Cademartiri F *et al.* Multi-detector row CT angiography in patients with abdominal angina. *Radiographics* 2004;**24**(4):969–984.

Romano S, Romano L, Grassi R. Multidetector row computed tomography findings from ischemia to infarction of the large bowel. *Eur J Radiol* 2007;**61**(3):433–441.

2.15 Spontaneous subcutaneous emphysema

Presence of air in the subcutaneous soft tissue of the chest, and neck; it can extend from head to thighs in severe cases. See Fig. 2.15.

Causes

Spontaneous, post-surgical, ruptured esophagus, trauma, tracheo-bronchial injury and ruptured lung parenchymal cyst.

Technique

Plain radiography is usually abnormal and diagnostic. Non-contrast chest CT is helpful in evaluating intra-thoracic causes. Oral contrast should be used in suspected esophageal rupture.

Findings

1. Subcutaneous and soft tissue air in the chest wall.
2. Pneumomediastinum.
3. Pneumothorax.
4. Pneumopericardium.

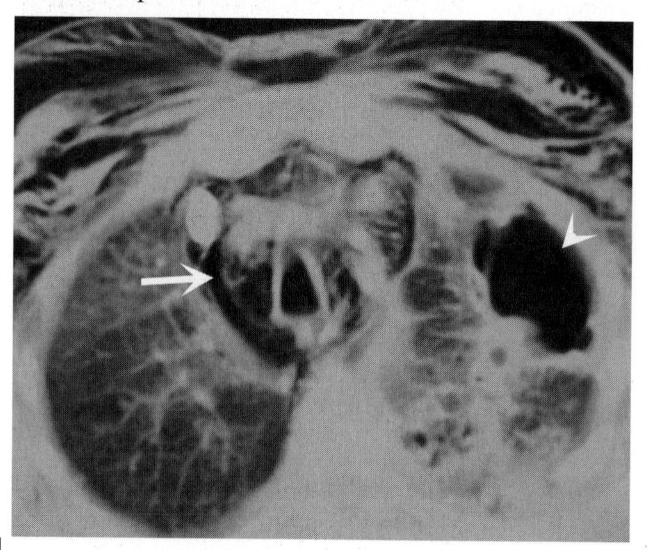

Fig. 2.15. Subcutaneous emphysema. Chest CT shows pneumomediastinum (arrow) and a large amount of air within the subcutaneous soft tissues of the chest due to a rupture of left upper lobe cavitary lesion (arrowhead).

5. Pulmonary interstitial emphysema (peri-bronchovascular hyperluceny/air).
6. Lung parenchymal cysts.
7. Tracheo-bronchial injury.
8. Fallen lung due to tracheo-bronchial rupture. This should be suspected when the pneumothorax fails to resolve after chest tube placement. Pneumoperitonium.
9. Extraluminal presence of oral contrast due to esophageal rupture.

Pearls

- Bronchoscopy and esophagogram/upper GI endoscopy have to be considered in patients with unexplained progressive surgical emphysema of unknown cause.
- On chest radiography, pneumothorax can be obscured in patients with severe overlying surgical emphysema.
- The presence of vomiting/retching prior to the onset of chest pain should suggest an esophageal tear. There should be a high index of suspicion.
- Blunt trauma causing duodenal injury can present with spontaneous subcutaneous emphysema.

Suggested reading

Zylak CM, Standen JR, Barnes GR, Zylak CJ. Pneumomediastinum revisited. *Radiographics* 2000;**20**(4):1043–1057.

2.16 Miscellaneous: Stridor

Stridor is an acute emergency. Causes include laryngeal and tracheal tumors, and foreign bodies. In acutely unwell patients with stridor, imaging is performed only after securing the airway. Contrast-enhanced CT of the neck extending down to the carina is helpful to rule out a mediastinal, tracheal or laryngeal mass. See Fig. 2.16.

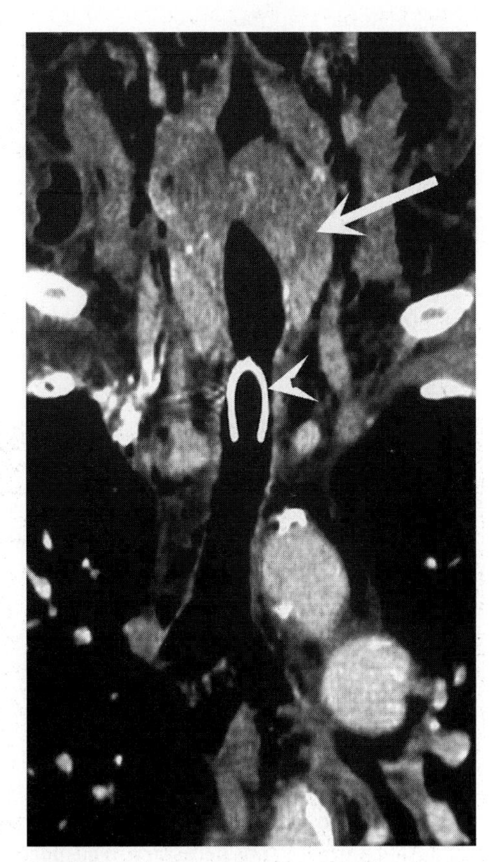

Fig. 2.16. Subglottic tumor. Coronal CT in a patient with stridor and emergency tracheostomy shows a large subglottic tumor surrounding, narrowing the superior trachea and a tracheostomy cannula (arrowhead).

Abdomen and pelvis

Mayil S. Krishnam

3.1 General principles

CT abdomen is increasingly performed in patients with acute abdominal pain. In most centers, CT is increasingly being used for the diagnosis of acute ureteric colic and suspected acute appendicitis. See Fig. 3.1.

Indications

Acute abdomen, acute pancreatitis, aortic dissection/rupture, hollow viscus perforation, fluid collections, diverticulitis/diverticular abscess, liver abscess, mesenteric infarcts, small bowel obstruction, abdominal trauma etc.

Technique

1. Intravenous contrast is necessary in most acute abdominal scanning. Oral contrast given via NG tube or by mouth at least 2 hours before the scan may be helpful in suspected GI tract perforation and in acute pancreatitis to delineate bowel loops. Water can be used as a negative oral contrast in cases of suspected pancreatitis.
2. Oral contrast is not necessary in suspected bowel obstruction, bowel ischemia and acute ureteric colic (in addition, no IV contrast is needed for ureteric colic).

3. In cases of suspected intra-abdominal collection, acute ureteric colic, appendicitis, obstructed bowel, pelvic trauma and retroperitoneal bleeding, thin section CT of the abdomen and pelvis is obtained.
4. Data are acquired in the portal venous phase.
5. Coronal reformats are useful at providing a panoramic "frontal" view of the abdomen.

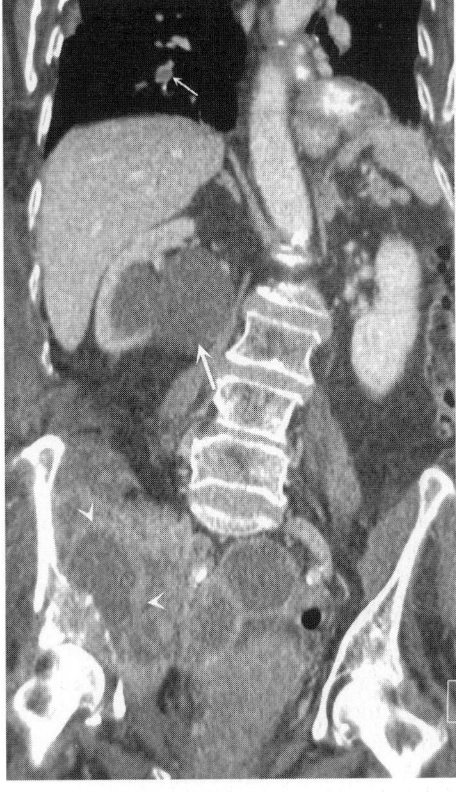

Fig. 3.1. Intra-abdominal abscess. CECT shows multi-loculated fluid collections in the right lower abdomen with thin peripheral enhancement (arrowheads). Note secondary right-sided hydronephrosis (arrow). Incidental pulmonary embolus in the right lower-lobe pulmonary artery (thin arrow).

Review areas in a "near-normal CT abdominal scan"

1. Aorta: Dissection, aneurysm.
2. Bowel: Ischemia, colitis, obstruction, hernia, diverticulitis, appendicitis.
3. Gallbladder: Cholecystitis, empyema.
4. Liver: Portal vein gas, duct dilation.
5. Pancreas: Pancreatitis.
6. Kidneys/Ureters: Stone, hydronephrosis, renal infarct.
7. Peritoneum: Free gas (this is best assessed by viewing the abdomen with lung windows at the workstation), collection, lesser sac collection, duodenal perforation.
8. Mesentery: Free gas, fat stranding.
9. Muscles: Psoas abscess, hematoma, rectus sheath hematoma.
10. Lung base for consolidation, collapse.
11. Diaphragm: Rupture.

3.2 Abdominal trauma – general principles

Blunt abdominal injury is one of the major causes of mortality and morbidity in patients with trauma. Compressive-type abdominal trauma causes vascular or solid organ injuries and deceleration-type trauma causes stretching or shearing vascular injuries. CT has an important role in triaging patients with suspected abdominal injury. See Fig. 3.2.

Clinical

Abdominal pain, abdominal bruise, hypotension, tachycardia etc. Hypotension at the time of presentation is often associated with serious intra-abdominal injury. It may be an indication for surgical or vascular intervention in the appropriate radiological and clinical settings.

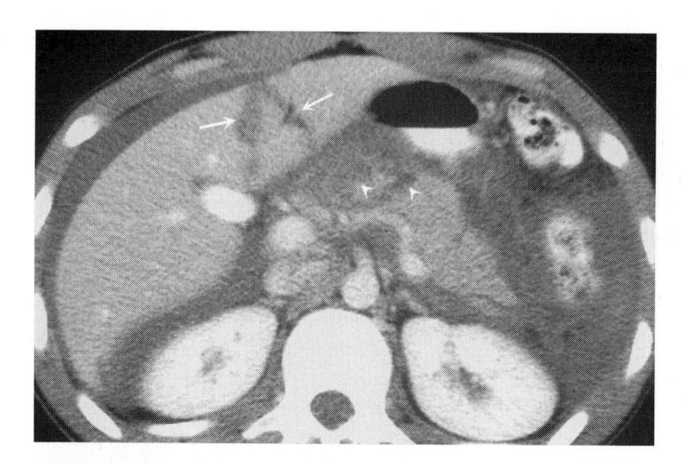

Fig. 3.2. Liver and pancreatic trauma. CECT of upper abdomen shows areas of reduced enhancement within the liver (arrows) and pancreatic body (arrowheads), with high-density fluid within the abdomen, consistent with traumatic parenchymal injury to the liver and pancreas with resultant intra-abdominal hemorrhage.

Technique

Oral contrast can be administered through a nasogastric tube, approximately 30 minutes before the scan which helps to delineate the proximal bowel from other organs such as the pancreas. The presence of extra-luminal contrast indicates bowel wall perforation. Intravenous contrast (120 ml of non-ionic contrast at 3 ml/s) should be given to all patients to evaluate for parenchymal and vascular injury. Portal venous phase (70-s delay) imaging should be performed. The urinary catheter should be clamped prior to imaging to look for bladder rupture. If there is a suspected bladder injury, then a CT cystogram (at least 200–350 ml of warm 30% solution of sodium diatrizoate and meglumine diatrizoate (Urografin) or iohexal (Omnipaque) is instilled via the urinary catheter into the bladder). Alternatively a scan of the pelvis after a 5–10 minute delay can be performed. Multislice axial acquisition of abdomen and pelvis with coronal and sagittal reformatting should be obtained. Images should be viewed on standard soft tissue settings and lung windows, or similar, to detect pneumoperitoneum.

Findings

1. Free fluid in the extra- and intraperitoneal spaces may indicate organ or bowel injury.
2. Density of the fluid assessed by the Hounsfield number is a reliable indicator of the nature of the fluid.
3. A low HU, less than 15, may be due to urine, bile, ascites and bowel secretions.
4. Acute arterial extravasation indicates active bleeding and requires immediate intervention. Venous contrast extravasation (a delayed scan may show more contrast leak) is seen as a vascular blush with a surrounding high density hematoma.
5. Free air indicates hollow viscus perforation (use wide window settings).
6. Extraluminal contrast is seen in the presence of upper or lower GI perforation.
7. Laceration, contusion or rupture of liver, spleen, pancreas and kidneys.
8. Assess aorta and mesenteric vessels for dissection, rupture, pseudoaneurysm or occlusion.
9. Osseous injury is assessed in sagittal and coronal reformatted images and is best viewed on bone windows.

Pearls

- Always look at the coronal and sagittal images.
- Small-sized aorta, collapsed IVC, diffuse hyper-enhancement of adrenals and enhancing bowel mucosa, and bowel wall thickening can occur in hypovolemic shock.
- HU: > 30 blood, 30–50 unclotted blood, 70 clotted blood.
- Look for diaphragmatic injury on sagittal and coronal images.
- Intraperitoneal spaces include subdiaphragmatic, paracolic gutters, Morison's pouch (the most dependent space, between liver and kidney – the hepatorenal space, fluid surrounds the liver edge), lesser sac and pelvis. Extra-peritoneal spaces include the anterior pararenal space, perirenal, posterior pararenal, and prevesical spaces.
- Seat belt injury: L2 or L3 horizontal vertebral body fracture involving spinous process and pedicles. Associated with bowel (free air and fluid), vascular and solid organ injuries.
- Adrenal injury: High-density blood (hematoma) within the enlarged gland and adjacent fat stranding.

Suggested reading

Linsenmaier U *et al.* Whole-body computed tomography in polytrauma: techniques and management. *Eur Radiol* 2002;12:1728–1740.

Novelline RA, Rhea JT, Bell T. Helical CT of abdominal trauma. *Radiol Clin N Am* 1999;37:591–612.

3.3 Spleen trauma

Following trauma, the spleen is the most commonly injured abdominal organ. See Fig. 3.3.

Clinical

May be associated abdominal bruising, abdominal pain, rib fractures and hemodynamic instability. Currently, conservative treatment is preferred over a surgical approach to preserve the spleen in patients with splenic trauma.

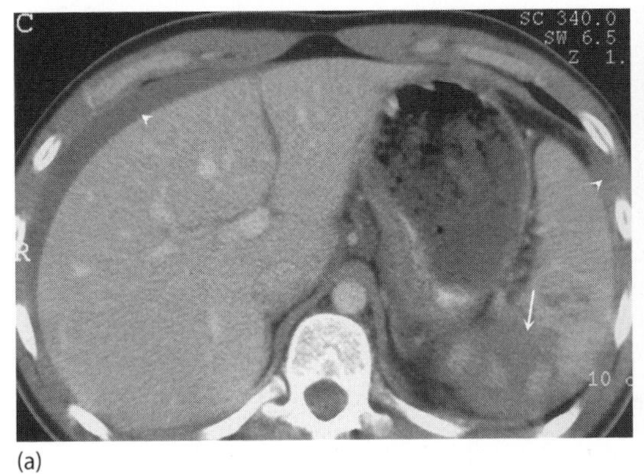

(a)

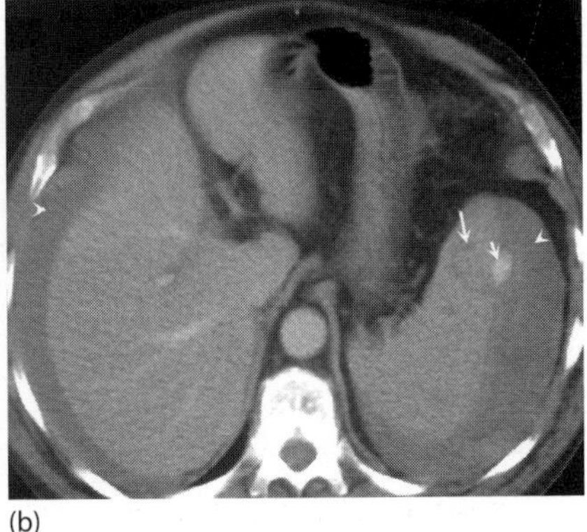

(b)

Fig. 3.3. (a) Splenic contusion. Axial CECT of abdomen shows irregular areas of reduced enhancement in the splenic parenchyma, consistent with splenic laceration (arrow). Hemoperitoneum is noted adjacent to the spleen and liver (arrowheads). (b) Splenic trauma. Axial CECT of abdomen shows perihepatic and perisplenic hemoperitoneum (arrowheads). Subtle heterogeneity of the splenic parenchyma anteriorly (large arrow), representing the site of organ trauma; immediately adjacent to this is a focus of contrast pooling (small arrow), consistent with active bleeding or pseudoaneurysm.

Technique

Contrast-enhanced MDCT is the modality of choice to identify splenic injury. Scans with a 60–70 s delay should be performed to evaluate the spleen. Note that the arterial phase images are difficult for interpreting splenic parenchyma because sinusoidal filling leads to marked heterogeneity of the parenchyma.

CECT findings

1. Laceration – seen as low-density linear irregular intraparenchymal lesions. They may be superficial or deep, extending from one margin to the other. They tend to be isodense on healing, a phenomenon that takes weeks to occur.
2. Hematoma – perisplenic and parenchymal. Perisplenic hematomas can be sub- or extra-capsular.
3. A subcapsular hematoma appears as a low-density (HU 40–70) lentiform collection deep to the capsule, having a well-defined outer margin, compressing the splenic edge medially. Peri- or extra-splenic hematomas and fluid are not well defined and do not compress the splenic margin.
4. Active bleeding – appears as high-density foci of active contrast extravasation in the splenic parenchyma or peri-splenic region (80–130 HU).
5. Vascular injuries – acute injuries include pseudoaneurysms, arteriovenous fistulae, and vascular pedicle disruption. Pseudoaneurysms will appear as contrast-filled, well-defined focal structures with subsequent wash-out on delayed images.
6. Delayed rupture – delayed appearance of multiple fragments of parenchyma following initial blunt injury.
7. Infarction appears as a peripheral wedge-shaped low-density area.

Pearls

- Preservation of the spleen rather than early surgery is the latest trend in the management of splenic trauma. Follow-up scans are very important to assess the stability of the injuries.
- Vascular injuries and active bleeding are emergencies which require urgent intervention.
- Splenic abscess and infarction are delayed complications.
- Look for associated organ injuries, rib fractures, pneumoperitoneum and free fluid.
- Grading splenic injuries on CT may be performed at some centers but is not reliable in predicting outcome in these patients.

Suggested reading

Becker CD *et al.* Blunt abdominal trauma in adults: role of CT in the diagnosis and management of visceral injuries. Part 1: Liver and spleen. *Eur Radiol* 1998;8(4):553–562.

3.4 Liver trauma

Following blunt trauma, the liver is the second most commonly injured organ in the body. See Fig. 3.4.

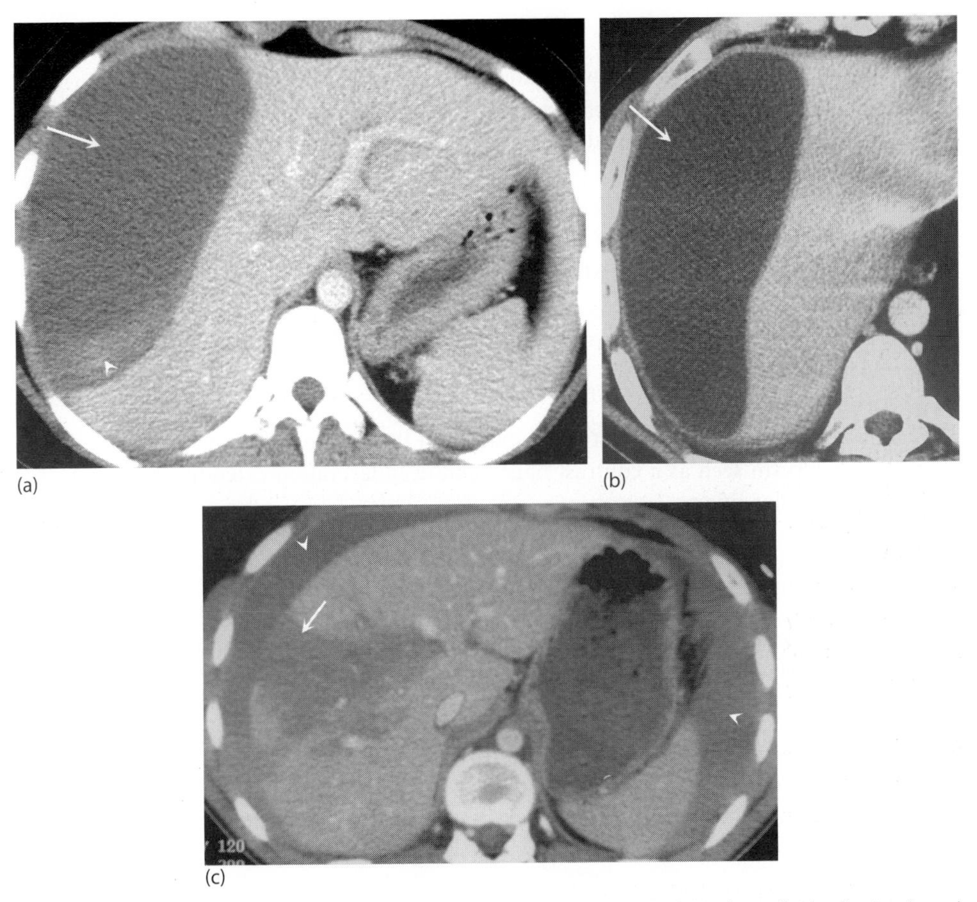

Fig. 3.4. (a) Subacute subcapsular hematoma. CECT shows a large lenticular hypodense fluid collection (arrow) with foci of high-density blood in the dependent portion (arrowhead) and resultant mass effect upon the subjacent liver, consistent with a subacute subcapsular hematoma. (b) Chronic subcapsular hematoma. CECT of abdomen shows a large lenticular hypodense fluid collection (arrow) displacing the subjacent liver parenchyma, representing a chronic subcapsular hematoma. (c) Liver laceration. CECT of abdomen shows well-defined areas of reduced enhancement within the liver (arrow), consistent with hepatic lacerations. High-density perihepatic and perisplenic hemoperitoneum (arrowheads). Note small calibre of the IVC and aorta due to severe hypovolemia.

Clinical

Abdominal pain, skin bruising, tachycardia, hypotension, shock. The majority of liver injuries are minor. The right lobe of the liver is more commonly injured than the left lobe. Active bleeding in the liver usually results in hemodynamic compromise.

Technique

Contrast-enhanced CT abdomen and pelvis. Enhanced CT readily demonstrates traumatic liver injuries. An unenhanced scan may show a high-density hematoma within the liver. Portal venous phase scan is useful in the assessment of the spleen.

CT findings

1. Contusion: Irregular area of low attenuation within the liver parenchyma.
2. Laceration: Irregular or well-defined linear low-density areas within the liver parenchyma. Deep lacerations that extend to vessels are more concerning and raise the possibility of vascular injury.
3. Subcapsular hematoma: Low density between the liver capsule and parenchyma. This causes compression of the liver parenchyma.
4. Intraparenchymal hematoma: Mixed or low density with relatively high-density collection in the parenchyma.
5. Free fluid: Hemoperitoneum around the liver produces a smooth hepatic margin.
6. Intraperitoneal fluid covers the undersurface of the liver edge and is contained within Morison's pouch.
7. Vascular injury: Active contrast extravasation in the liver parenchyma, pseudoaneurysm seen as a contrast blush, and deep laceration extending to vessel indicate vascular injury.

Pearls

- Always perform a contrast-enhanced abdominal CT in evaluating trauma patients. Look for associated injuries to spleen, pancreas, bowel, kidneys, adrenals, bones, diaphragm, and for pneumoperitoneum. Limited non-contrast imaging in the context of high-velocity bullet injuries may be helpful.
- Differentiate between subcapsular and perihepatic hematoma. An extracapsular hematoma is seen as less-demarcated perihepatic fluid collection without significant mass effect.
- GB injury: Intra-luminal high-density blood, wall thickening, interrupted wall with adjacent blood or bile.

Suggested reading

Refer to Section 3.3.

Yoon W *et al.* CT in blunt liver trauma. *RadioGraphics* 2005;**25**(1):87–104.

3.5 Renal trauma

Urinary tract injury occurs in 10% of patients with abdominal trauma. CT is indicated in patients with suspected renal injury or in the presence of gross hematuria, hypotension, lower rib fractures, lumbar spine fracture or major abdominal trauma. See Fig. 3.5.

Clinical

Hematuria, hypotension, tachycardia and abdominal bruising. Causes include blunt trauma, penetrating injury, and iatrogenic due to interventional procedures such as biopsy.

Technique

Contrast-enhanced MDCT angiography of the abdomen and pelvis; arterial phase, and delayed parenchymal phase. If there is a suspicion of uretero-pelvic injury a further

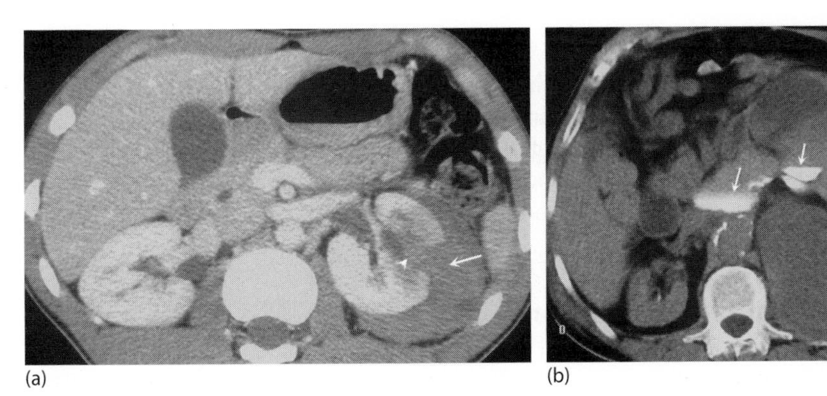

Fig. 3.5. (a) Renal trauma. CECT of abdomen shows a left perirenal hematoma (arrow) and focal renal parenchymal hypoenhancement (arrowhead) consistent with renal laceration. (b) Ureteric injury. Delayed post-contrast CT scan in a patient with abdominal swelling following AAA repair shows renally excreted contrast material pooling (arrows) within the perirenal fluid collections, consistent with large urinomas resulting from traumatic ureteral injury during aortic repair.

delayed scan may be helpful. Arterial phase can be performed by bolus tracking with a region of interest (ROI) placed on the abdominal aorta.

Findings

1. Laceration.
2. Contusion.
3. Subcapsular hematoma.
4. Perirenal hematoma.
5. Fractured or shattered renal parenchyma due to multiple deep lacerations.
6. Avulsion of renal pedicles.
7. Renal infarction.
8. Complete absence of parenchymal enhancement.
9. Pseudoaneurysms.
10. Urinoma and/or urinary contrast extravasation.

Pearls

- Renal pelvic disruption, shattered kidney, renal artery pseudoaneurysm, active bleeding, renal pedicle avulsion, complete renal infarction, expanding subcapsular hematoma, urinary extravasation are suggestive of major injuries and immediate intervention may be indicated.
- Liaise with an interventional radiologist and referring physician if there is a sign of major injury.
- Findings of renal collecting system injury are absent, renal parenchymal enhancement and urinoma (extra-luminal urinary contrast).

Suggested reading

Harris AC *et al.* CT findings in blunt renal trauma. *RadioGraphics* 2001;**21**:S201–S214.

Kawashima A *et al.* Imaging of renal trauma: a comprehensive review. *RadioGraphics* 2001;**21**: 557–574.

3.6 Pancreatic trauma

Pancreatic injury is due to the compression of the pancreas against the vertebral bodies, usually associated with seat-belt injuries and polytrauma. This is rarely seen in the setting of trauma (< 3%). It is associated with a high degree of morbidity due to a delay in the initial diagnosis. There is an increased incidence of associated liver and duodenal injuries in adults. The neck of the pancreas is the commonest site of injury. See Fig. 3.6.

Clinical

Abdominal pain, skin bruising, tachycardia, raised serum amylase etc.

Technique

Contrast-enhanced CT of the abdomen.

CT findings

1. Contusion: Focal mild swelling of pancreas with loss of normal septa.
2. Laceration: Seen as a vertical low-density tear in the pancreas. This can be associated with duct injury if the tear extends more than 50% of the width of the pancreas.
3. Fracture: Multiple fragments of pancreas. This is always associated with the presence of peri-pancreatic fluid and duct injury.
4. Duct injury: Associated with deep laceration and pancreatic fracture.
5. Peripancreatic fluid collection with HU less than 10.
6. Free fluid: Seen in the anterior pararenal space. High-density blood may be present. Low-density fluid due to duct disruption or associated pancreatitis.
7. Fluid also seen in the retroperitoneal space.
8. Associated injury to duodenum and pleural effusion.

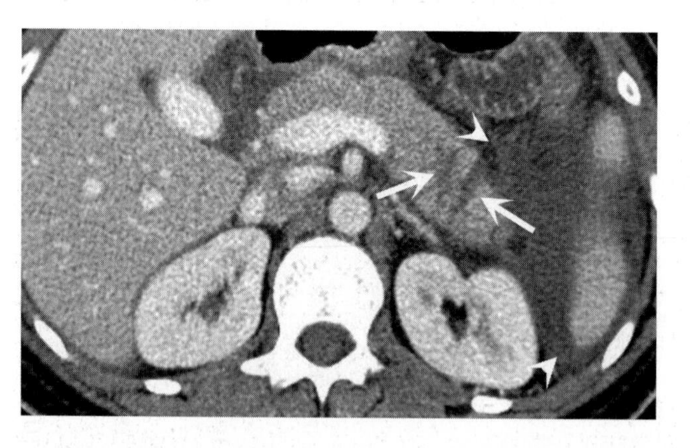

Fig. 3.6. Pancreatic trauma. CECT of abdomen in a trauma patient shows two linear areas of reduced enhancement within the pancreatic tail (arrows), indicating laceration. Note hemorrhage adjacent to the pancreas and spleen (arrowheads).

Pearls

- Grading is generally not indicated but some centers do (follow local policy). Duct injury, major laceration, pancreatic rupture and duodenal injury are associated with a worse prognosis.
- Pancreatic pseudocyst and abscess are delayed complications.

- Pancreatic duct injury is an emergency requiring urgent intervention. CT is not sensitive enough to detect direct injury. ERCP or MRCP can confirm the ductal disruption.
- Always check the HU of free fluid.
- Asymmetry with loss of pancreatic septa is a feature of isoattenuating pancreatic contusion on CT.

Suggested reading

Gupta A, Stuhlfaut JW, Fleming KW, Lucey BC, Soto JA. Blunt trauma of the pancreas and biliary tract: a multimodality imaging approach to diagnosis. *RadioGraphics* 2004;24(5):1381–1395.

Patel SV, Spencer JA, el-Hasani S, Sheridan MB. Imaging of pancreatic trauma. *Br J Radiol* 1998;71:985–990.

3.7 Bladder trauma

Bladder injury is seen in 5–10% of patients with pelvic trauma either due to a penetrating bone injury or increased pressure on a full bladder. See Fig. 3.7.

Clinical

Intraperitoneal rupture – urgency and hesitancy. Peritoneal sepsis is a serious complication in unrecognized cases, occurring about 24 hours after the injury.
Extraperitoneal rupture – hematuria, uralgia, suprapubic hematoma.

Techniques

1. A foley catheter can be inserted into the bladder and can be clamped for 30–60 minutes prior to the scan to achieve a full bladder. Following an initial contrast-enhanced CT scan of the abdomen and pelvis, a delayed 20-minute limited scan can be performed through the lower abdomen and pelvis to demonstrate contrast extravasation.

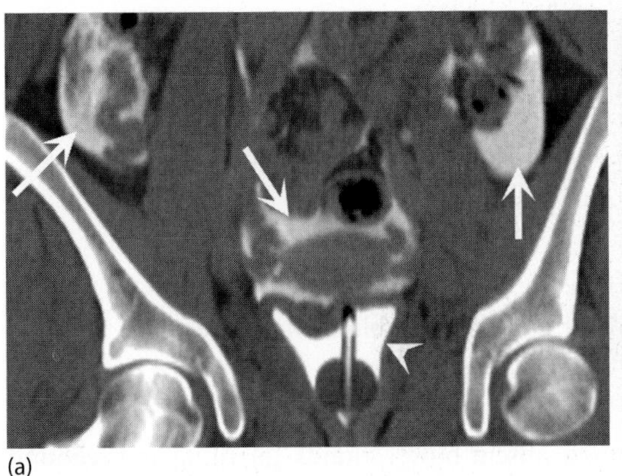

(a)

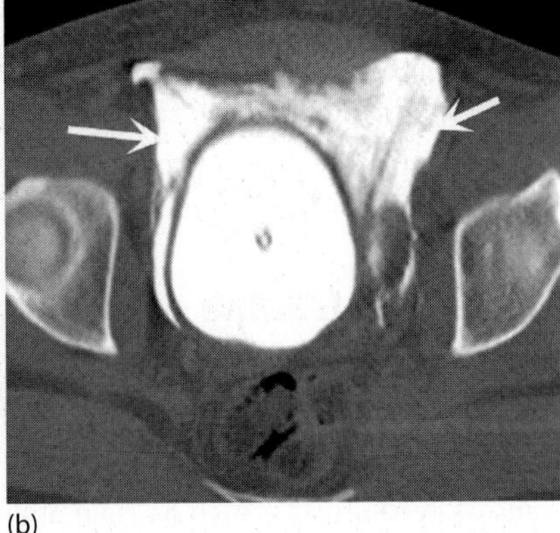

(b)

Fig. 3.7. (a) Intraperitoneal bladder rupture. Coronal CT cystogram image in a trauma patient shows the leakage of contrast (arrows) from the bladder (arrowhead) into the peritoneal cavity surrounding loops of bowel. (b) Extraperitoneal bladder rupture. Axial image following CT cystogram in a different patient with pelvic trauma, showing leakage of contrast material from the bladder into the pelvis, outlining both sides of the bladder wall – "molar tooth sign" (arrows).

2. CT cystogram. Foley catheter is inserted into the bladder. Urine is drained. Then 350–500 ml of 30% solution of sodium diatrizoate and meglumine diatrizoate (Urografin) or iohexal (Omnipaque) is instilled slowly via the catheter to fill the bladder. Warm the contrast medium to body temperature to avoid ureteral spasms. CT of the abdomen and pelvis is performed. This is a reliable method to rule out bladder injury.

Findings

1. Rupture.
2. Extravasation of contrast.
3. Intraperitoneal: Contrast seen as a triangular density layering in the mesenteric recesses. Free intraperitoneal collection – Urinoma – check Hounsfield unit.
4. Extraperitoneal: Usually fills the perivesical space (molar tooth sign) and tracks along the anterior abdominal wall; extends to pelvic wall, scrotum and anterior thigh. It can also be seen in the anterior pararenal space.
5. Contusion.
6. Hematocrit level in the posterior bladder.
7. Bladder wall hematoma.

Pearls

- Extraperitoneal rupture is managed conservatively whereas intraperitoneal rupture needs surgery.
- Extraperitoneal spaces include anterior pararenal space, perirenal, post-pararenal and prevesical.
- Intraperitoneal spaces include subdiaphragmatic, paracolic gutters, Morison's pouch (the hepato-renal space, the most dependent space, between liver and kidney). Fluid surrounds the liver edge, lesser sac and pelvis.

Suggested reading

Pao DM, Ellis JH, Cohan RH, Korobkin M. Utility of routine trauma CT in determination of bladder rupture. *Acad Radiol* 2000;7:317–324.

Vaccaro JP, Brody JM. CT cystography in the evaluation of major bladder trauma. *RadioGraphics* 2000;**20**:1373–1381.

3.8 Bowel trauma

Small bowel injury is seen in less than 6% of patients with blunt trauma. See Fig. 3.8.

Clinical

Signs of peritonism – such as rigid abdomen, absent bowel sounds, guarding and rebound tenderness – are often difficult to elicit in trauma patients.

Technique

MDCT of abdomen and pelvis with intravenous contrast. Oral contrast is not necessary.

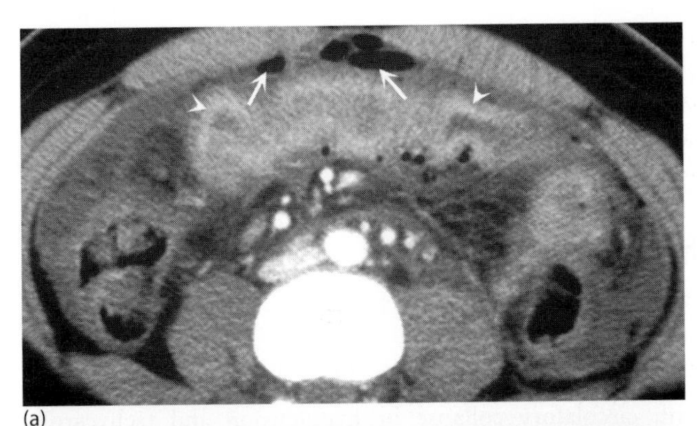
(a)

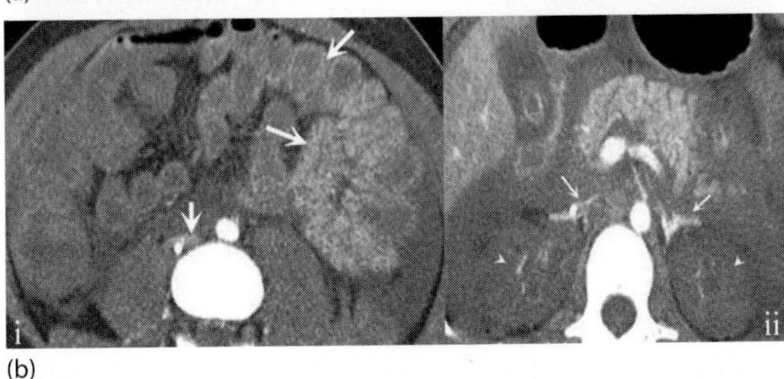

(b)

Fig. 3.8. (a) Bowel injury. CECT image demonstrates free intraperitoneal air (arrows), free fluid and ill-defined thickening and enhancement of bowel wall (arrowheads), consistent with traumatic bowel injury with perforation. (b) Shock bowel. CECT (i) in a patient with severe hypotension shows diffuse small bowel wall thickening, high-density bowel wall (arrows), flat IVC (short arrow) and small calibre aorta. Image (ii) shows high-density pancreas, and adrenals (thin arrows), and diffusely hypo-enhancing kidneys (arrowheads); features are consistent with shock bowel ischemia. Note is also made of pancreatic tail contusion.

Findings

1. Bowel injury.
   Bowel wall thickening of more than 4 mm.
   Apparent bowel wall defect – difficult to see.
   Extraluminal oral contrast or bowel contents.
   Extraluminal air.
   Intramural air or hematoma.
2. Mesenteric injury.
   Mesenteric hematoma.
   Active bleeding seen as extravasation of contrast.
   Bowel wall thickening.
   Mesenteric fat stranding.

Pearls

- Traumatic bowel injury is associated with focal/segmental bowel wall thickening.
- Shock bowel (hypoperfusion complex) and overhydration following resuscitation result in diffuse bowel wall thickening. Periportal edema and dilated IVC are seen in overhydration following resuscitation.
- Signs of shock bowel ischemia are dilated fluid-filled small bowel, diffuse small bowel wall thickening (may be > 11 mm), high-density bowel wall (due to poor capillary return), dense pancreas and adrenals, flat IVC (AP diameter usually < 9 mm), diffusely low-density (hypoperfused) spleen and kidneys, small aorta, normal large bowel, and usually reversal of signs following correction of fluid status.

Suggested reading

Brody JM, Leighton DB. CT of blunt trauma bowel and mesenteric injury: typical findings and pitfalls in diagnosis. *RadioGraphics* 2000;**20**:1525–1536.

Brofman N *et al.* Evaluation of bowel and mesenteric blunt trauma with multidetector CT. *RadioGraphics* 2006;**26**(4):1119–1131.

3.9 Intra-abdominal hemorrhage

Spontaneous or traumatic intra-abdominal bleeding. See Fig. 3.9.

Clinical

Abdominal pain associated with circulatory collapse or hypotension and tachycardia. Patients receiving anti-coagulation are at increased risk of bleeding due to over-coagulation. Ruptured aortic aneurysm, blunt trauma and falls are associated with intra-abdominal hemorrhage.

Indications: Acute abdominal pain, unexplained tachycardia and hypotension, low hemoglobin, suspected intra-abdominal hemorrhage, known AAA with abdominal pain and hypotension.

Technique

Non-contrast 5 mm images of the abdomen and pelvis. Contrast-enhanced CT angiography of the abdomen and pelvis using 1.5 mm collimation. 80–120 ml of intravenous contrast given at 3 ml/s.

Findings

1. Usually well-defined whorled collection of intermediate to high density.
2. Extravasation of contrast seen in active bleeding.
3. Origin of extravasation from vessels like the aorta, splenic artery or small vessels.

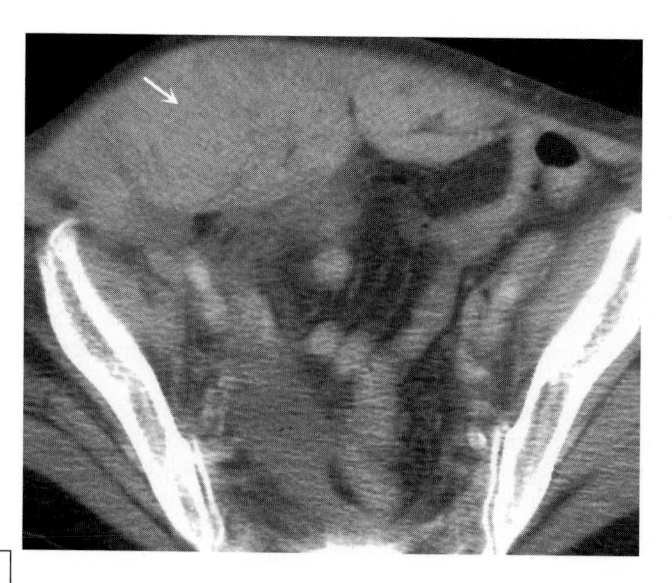

Fig. 3.9. Rectus sheath hematoma. Axial CT demonstrates marked heterogeneous thickening of the right aspect of the rectus abdominis (arrow), consistent with a rectus sheath hematoma.

4. Hematocrit level in the dependent portion (usually seen when coagulopathy is the underlying cause).
5. No definite enhancement of the wall of the hematoma following IV contrast.

Pearls

- Always check the rectus sheath psoas, iliacus and obturator internus muscles for hematomas, which are typically seen in patients who are over anti-coagulated.
- Measure the Hounsfield unit of any collection – high density suggests hematoma.
- Low-density fluid within the hematoma occurs in lysis (liquefication process of hematoma seen in subacute or chronic hematoma) and in super-added infection.
- Calcification of the hematoma indicates chronicity.

Suggested reading

Davies RS, Goh GJM, Curtis JM *et al.* Abdominal wall hematoma in anticoagulated patients: the role of imaging in diagnosis. *Australasian Radiology* 1996;**40**(2):109–112.

Lubner M, Menias C, Rucker C *et al.* Blood in the belly: CT findings of hemoperitoneum. *RadioGraphics* 2007;**27**(1):109–25.

3.10 Intra-abdominal collection

Intra-abdominal abscesses are an important cause of sepsis and represent clinical and radiological emergencies. See Fig. 3.10.

Clinical

Usually presents with fever, and other signs of infection.

Causes include inflammatory processes – appendicitis, diverticulitis, inflammatory bowel disease, pancreatitis, cholecystitis or post-surgical. Most hepatic abscesses are pyogenic, although fungal and amebic are also possible.

The site of abscess formation is in solid organs such as the liver, kidneys, spleen and gallbladder or in the intra- or extra-peritoneal spaces including mesentery.

Technique

Ultrasound may be limited in its ability to reliably rule out a small abscess in the peritoneal space. On ultrasound, dilated atonic fluid-filled bowel is more often mistaken for an abscess in the sick post-operative patient. However, contrast-enhanced CT has a high sensitivity, specificity and negative predictive value. Coronal reformats can be very useful.

Findings

1. Focal fluid-filled, walled-off lesion. Intermediate density of fluid.
2. Gas pockets within the fluid due to gas-forming organisms.
3. Wall enhancement.
4. Adjacent mesenteric fat stranding.

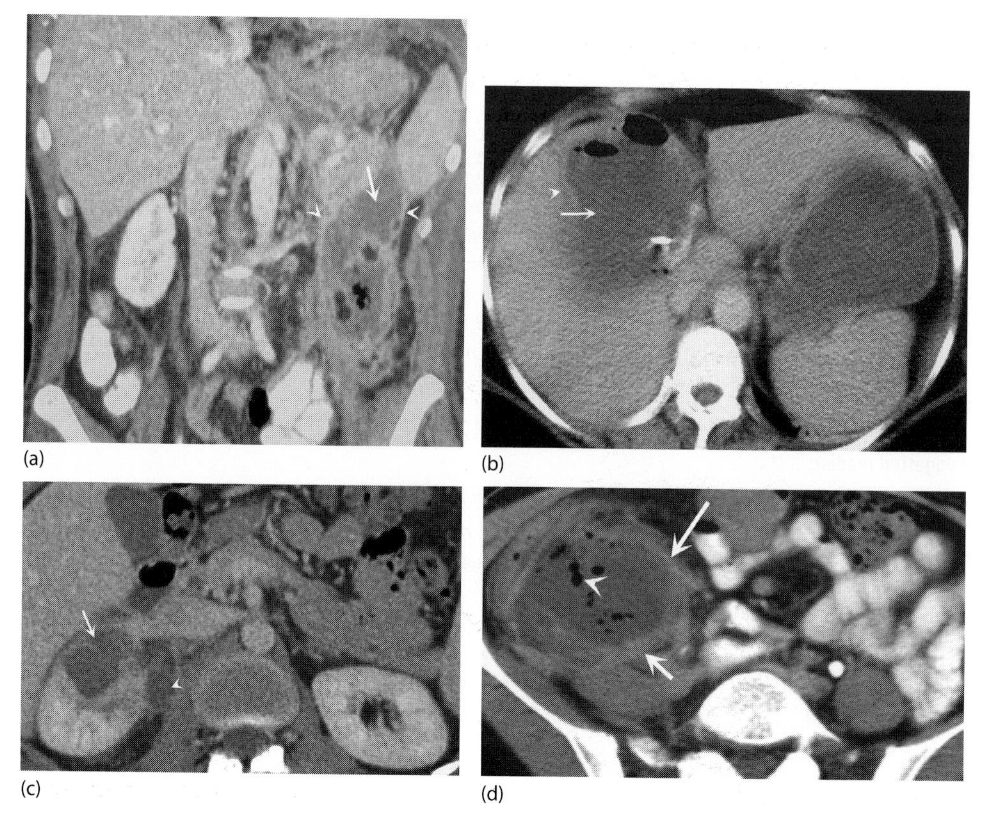

Fig. 3.10. (a) Mesenteric abscess. Coronal CE CT shows a fluid collection (arrow) in the left abdomen with thick irregular peripheral enhancement (arrowheads), adjacent stranding and internal gas. (b) Liver abscess. Axial CECT shows a large poorly circumscribed low-attenuation lesion (arrow) within the liver that contains internal foci of gas, representing hepatic abscess. Note the "double target sign" of peripheral enhancement and surrounding hypodensity (arrowhead). (c) Renal abscess. Axial CECT shows peripherally enhancing but centrally necrotic lesion in the upper pole of the right kidney, consistent with renal abscess (arrow). There is a small abscess adjacent to right psoas muscle (arrowhead). Culture of the drained fluid was positive for mycobacterium tuberculosis. (d) Appendix abscess. Axial CECT shows a large right iliac fossa fluid collection (arrow) with gas pockets (arrowhead) and associated peripheral enhancement (small arrow) and stranding of the adjacent fat, consistent with perforated appendicitis and organizing abscess.

5. Measure the Hounsfield units: 0–10 usually indicates simple fluid but does not rule out infected fluid.
6. Look for vascular filling defects in cases of thrombosis, since sepsis is a prothrombotic condition.

Pearls

- It is important to scroll through the abdomen and pelvis for all peritoneal reflections, which include subdiaphragmatic, subhepatic, Morison's pouch (right subhepatic space, the deepest dependent space), lesser and greater sacs, anterior pararenal space and retroperitoneal space.

- Look out for signs of GB empyema, liver abscess, tubo-ovarian abscesses, diverticulitis, appendicitis, ureteric calculus, pyonephrosis and paravertebral collection. Never forget to look closely at the psoas and iliacus muscles.
- Evaluate the hip joints for infection, which is associated with bone destruction, osteopenia, soft tissue edema and fluid collection. Typically there is involvement of bones adjacent to a joint.

Suggested reading

Bydder GM, Kreel L. Computed tomography in the diagnosis of abdominal abscess. *J Comput Tomogr* 1980;4(2):132–145.

Gazelle GS, Mueller PR. Abdominal abscess. Imaging and intervention. *Radiol Clin North Am* 1994; 32(5):913–932. Review.

3.11 Acute appendicitis

Inflammation of the appendix. Multi-slice spiral CT plays a major role in the diagnosis of appendicitis and its related complications. See Fig. 3.11.

Clinical

Acute appendicitis is one of the most common causes of acute abdominal pain, especially in an adult. Typically it presents with abdominal pain (colicky abdominal pain, initially central, moving subsequently to RIF), vomiting and rarely fever. Major complications include perforation, abscess, small bowel obstruction, portal vein pyemia, mesenteric vein occlusion and peritonitis.

Technique

Multi-slice CT of the abdomen and pelvis with intravenous and oral contrast. Colonic (rectal) contrast may be used to opacify the ileocecal area in an emergency setting. Thin section images, ideally less than 5 mm, should be obtained. Coronal reformatted images are very useful for panoramic views of the abdomen and pelvis.

Findings

1. Unopacified dilated appendix greater than 6 mm in diameter.
2. Thickening of the appendix wall.
3. Periappendicial fat stranding and clouding.
4. Cecal pole thickening.
5. Appendicolith with adjacent soft-tissue inflammation.
6. Wall enhancement with a focal defect when there is necrosis.
7. Bowel obstruction.

Complications

Local abscess – walled-off collection with enhancing wall and air–fluid level within the collection. Surrounding air could relate to a perforated appendix. Small bowel ileus or

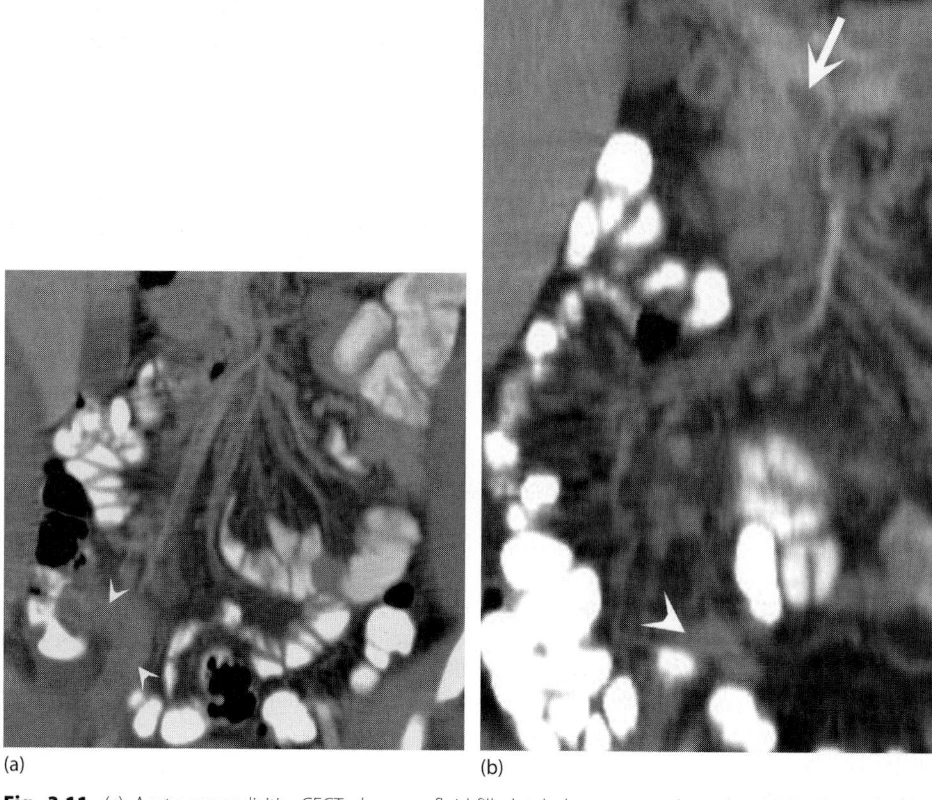

(a) (b)

Fig. 3.11. (a) Acute appendicitis. CECT shows a fluid-filled tubular structure (arrowheads) in the right lower quadrant extending from the cecum, with thickened enhancing walls and stranding of the adjacent fat, representing acute appendicitis. (b) Pylephlebitis. Coronal CECT images show a hypodense filling defect within the superior mesenteric vein (arrow), consistent with SMV thrombosis in a patient with appendicitis. Note thickening of appendix (arrowhead).

obstruction, bowel wall thickening, portal vein gas and liver abscesses. Ascending pylephlebitis can result in mesenteric vein thrombosis.

Pearls

- Ultrasound is contributory in patients with less abdominal adipose tissue, and in pregnancy and children.
- Aim for reconstruction with less than 5 mm. Greater than 5 mm reconstruction images of CT are associated with false negatives due to partial volume averaging.
- Identification of the anatomical position of the cecal pole is helpful in identifying the appendix. Normal diameter appendix with contrast filling its entire lumen is necessary to exclude appendicitis.
- Absence of appendix but presence of mesenteric or portal vein gas or occlusion, remote bowel wall thickening in pelvis and cloudy mesentery should raise the suspicion for a perforated appendix.

- Good bowel distension with intraluminal contrast is important to avoid false positive or negative appendicitis.
- Normal opacified vessels such as the right colic artery can simulate a normal appendix. Unopacified small bowel loops can mimic an abnormal appendix; beware of these caveats!

Suggested reading

Hoeffel C *et al.* Multi-detector row CT: spectrum of diseases involving the ileocecal area. *Radiographics* 2006;**26**(5):1373–1390.

Urban BA, Fishman EK. Targeted helical CT of the acute abdomen: appendicitis, diverticulitis, and small bowel obstruction. *Semin Ultrasound CT MR* 2000;**21**:20–39.

3.12 Acute pancreatitis

Acute inflammation of the pancreas. See Fig. 3.12.

Clinical

Alcohol and gallstones are the most common causes of pancreatitis. Abdominal pain radiating to the back is the main symptom and in severe cases patients may present with shock. Serum amylase and lipase are typically elevated.

Indications

Acute abdominal pain. CT plays a role in the diagnosis, and to assess the degree of necrosis, and in the follow-up to evaluate for complications.

Technique

Unenhanced CT scan of the pancreas. Contrast-enhanced dual phase CT scan of the abdomen; pancreatic (40 s delay) and portal-venous phases. Venous phase should cover the whole abdomen and pelvis. In a sick patient the portal venous phase alone is usually sufficient.

Findings

1. Diffuse swelling of the pancreas with obscuration of the serrated margin.
2. Reduced attenuation of pancreas due to necrosis: increased foci of high attenuation suggest active bleeding in hemorrhagic pancreatitis.
3. Peripancreatic inflammatory change (phlegmon).
4. Thickening of latero-conal fascia and Gerota's fascia.
5. Collection – look for gas pockets.
6. Look for causes: Gallstones, pancreatic head tumor, and pancreatic calcifications. Presence of gallstones cannot be excluded on CT. Patients require GB ultrasound.

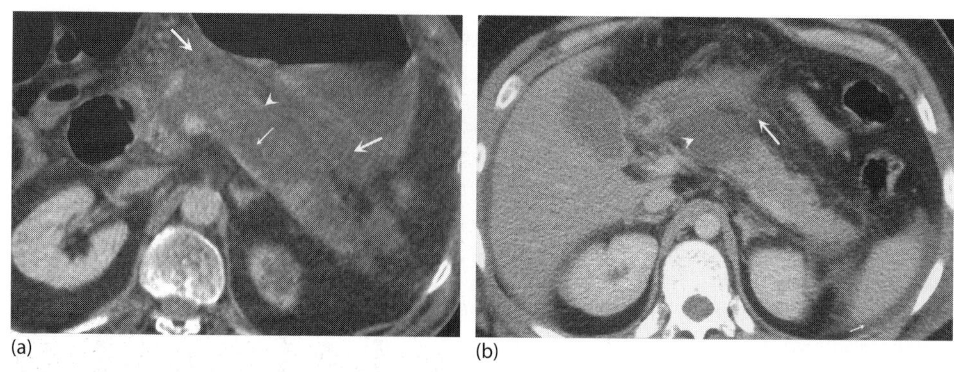

Fig. 3.12. (a) Acute pancreatitis with necrosis. CECT shows peripancreatic fluid, fat stranding (arrows) with obscuration of pancreatic margins (arrowhead), consistent with acute pancreatitis. Note diffuse low-attenuation change in the pancreas (thin arrow), suggestive of pancreatic necrosis. (b) Acute pancreatitis. CECT shows mild peripancreatic stranding (arrow) consistent with acute pancreatitis, and associated perisplenic fluid (thin arrow). There is reduced attenuation in the pancreatic body due to necrosis (arrowhead).

Pearls

- Mild thickening of pancreas with mild peripancreatic fat stranding, should raise the suspicion of early pancreatitis, and a correlation with serum amylase is indicated. Thickening of the latero-conal and Gerota's fasciae are also early findings in pancreatitis.
- The degree of necrosis, denoted by reduced enhancement of the pancreas correlated with prognosis. Higher degree of pancreatic necrosis is associated with worse prognosis.
- Always look for a potential cause and for complications of pancreatitis. Parenchymal calcification in chronic and hereditary type of pancreatitis; the latter is a cause in pediatric age groups.
- A peripancreatic collection persisting for at least 4 weeks is called a pseudocyst. Enhancement of the wall with gas or air–fluid level of the collection is suggestive of an abscess. A bowel fistula should also be considered.
- Complications: Pleural effusion, pseudocyst, collection, abscess (gas pockets), venous thrombosis and splenic artery aneurysm.

Suggested reading

Nichols MT, Russ PD, Chen YK. Pancreatic imaging: current and emerging technologies. *Pancreas* 2006;**33**(3):211–220. Review.

Procacci C *et al.* Non-traumatic abdominal emergencies: imaging and intervention in acute pancreatic conditions. *Eur Radiol* 2002;**12**:2407–2434.

3.13 Acute renal/ureteric colic

Acute renal colic typically causes severe excruciating abdominal pain, which waxes and wanes, radiating from flank to groin. Non-contrast CT has higher sensitivity and specificity than ultrasound or KUB radiograph in diagnosing acute obstruction due to renal or ureteric calculi. See Fig. 3.13.

Clinical

Severe excruciating waxing and waning pain radiating from loin to groin and to testes or labium. Diaphoresis. Patients may roll on the bed with pain.

Technique

Imaging is important in evaluating stones and obstruction.

Non-contrast enhanced axial CT of the abdomen and pelvis. Intravenous contrast is not essential; contrast may mask the presence of a urinary tract stone.

Findings

1. High-density calcific focus in the ureter or renal tract.
2. Perinephric fat stranding.
3. Periureteric fat stranding.
4. Hydronephrosis.
5. Ureteric wall thickening with central high-density calculus – "ureteric rim sign."
6. Perinephric fluid.

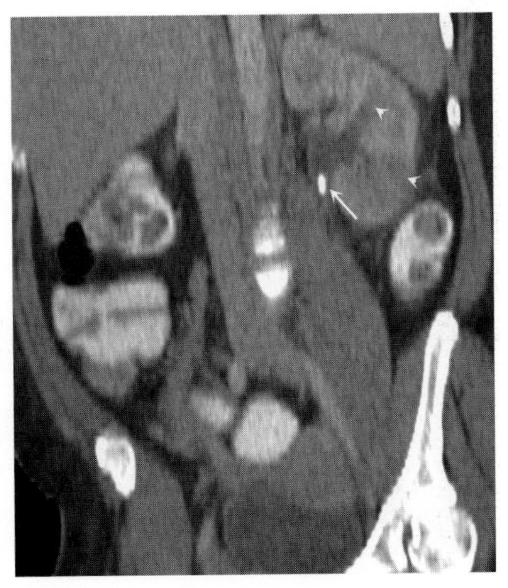

Fig. 3.13. Pyonephrosis. CECT scan performed to rule out appendicitis shows an obstructing left uretero-pelvic junction stone (arrow) with resultant mild left hydronephrosis. Note also the wedge-shaped areas of cortical hypoenhancement (arrowheads) and associated perinephric stranding, consistent with pyelonephritis. Emergency nephrostomy drainage showed pyonephrosis. (Photo courtesy of Dr. A Sassani MD, Radiology Fellow, UCLA.)

Pearls

- Look for other acute abnormality.
- Air pockets and septations within the hydronephrosis are suggestive of pyonephrosis. US can be performed to further evaluate. Hydro- or pyonephrosis is a radiological emergency, requiring an urgent nephrostomy drainage tube insertion.

Suggested reading

Dalrymple NC, Casford B, Raiken DP, Elsass KD, Pagan RA. Pearls and pitfalls in the diagnosis of ureterolithiasis with unenhanced helical CT. *RadioGraphics* 2000;**20**:439–447.

Rickards D. Non-traumatic abdominal emergencies: imaging and intervention in acute urinary conditions. *Eur Radiol* 2002;**12**:2435–2442.

3.14 Bowel perforation

In suspected perforation, if the erect chest radiograph is normal, a CT abdomen may be obtained to exclude, or confirm, pneumoperitoneum. See Fig. 3.14.

Clinical

Causes are perforated ulcer, usually duodenal hollow viscus perforation, bowel obstruction, necrotic tumor, bowel ischemia, immunosuppression, active colitis and recent instrumentation.

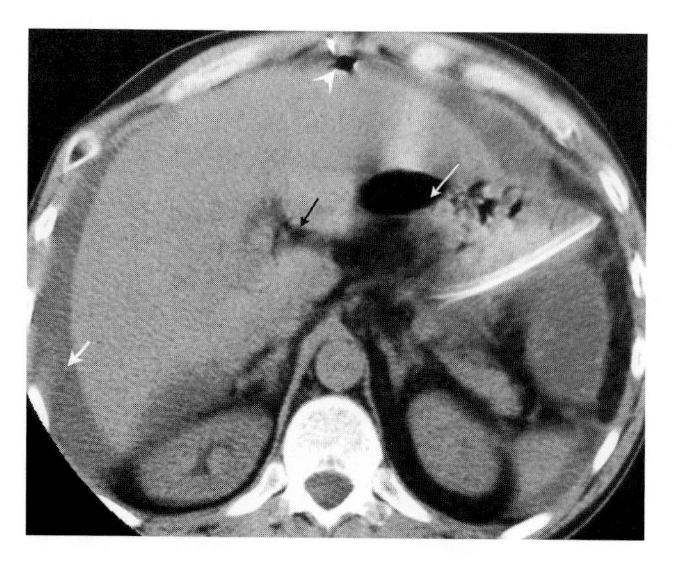

Fig. 3.14. Duodenal perforation. Axial CT shows a small amount of pneumoperitoneum anterior to the left lobe of the liver (arrowhead). Note ascites (short white arrow), gas in the hepato-duodenal ligament (black arrow) and associated lesser sac abscess (long white arrow).

Abdominal pain, tenderness, rigid abdomen, guarding and rebound tenderness (peritonism).

A small pneumoperitoneum is easy to miss and is usually due to small bowel perforation whereas a large pneumoperitoneum is usually due to colonic or gastro-duodenal perforation.

Technique

Whole abdomen and pelvic CT with IV and oral contrast. Non-ionic oral contrast in cases of suspected perforation.

Intravenous contrast may be useful in detecting associated pathologies like necrotic bowel tumor, ischemic bowel and abscess. Oral contrast may demonstrate extra-luminal leak especially in upper GI perforation.

Findings

1. Small pockets of free gas (–1000 HU) collect around the liver and stomach. A large collection of gas is readily detected but may be confused with bowel gas.
2. Mesenteric free gas.
3. Extra-luminal contrast leak suggests bowel perforation.
4. Look for underlying causes like necrotic tumor, bowel ischemia, colitis, obstruction/strangulation and for associated complications, e.g. abscess formation.

Pearls

- Acute abdominal scan should always be reviewed on lung settings at the modality or PACS workstation to detect subtle pneumoperitoneum.
- A lesser sac abscess with free gas in the hepato-duodenal ligament suggests duodenal perforation.

- Benign pneumoperitoneum is seen in immunocompromised individuals as intramural air (pneumatosis coli). No free air in the abdomen.
- Is it bowel or free gas? Absence of feces and mucosal folds favors free gas. Absence of continuity of gas with the bowel loops in a large pneumoperitoneum (use workstation).

Suggested reading

Ghekiere O *et al.* Value of computed tomography in the diagnosis of the cause of nontraumatic gastrointestinal tract perforation. *J Comput Assist Tomogr* 2007;**31**(2):169–176.

Kasznia-Brown J, Cook C. Radiological signs of pneumoperitoneum: a pictorial review. *Br J Hosp Med (Lond)* 2006;**67**(12):634–639. Review.

3.15 Acute inflammatory bowel disease

Acute inflammation of the small and/or large bowel. See Fig. 3.15.

Clinical

Common etiologies include ischemia, Crohn's disease, ulcerative colitis (UC), pseudomembranous colitis, neutropenic colitis, graft versus host disease, and infectious colitis. Acute abdominal pain, altered bowel habit, e.g. diarrhea, lower GI bleed, abdominal tenderness.

Technique

Contrast-enhanced CT scan with administration of oral contrast prior to scan. If there are clinical signs of bowel obstruction, then the administration of oral contrast can be avoided. Intraluminal fluid and air act as a negative contrast.

Technique can vary depending upon the indication. Arterial phase scan is important in suspected bowel ischemia. Otherwise, delayed portal venous phase scan is ideal in the emergency situation. In suspected appendicitis, oral contrast to opacify the cecum is suggested.

Findings

Appendicitis

Dilated, thickened, fluid-filled and non-opacified appendix with periappendicial and pericecal thickening.

Please refer to Section 3.11 on appendicitis.

Epiploic appendagitis

This is due to torsion or spontaneous thrombosis of appendageal epiploica (pockets of fat along the colonic wall adjacent to teniae coli).

Conservative management. A well-defined fat-containing oval lesion with an enhancing peripheral rim is usually seen adjacent to the large bowel with pericolonic fat standing. Central high-attenuation dot may be seen, which is likely due to thrombosed vein. Segmental omental infarction can simulate as epiploic appendagitis.

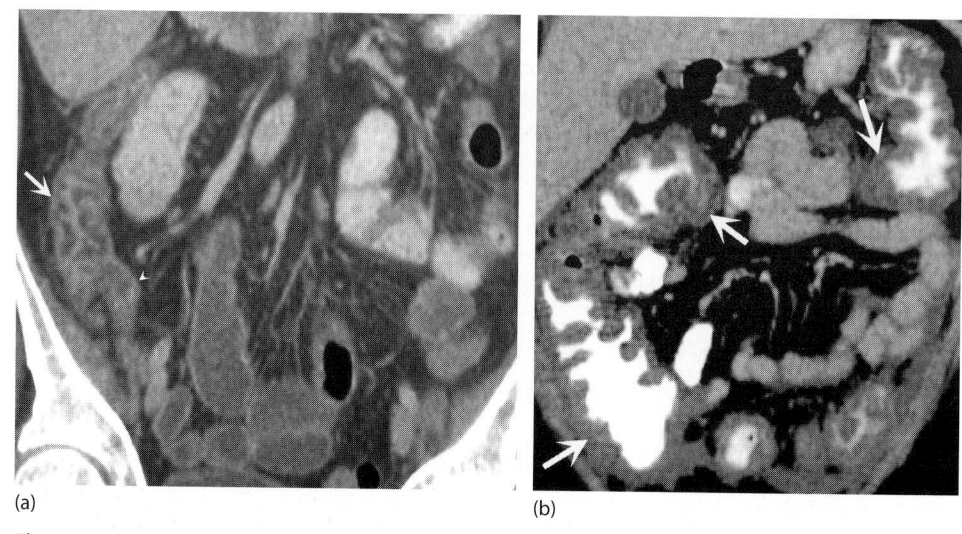

Fig. 3.15. (a) Acute Crohn's disease. Coronal image shows segments of large bowel wall thickening (arrow). Colonoscopy and biopsy showed Crohn's disease of large bowel. (b) Pseudomembranous colitis. CECT shows dilated large bowel, and diffuse marked eccentric colonic wall thickening (arrows) with typical paucity of pericolonic fat stranding in a patient with confirmed pseudomembranous colitis.

Acute Crohn's and ulcerative colitis

Acute Crohn's disease usually involves the right-side colon and/or small bowel, with bowel wall thickening, mucosal ulceration, skip lesions, and pericolonic fat stranding.

Acute UC usually affects the distal colon without skip lesions and with involvement of the rectum. There may be so-called "rectal-sparing" in patients treated with steroid enemas. Increased mucosal edema and ulceration, mucosal thumb printing and dilatation.

Pseudomembranous colitis

Usually there is a diffuse involvement of the colon with increased irregular, eccentric bowel-wall thickening (degree of thickening is greater than other colitis), mucosal edema and less pericolonic inflammatory changes. Colonic wall may have low attenuation due to edema or high density after intravenous contrast due to hyperemia.

Typhilitis

Abnormal dilatation of the cecum (>9 cm) with circumferential wall thickening, low attenuation wall edema and pericecal mesenteric fat stranding, especially in immunocompromised neutropenic patients. Presence of intramural air, free air and collection requires surgery.

Infectious colitis

Diffuse (*E. coli*, CMV) or segmental bowel-wall thickening with homogeneous enhancement due to hyperemia. Low-attenuation bowel edema can occur. Dilated loops of bowel with increased fluid. Pericolonic fat stranding. Commonly right-sided involvement (*Shigella* and *Salmonella* but left-sided colonic involvement in schistosomiasis).

Ischemic colitis

Usually there is segmental involvement of the bowel in the arterial territory. Watershed areas such as splenic flexure and rectosigmoid are more prone to the effects of ischemia. In elderly people, the left-side colon is more commonly involved but when ischemic colitis involves younger patients the right colon tends to be involved. Please refer to Section 3.16 on bowel ischemia.

Circumferential, symmetrical, wall thickening associated with fold thickening and the target sign.

Hypo- or hyper-attenuating bowel wall. Hyper-attenuating bowel wall occurs because of poor capillary return.

Intramural air suggestive of necrosis.

Mesenteric venous or arterial thrombosis in occlusive bowel ischemia.

Pearls

- In general, bowel dilatation, bowel wall thickening, bowel wall edema, hypo- or hyper-enhancement of bowel wall and pericolonic mesenteric fat stranding indicates colitis.
- Segmental involvement is usually due to Crohn's disease or ischemic bowel.
- Diffuse involvement of the bowel is likely due to UC, pseudomembranous colitis or in certain types of infectious colitis.
- Presence of pneumatosis (may indicate bowel necrosis/infarction), pneumoperitoneum, and focal collections may indicate the need for surgical intervention.

Suggested reading

Hoeffel C *et al.* Multi-detector row CT: spectrum of diseases involving the ileocecal area. *RadioGraphics* 2006;**26**(5):1373–1390.

Horton MD, Corl MS, Fishman E. MD CT evaluation of the colon: inflammatory disease. *RadioGraphics* 2000;**20**(2):399–418.

3.16 Bowel ischemia

Bowel ischemia is one of the most common causes of an acute abdomen where CT scan plays an essential role to confirm or exclude the diagnosis. It represents a decreased or absent blood supply to the bowel due to occlusive or non-occlusive arterial or venous disease. See Fig. 3.16.

Clinical

Causes include arterial thromboembolism, venous occlusive disease, severe hypotension and shock. It is commonly associated with atherosclerosis, atrial fibrillation, post-operative cholesterol emboli, venous stasis due to bowel dilatation, vasculitis and bowel obstruction. In elderly patients, the left hemi-colon is affected more commonly; however, in young individuals the right-side colon is involved. Usually there is segmental involvement of the bowel in the arterial territory.

Technique

Non-contrast CT scan to evaluate for high-density bowel wall due to intra-mucosal hemorrhage and hyper-attenuating intravascular thrombi. Arterial phase scan to evaluate

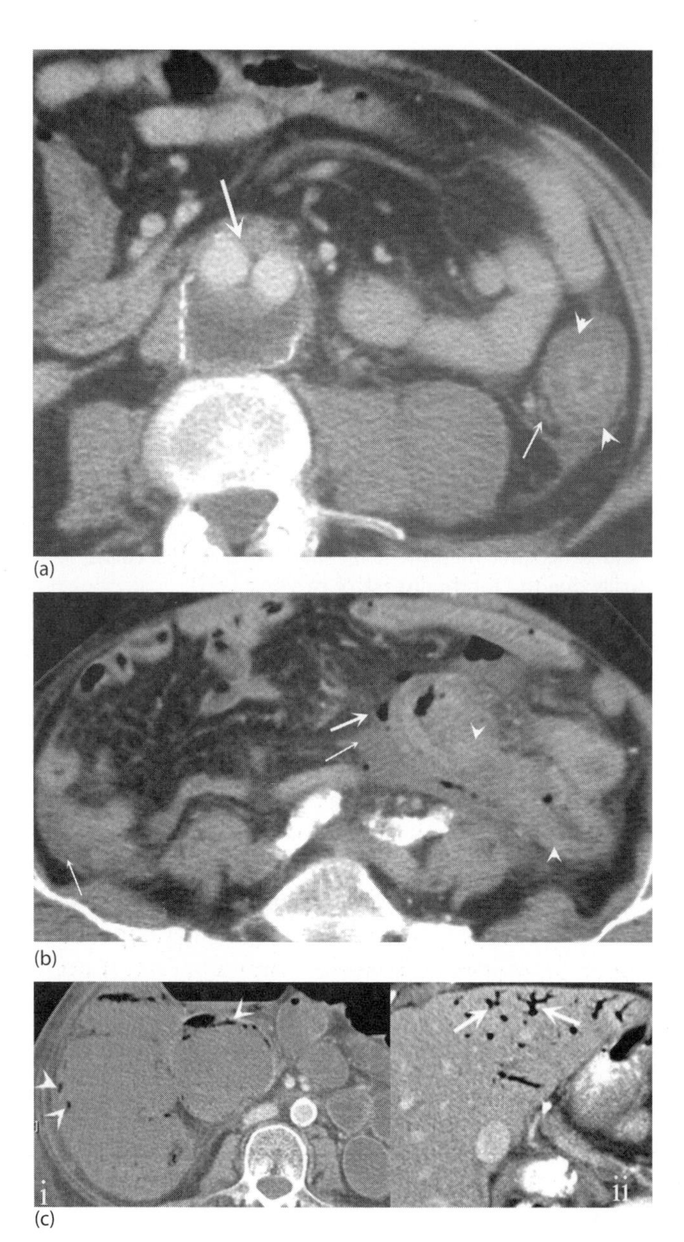

Fig. 3.16. (a) Bowel ischemia. Axial CECT shows surgical repair of AAA (arrow), thickening/edema of the descending colonic wall (arrowheads) and mild pericolic stranding (thin arrow), consistent with bowel ischemia. Note the alternating layers of high and low attenuation ("target sign") in the colonic wall. (b) Segmental bowel ischemia. CECT shows marked segmental large bowel wall thickening (arrowheads) and associated pericolonic stranding, free fluid (thin arrows) and some free air in the adjacent mesentery (arrow), consistent with segmental ischemic colitis complicated by local perforation. (c) Colonic ischemia. CECT shows dilated loops of small and large bowel and gas within the colonic wall (i – arrowheads). Peripheral small lucent branchings in the liver represent portal venous gas (ii – arrows).

for mesenteric vascular thrombo-emboli. Portal venous phase scan (70 s delay) is helpful to assess the mesenteric arteries and veins, to better evaluate the bowel wall for enhancement. It also helps to identify associated abscess and to exclude other causes of acute abdomen.

Oral contrast is not necessary but water can be used as a negative contrast if the bowel is not dilated and fluid-filled. Positive oral water-soluble contrast may be helpful in identifying the site of transmural perforation.

Findings

Unenhanced scan

1. Hyper-attentuating bowel wall, high-density intravascular clot in the celiac or SMA vessels.
2. Free air is suggestive of transmural necrosis.

Enhanced scan

1. Bowel wall thickening
2. Mucosal hyperemia and hyperperfusion with edema, causing the target sign.
3. Intramural hemorrhage is seen as high density.
4. Lack of bowel wall enhancement.
5. Abnormally dilated fluid-filled bowel.
6. Pneumatosis intestinalis: seen as intra-mural bubbles or linear lucencies in both the dependent and non-dependent bowel wall.
7. Porto-mesenteric gas: Gas tracking into mesenteric draining veins especially seen adjacent to the abnormal bowel. Gas is also seen in major veins like SMV.
8. Portal vein gas is seen as a small peripheral branching pattern extending to the periphery of the liver. Gas may also be noted in the main portal vein.
9. Mesenteric stranding, fluid and ascites.
10. Evidence of thrombo-emboli within the celiac, superior and inferior mesenteric arteries or veins.

Pearls

- Review the coronal and sagittal reformatted images.
- Mucosal edema is relatively pronounced in venous infarction due to impaired venous drainage.
- Ischemia can present predominantly with fluid-filled dilated bowel without wall thickening.
- Pneumatosis and portomesenteric gas represents bowel-wall necrosis but this is not always due to infarction. Bowel luminal dilatation likely represents irreversible damage.
- Normal colonic collapse has to be differentiated from ischemic colitis.
- Always look for associated abscess, perforation, bowel obstruction etc. Infarction can involve a single or multiple segments of the bowel.
- Watershed areas such as splenic flexure and rectosigmoid are more prone to be affected in ischemia.
- Always look at the mesenteric vessels in ischemic bowel.

Suggested reading

Chou CK. CT manifestations of bowel ischemia. *Am J Roentgenol* 2002;**178**:87–91.

Frauenfelder T, Wildermuth S, Marincek B, Boehm T. Nontraumatic abdominal vascular conditions: advantage of multi-detector row CT and three-dimensional imaging. *Radiographics* 2004;**24** (2):481–496.

Rha SE *et al.* CT and MR imaging findings of bowel ischemia from various primary causes. *RadioGraphics* 2000;**20**:29–42.

Wiesner W, Khurana B, Ji H, Ros PR. CT of acute bowel ischemia. *Radiology* 2003;**226**:635–650.

3.17 Small bowel obstruction

Abnormal dilatation of small bowel loops may be due to mechanical or adynamic obstruction. Small bowel obstruction comprises 80% of all bowel obstruction. Causes of mechanical obstruction include: adhesions (most common, 75% of all causes), hernias, tumors, small bowel volvulus, inflammatory bowel disease, gallstone ileus, and mesenteric infarction/ischemia. See Fig. 3.17.

Clinical

Presents with acute abdominal pain, bilious vomiting, abdominal distention. Common causes: Ileus, adhesion, hernias, tumor, intussusception, stricture, large bowel obstruction. Gallstone ileus in the elderly.

Technique

The supine abdominal radiograph will demonstrate small bowel dilatation. Urgent CT abdominal scan may be indicated to exclude a mechanical obstruction and to determine the site, level and cause of obstruction in order to plan for further management.

Multi-slice spiral CT abdomen and pelvis with IV contrast. Fluid within the dilated bowel acts as a negative contrast therefore no oral contrast is usually needed.

The scan should include pelvis and the inguinal orifices.

Findings

1. Abnormal dilatation (> 2.5 cm) of fluid-filled small bowel loops.
2. Presence of transition zone (change in the bowel calibre) indicates site of obstruction due to mechanical obstruction. The following changes at the transition zone suggest different pathologies:
   Angulated and kinked bowel = Adhesions.
   Irregular soft tissue (+/– nodular) wall thickening = Tumor.
   Transmural wall thickening with skip lesions = Crohn's disease.
   Mucosal edema with bowel wall thickening over a long distance = ischemia.

Caption for Fig. 3.17 (a) Gallstone ileus. (i) CECT shows dilated small bowel loops (arrowheads). The transition point (the junction between non-dilated collapsed (thin arrow) and dilated bowel) is found to be in the distal small bowel, where a laminated gallstone is seen within the bowel lumen (arrow) (ii). Note pneumobilia (arrow) (iii). This image shows a fistulous track (arrowhead) between the collapsed and edematous gallbladder (arrow) and the duodenum. (b) Meconium ileus. Axial CT of an adult patient with cystic fibrosis (CF) shows marked dilatation of small bowel (arrow) secondary to obstruction of the distal ileum with abnormally viscid bowel contents (thin arrows), called "meconium ileus-equivalent syndrome" or distal intestinal obstruction syndrome. (c) Adhesions. Coronal CECT shows multiple dilated bowel loops (arrows) consistent with small bowel obstruction. There is a transition zone showing kinking and beaking of the bowel (arrowhead) with resultant proximal dilatation and distal collapse of small bowel loops (small arrow). (d) Bowel carcinoma. CECT shows multiple dilated loops of small bowel with a peripherally enhancing necrotic soft tissue mass in the cecum (arrowhead). A few loops of bowel are also seen within the left abdominal wall (arrows). (e) Intussusception. CT abdomen shows dilated small bowel loops, an abnormal loop of bowel in the right lower quadrant (arrow) with mesenteric fat (thin arrow) and vessels and accompanying a telescoped loop of bowel – intussusceptum (arrowhead). The portion of intestine that receives this loop is called the intussuscipiens. (f) Obstructed obturator hernia. CECT images show multiple dilated small bowel loops (i – arrows). A loop of bowel with thickened wall is interpositioned between the left pectineus muscle anteriorly and the obturator muscles posteriorly (ii – arrowhead).

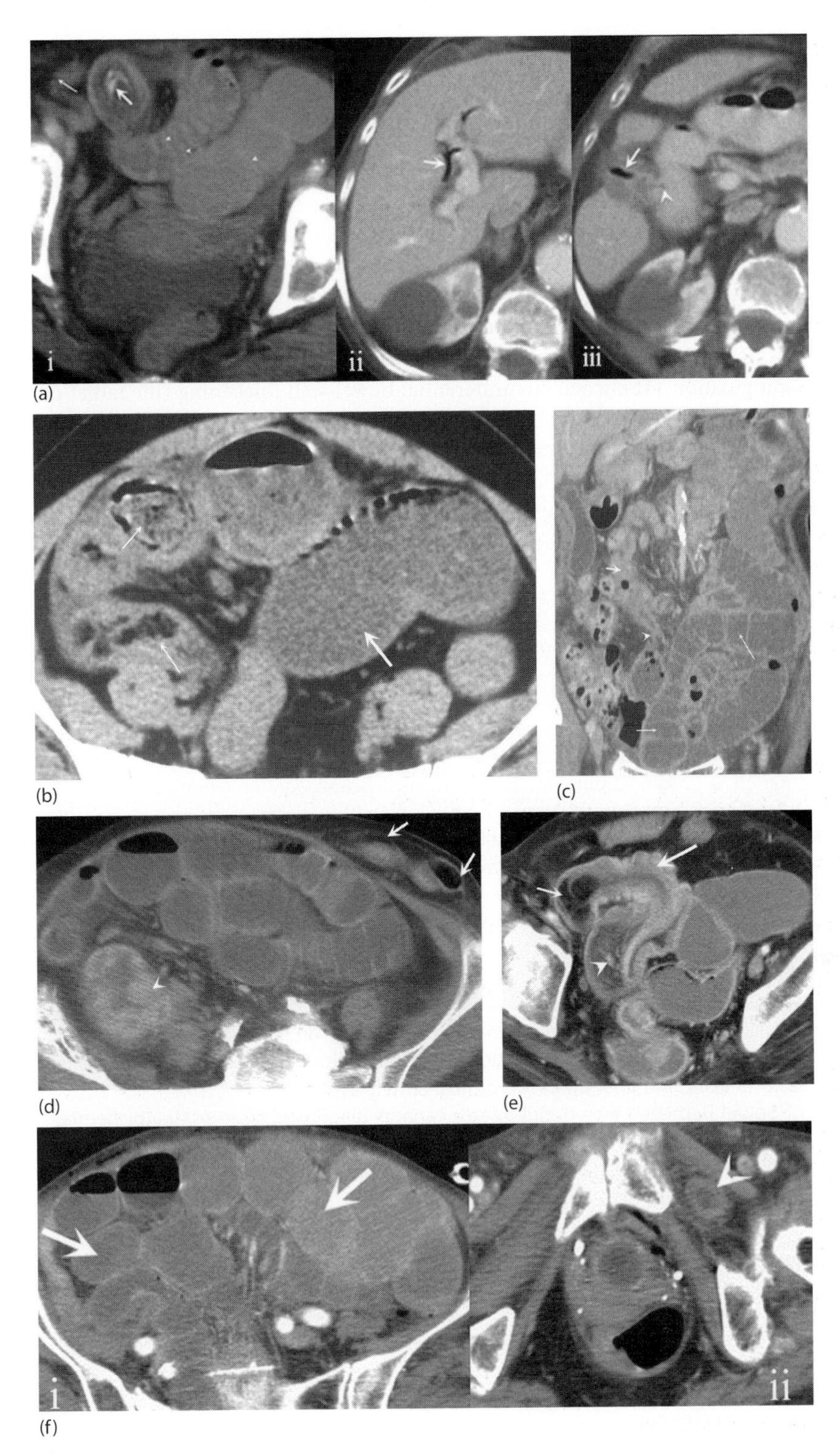

Fig. 3.17.

Associated with C or U shaped dilated bowel and crowding of mesentery towards the site of obstruction (whirl sign) = closed loop obstruction.
Transition zone in the hernial orifices = obstructed hernia.
Doughnut sign (Bowel within a bowel) = intussusception.
Gallstone(s) in small bowel = GB ileus (look for pneumobilia). Rigler's triad = ectopic gallstone, pneumobilia and small bowel obstruction.
Smooth mucosal bulge into the lumen in bowel – hematoma is a rare cause.

3. Pseudofeces sign: Presence of feces within the small bowel indicates mechanical obstruction (e.g. meconium equivalent syndrome due to cystic fibrosis).
4. Diffuse dilatation of small bowel without evidence of colonic collapse is likely due to ileus.
5. Signs of strangulation: Abnormal circumferential bowel-wall thickening (the target or halo sign), absence or asymmetric bowel-wall enhancement, pericolonic high-density mesenteric fluid or hemorrhage, mesenteric clouding, pneumatosis intestinalis, mesenteric and portal vein gas.
6. Look for locally perforated cecal tumor and appendix.

Pearls

- Bowel should be inspected retrogradely from the rectum to duodenum in order to identify the transition zone.
- Multi-planar coronal reformatted images should be routinely performed and reviewed.
- Adhesive bands due to prior surgery are not usually seen on CT. They represent the commonest cause of closed loop obstruction.
- Obstruction in a "virgin abdomen", complete obstruction, strangulation, closed loop obstruction need urgent surgical intervention.
- Pseudo-obstruction is seen as dilated small and large bowel without evidence of mechanical obstruction. Commonly seen in moribund patients with COPD or electrolyte disturbance.
- Closed loop obstruction is an emergency mechanical obstruction, which can cause volvulus and strangulation. It is due to obstruction of two segments of the bowel at a single site.
- Pneumobilia is differentiated from portal venous gas by the location of the gas: pneumobilia is typically seen centrally while portal venous gas is seen in the periphery of the liver.
- Causes of gas in the gallbladder and/or biliary tree include an incompetent sphincter of Oddi, emphysematous cholecystitis, a duodenal ulcer perforating into the common bile duct, gallstone ileus, and post-operative or post-sphincterotomy.
- A loop of bowel herniated into the obturator canal is diagnostic of an obturator hernia, a rare form of hernia with a high rate of mortality secondary to strangulation. Clinical diagnosis is often delayed, although CT findings are diagnostic.

Suggested reading

Boudiaf M *et al.* CT evaluation of small bowel obstruction. *Radiographics* 2001;**21**:613–624.

Khurana B, Ledbetter S, McTavish J, Wiesner W, Ros PR. Bowel obstruction revealed by multidetector CT. *Am J Roentgenol* 2002;**178**:1139–1144.

Taourel P *et al.* Non-traumatic abdominal emergencies: imaging of acute intestinal obstruction. *Eur Radiol* 2002;**12**:2151–2160.

3.18 Diverticulitis and diverticular abscess

Inflammation or infection of colonic diverticulosis. Diverticulosis is due to mucosal and submucosal herniation through the muscularis propria at the site of the nutrient arteries. Hard and dehydrated inspissated fecal matter trapped in diverticula may lead to mucosal erosion and inflammation/diverticulitis. Intramural tracking and localized perforation can occur with subsequent pericolonic abscess formation. See Fig. 3.18.

Clinical

Abdominal pain (left iliac fossa): May have symptoms of large bowel obstruction.

Pyrexia, localized tenderness, rectal bleeding.

Technique

CT abdomen and pelvis with oral/rectal and intravenous contrast.

Findings

1. Colonic outpouching typically involving sigmoid colon: Diverticulosis.
2. Long segment colonic wall thickening and pericolonic mesenteric fat stranding and vessel engorgement favor diverticulitis.
3. Local perforation or pneumoperitoneum.
4. Walled-off collection: Diverticular abscess.
5. Bowel obstruction is not common with diverticular disease.

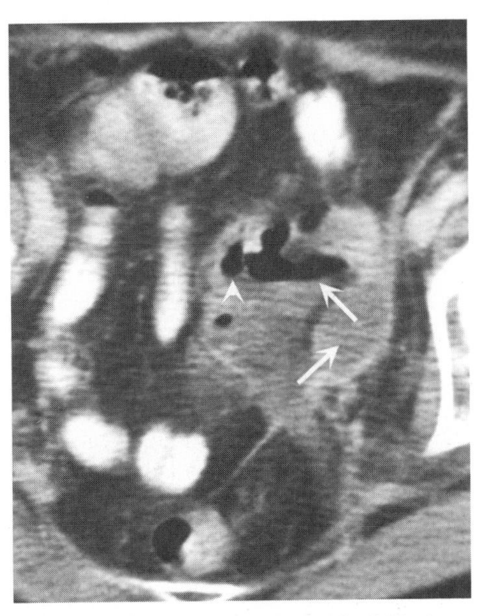

Fig. 3.18. Diverticular abscess. Axial CECT shows a gas/fluid collection (arrows) with adjacent fat stranding in the region of the sigmoid colon diverticula (arrowhead), representing an abscess associated with diverticulitis.

Pearls

- Severe eccentric bowel wall thickening of sigmoid due to diverticulitis can mimic colonic carcinoma.
- Pericolonic mesenteric fat stranding and vascular congestion are more likely due to diverticulitis but perforated carcinoma can cause similar features.
- Carcinoma is more likely associated with larger inflammatory mass and bowel obstruction than diverticulitis.
- Focal shelf like bowel wall thickening favors carcinoma.
- Look for air in the bladder/vagina due to colovesical/vaginal fistula.

Suggested reading

Macari M, Balthazar EJ. CT of bowel wall thickening: significance and pitfalls of interpretation. *Am J Roentgenol* 2001;**176**:1105–1116.

Wittenberg J *et al.* Algorithmic approach to CT diagnosis of the abdominal bowel wall. *RadioGraphics* 2002;**22**:1093–1109.

Section 2 Chapter 4

Other emergencies

Ultrasound

Jolanta Webb and Swati P. Deshmane

4.1 General principles

Portable ultrasound machine

Familiarize yourself with the portable ultrasound (US) machine used on-call in your department.

On/off switch, selecting probes (curvilinear, linear) and settings (abdomen, pelvis, small parts), adjusting depth, focus and gain, entering patients' details and annotations, printing. See Fig. 4.1.

Alternative arrangements for scanning

Consider using the stationary machine for scanning patients who are stable enough to be brought into the department.

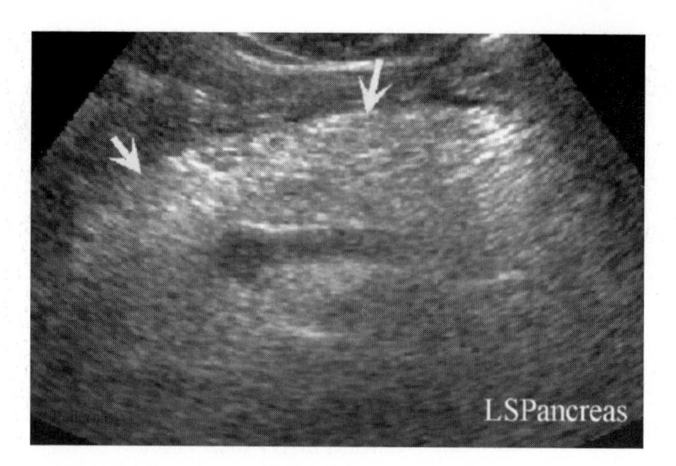

Fig. 4.1. Acute pancreatitis. US abdomen in a patient with acute abdominal pain and raised serum amylase shows diffuse swelling of pancreas with obscuration of its normal serrated margins (arrows) due to acute pancreatitis. (Photo courtesy of Dr. Sonali Maniar, Wockhardt Hospital, Mumbai.)

Purpose

Remember you are being asked for a prompt answer to a fairly specific question in a sick patient.

In many conditions US makes a vital contribution to the immediate patient management and has to be performed without delay.

Potential controversies

Appendicitis – not used widely outside pediatric population; may be useful in a slim patient if the operator is experienced in performing it. Leaking abdominal aortic aneurysm and testicular torsion – clinical diagnoses requiring emergency surgery, but sometimes clinical picture is unclear and ultrasound may be useful in excluding other causes. Psoas abscess/hematoma – CT is superior, but US may be adequate in a slim patient.

Suggested reading

Meire H, ed. *Clinical Ultrasound. A Comprehensive Text. Abdominal and General Ultrasound.* Churchill Livingstone, 2001.

4.2 Abdominal trauma

Abdominal trauma results from blunt or penetrating injuries. See Fig. 4.2.

Clinical

Ultrasound is very good at detecting free intraperitoneal fluid as an indirect sign of trauma but inferior to CT at showing solid organ laceration/hematoma.

Focused Assessment with Sonography For Trauma (FAST)

FAST is a useful technique for evaluation of free fluid or bleeding following blunt and penetrating trauma.

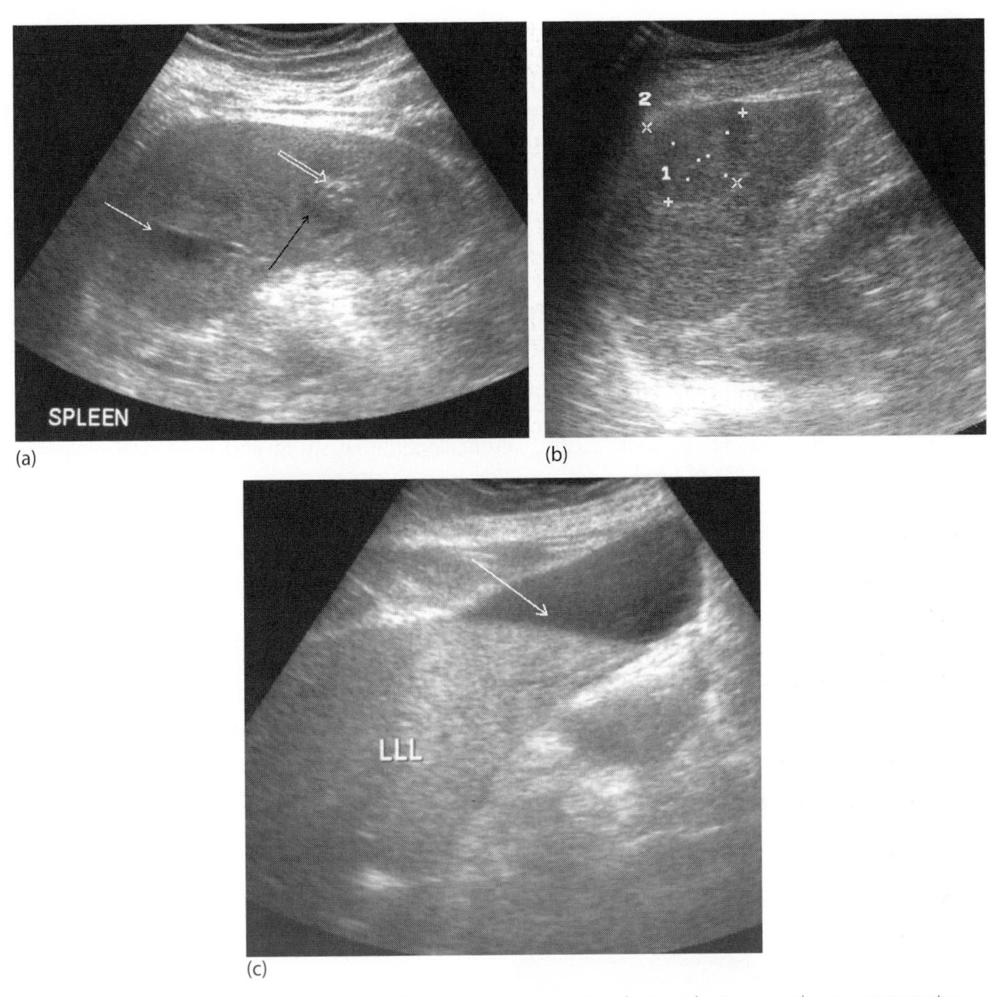

(a) (b) (c)

Fig. 4.2. (a) Splenic trauma. A linear anechoic focus seen posteriorly in splenic parenchyma, representing laceration (solid white arrow). There is a rounded area in the anterior spleen (black arrow) of mixed echogenicity with a high echogenicity component (open white arrow), representing fresh blood. Note that trauma to liver, kidneys or pancreas will produce a similar appearance. (b) Splenic hematoma. Rounded decreased echogenicity region in splenic parenchyma (between calipers), representing hematoma following a fall a few weeks prior to the scan. (c) Hemoperitoneum. Abdominal intraperitoneal free fluid anterior to left lobe of liver (arrow) following trauma.

Technique

Limited 4–6 views scan for detection of free intraperitoneal fluid as a marker of injury. Performed parallel to resuscitation, after primary survey. Orthogonal images should be used to increase the sensitivity of the scan.

Views: Morison's pouch, perisplenic space, suprapubic, pericardial (subcostal), bilateral paracolic (optional).

Extended FAST views: Pleural space (anterior view for pneumothorax); subcostal or parasternal and apical views for hemopericardium.

Findings

1. Hemoperitoneum: Anechoic fluid if fresh blood; fluid with internal echoes if clotted blood, accumulating in a dependent position.
2. Laceration: Low-echogenicity elongated irregular area within a parenchymal organ.
3. Hematoma: Central or subcapsular fluid collection.
4. Intraperitoneal gas: Multiple short linear echogenic foci with posterior shadowing due to reverberation artefact (comet-tail artefact or ring-down artefact).

Pearls

- Hemoperitoneum has to be of sufficient duration and volume to be detected by FAST.
- Up to 3 cm of anechoic fluid in the cul-de-sac of premenopausal women in isolation can be physiological.
- Pathological conditions such ascites, ventriculoperitonal shunt and peritoneal dialysis limit the usefulness of FAST.
- FAST remains the first-line examination in trauma. If FAST is negative and there is high clinical suspicion of significant injury – proceed to CT.

Suggested reading

Bahner D *et al.* AIUM practice guideline for the performance of the focused assessment with sonography for trauma (FAST) examination *J Ultrasound Med* 2007;**27**:313–318.

Dolich MO, McKenney MG. Ultrasound for blunt abdominal trauma. *J Trauma* 2001;**50**(1):108–112.

4.3 Pleural empyema

Fluid in pleural space (sterile in non-infective pleural effusion or infected in empyema). See Fig. 4.3.

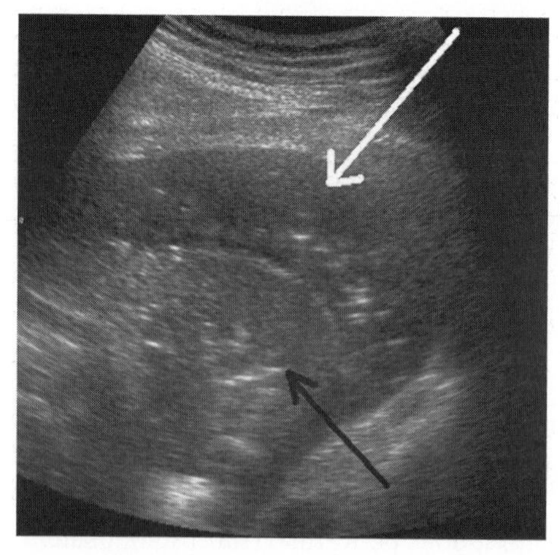

Fig. 4.3. Pleural empyema. Echogenic fluid in pleural space (white arrow) consistent with empyema in a patient with recent pneumonia. Left lower consolidation is seen (black arrow).

Clinical

Refer to Section 2.10.

Technique

3.5–5 MHz curvilinear transducer for wider survey.

7.5–10 MHz linear transducer for detail of superficially located abnormalities.

Patient in sitting position for posterior chest; in decubitus position for anterior and lateral chest.

Combine with US guided needle aspiration (sample for cell count, Gram stain, culture and biochemistry – pH < 7.1 suggests infection) and insertion of pig-tail catheter (≥ 8 Fr).

Findings

1. Anechoic fluid.
2. Fluid containing variable amount of internal echoes in empyema; may be loculated and/ or septated.

Pearls

- It is not possible to differentiate between sterile and infected effusion on US (anechoic fluid may be sterile or infected; echogenic fluid is usually infected).
- Pus may be too thick to aspirate.

Suggested reading

Koh DM, Burke S, Davies N, Padley SPG. Transthoracic US of the chest: clinical uses and applications. *RadioGraphics* 2002;22:e1.

4.4 Acute cholecystitis

Acute inflammation of gallbladder (GB) as a result of complication of stone disease in majority of patients, but sometimes no gallstones can be seen (acalculous cholecystitis; typically in intensive-care unit patients who have not received enteral feeding). See Fig. 4.4.

Clinical

Right upper quandrant/epigastric pain, vomiting, fever, may be jaundiced.

Technique

3.5–5 MHz curvilinear transducer. Preparation – fast 6 hours (if not fasted, GB may be contracted, with artefactually thickened wall).

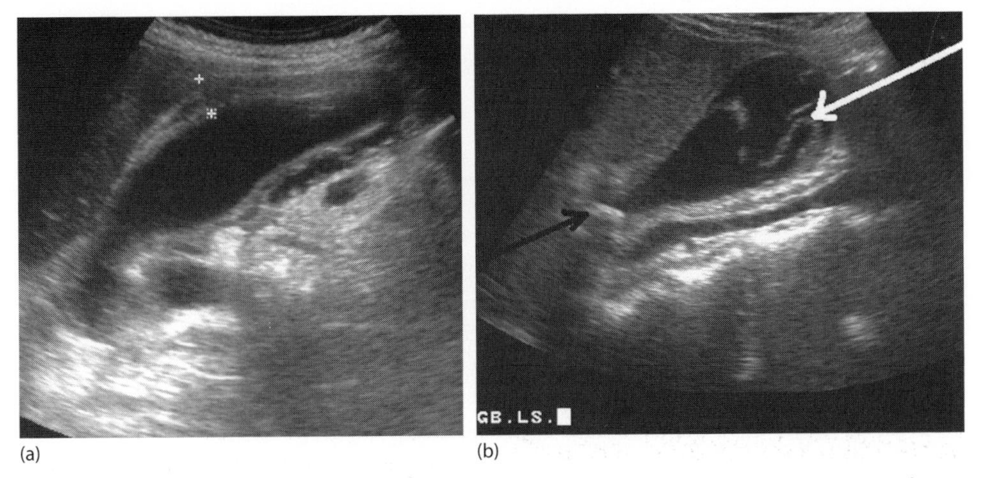

(a) (b)

Fig. 4.4. (a) Acute cholecystitis. Thickening of gallbladder wall > 3 mm (between calipers) is a non-specific sign seen in acute cholecystitis. (b) Gangrenous cholecystitis. US of gall bladder shows internal echoes resembling membranes (white arrow), representing sloughing of the mucous membrane in a patient with gangrenous cholecystitis. Gallstone impacted in GB neck (black arrow).

Findings

1. Presence of gallstones (unless acalculous), especially blocking the neck of the GB.
2. Thickened GB wall (> 3 mm; use anterior wall to perform the measurement).
   NB: In isolation it is a non-specific sign.
3. Poorly defined GB wall.
4. Abnormal appearance of GB wall – either a three-layer appearance (with low echogenicity middle layer representing edema) or two-layer appearance (with outer low echogenicity layer representing pericholecystitic fluid); specific for acute cholecystitis (unlike isolated wall thickening).
5. GB may be distended (> 10 × 4 cm, rounded in shape).
6. Positive sonographic Murphy's sign (marked tenderness on scanning over GB).

Delay in treatment may lead to gangrenous cholecystitis.

Findings: gangrenous cholecystitis

1. Markedly irregular thick wall representing ulceration of GB mucosa, necrosis and hemorrhage.
2. High echogenicity foci in the wall (microabscesses).
3. Internal echoes – coarse, forming membrane-like structures.

Specific form of cholecystitis in diabetic patients – emphysematous cholecystitis.

Findings: emphysematous cholecystitis

1. High-echogenicity arcuate-shaped structures in the GB wall, due to intramural gas.
2. May resemble a bowel loop.

Pearls

- GB wall thickening alone is not diagnostic of acute cholecystitis.
- Acute cholecystitis may be present in the absence of gallstones.

Suggested reading

Refer to Section 4.1.

Bertoff GA *et al.* Gallbladder stones: imaging and intervention. *RadioGraphics* 2000;**20**:751–766.

4.5 Gallbladder empyema

Pus in the gallbladder (GB).
Complication of acute cholecystitis. See Fig. 4.5.

Clinical

As acute cholecystitis + palpable right upper quadrant mass.

Technique

3.5–5 MHz curvilinear transducer.
Fast 6 hours (but patient usually too ill to eat anyway).

Findings

1. Distended GB (subjective assessment; size $> 10 \times 4$ cm and a rounded shape are suggestive).
2. Intraluminal echoes representing purulent debris/exudate.
3. Similar to sludge (may be impossible to distinguish) but no layering/movement with change in patient's position.

Pearls

- GB empyema requires emergency drainage to prevent perforation.

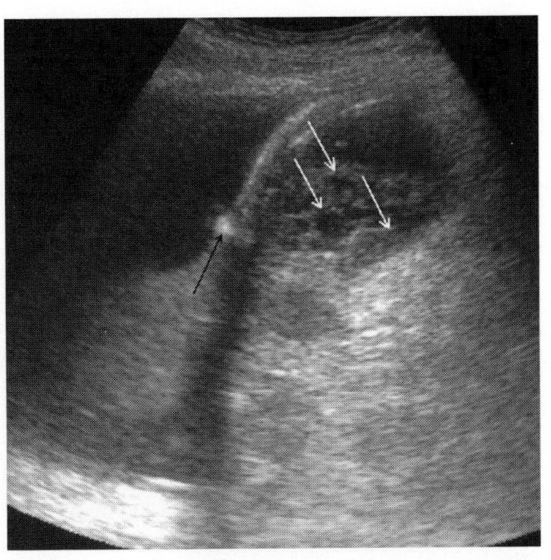

Fig. 4.5. Gallbladder empyema. US abdomen in a patient with recent acute cholecystitis shows a distended gallbladder with numerous internal echoes (white arrows), consistent with gallbladder empyema. Note an impacted stone in the GB neck (black arrow).

Suggested reading

Refer to Section 4.1.

Kane RA. Ultrasonographic diagnosis of gangrenous cholecystitis and empyema of the gallbladder. *Radiology* 1980;**134**:191–194.

4.6 Liver abscess

Localized collection of pus in liver parenchyma. See Fig. 4.6.

Clinical

Fever, rigors, malaise, anorexia, vomiting, weight loss, abdominal pain, jaundice, shock.

Technique

3.5–5 MHz curvilinear transducer.

Findings

1. Single or (less commonly) multiple low-echogenicity lesions.
2. Preferential location – in the dome/posterior aspect of the right lobe.
3. Exact appearance depends on its age (therefore serial scanning will demonstrate rapid evolution of appearances).

Early

1. Poorly defined, only slightly lower echogenicity than surrounding liver.
2. Surrounding hypoechoic halo.
3. Right pleural effusion.

Late

1. Well-defined hypoechoic lesion, with perceivable high-echogenicity wall.
2. Internal echoes representing debris or gas.

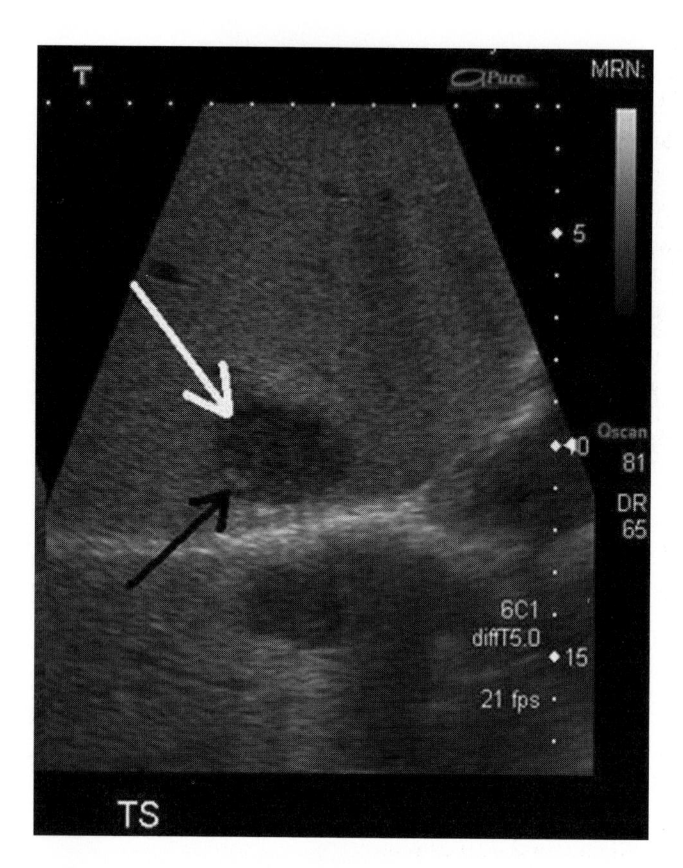

Fig. 4.6. Liver abscess. TS of liver shows small amount of solid debris (black arrow) in predominantly anechoic abscess (white arrow).

Pearls

- It is not possible to distinguish between different etiologies (e.g. bacterial vs amebic) on ultrasound grounds.
- Look for clues to the underlying cause e.g. biliary obstruction, appendicitis, diverticulitis.

Suggested reading

Dewbury KC *et al.* Ultrasound in the diagnosis of the early liver abscess. *Br J Radiol* 1980;53:1160–1165.

4.7 Obstructive jaundice

Presence of jaundice due to blockage of bile drainage. See Fig. 4.7.

Clinical

Features of jaundice, features of underlying condition (e.g. biliary colic in stone disease, weight loss in pancreatic malignancy).

Technique

3.5–5 MHz curvilinear transducer.
Also endoscopic ultrasound (during ERCP).

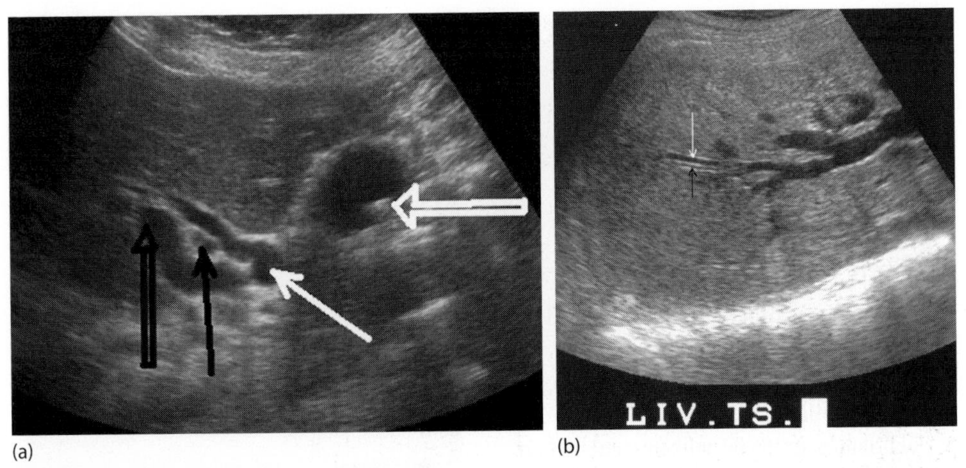

(a) (b)

Fig. 4.7. (a) Biliary duct dilatation. Dilated common duct (white arrow) and gallbladder stone (open white arrow) are noted in a patient with common duct stone (not shown). Hepatic artery (black arrow) and portal vein (open black arrow) are depicted. (b) Intrahepatic bile duct dilatation. Parallel channels in the peripheral liver parenchyma, one representing dilated intrahepatic bile duct (white arrow), the other a normal portal vein branch (black arrow). Spider-like configuration of prominent intrahepatic bile ducts at the porta hepatis is noted.

Findings

1. Dilated common duct, measured at the level of hepatic artery, > 6 mm in ≤ 60-year-olds, adding 1 mm per decade; > 10 mm post-cholecystectomy).
2. "Parallel channel"/"double barrel" sign (in LS and TS respectively) – intrahepatic bile ducts become visible alongside portal vein branches.
3. Stellate appearance at the porta due to duct dilatation.
4. Coexisting dilatation of pancreatic duct (≥ 3 mm) in obstruction at the level of the ampulla of Vater.
5. Look for intraductal stones, pancreatic or ampullary tumor.

Pearls

- There may be lack of detectable dilatation early on – rescan in 2 days.
- Lack of dilatation of intrahepatic bile ducts in the presence of dilatation of extrahepatic common ducts suggests obstruction by a stone.

Suggested reading

Refer to Section 4.1.

Razzaq R, Sukumar SA. Imaging of the jaundiced adult. *Imaging* 2004;**16**:287–300.

4.8 Biliary stent

Treatment of biliary obstruction. See Fig. 4.8.

Clinical

To relieve biliary obstruction and prevent obstructive cholangitis.
Inserted at ERCP or PCT.

Plastic or metallic.
Recurrent dilatation of proximal bilary tree suggestive of blockage.

Technique

5 MHz curvilinear transducer.

Findings

1. Hyperechoic tube in common bile duct/ proximal intrahepatic ducts.
2. Echogenic intrahepatic bile ducts due to pneumobilia if stent is patent.
3. Echogenic material within stent which may represent tumor or stones (depending on initial reason for stent placement).

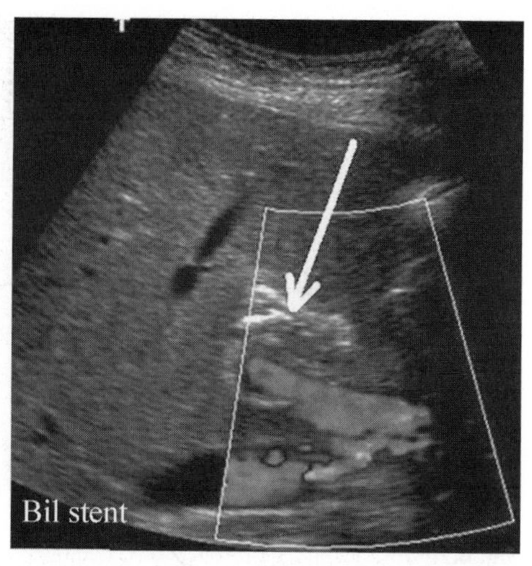

Fig. 4.8. Biliary stent. Hyperechoic tubular structure within the common duct is consistent with biliary stent (white arrow).

Pearls

- Compare with pre-stent imaging to establish whether stent effective in relieving biliary obstruction.

Suggested reading

Phillips-Hughes J. Invasive and interventional uses of endoscopic ultrasound. *Br J Radiol* 2007;**80**:1–2.

4.9 Transjugular intrahepatic portosystemic shunt (TIPSS)

Communication created between a branch of the portal vein and hepatic vein via a percutaneous transjugular approach, aimed at alleviation of portal hypertension. See Fig. 4.9.

Clinical

Failure of TIPSS can result in progressive jaundice, variceal bleeding and hepato-renal failure.

Technique

3.5–5 MHz curvilinear transducer; color, spectral and power Doppler.
High rate of stenosis/occlusion, which may be detected early with regular US follow-up (day 1, 7, then 3 monthly in 1st year, 6 monthly thereafter).

Findings

Patent TIPSS

1. Presence of a spectral waveform and color flow signal within the shunt.
2. High intrashunt velocity (200–300 cm/s).

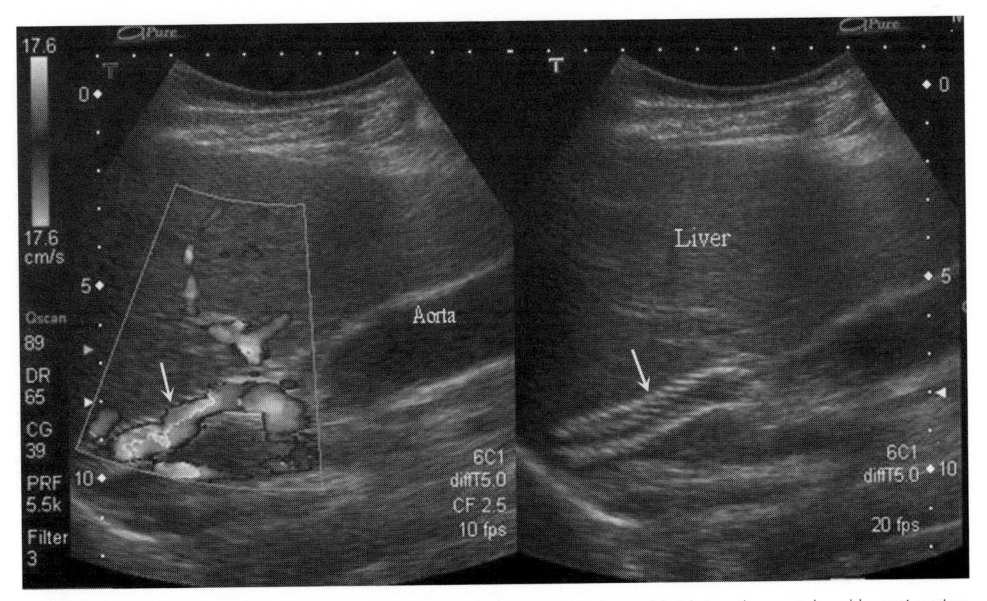

Fig. 4.9. Patent TIPSS. US liver shows an echogenic tubular structure (arrow) bridging the portal and hepatic veins, with high velocity flow towards the liver. No internal debris or echoes within the stent.

3. Maximum velocity in the portal 1/3 of TIPSS (Vmax) > 50 cm/s.
4. Hepatofugal intraparenchymal portal venous flow.

Stenosed TIPSS

1. Vmax < 50 cm/s.
2. Change in intraparenchymal portal venous flow from hepatofugal to hepatopetal.

Occluded TIPSS

1. No detectable flow.

Pearls

- Regular surveillance post-TIPSS placement required to promptly relieve occlusion.

Suggested reading

Feldstein VA *et al.* Transjugular intrahepatic portosystemic shunts: accuracy of Doppler US in determination of patency and detection of stenoses. *Radiology* 1996;**201**:141–147.

4.10 Hydro/pyonephrosis

Dilatation of urinary tract due to presence of obstruction. See Fig. 4.10.

Clinical

Flank pain, pyrexia and unwell in pyonephrosis.

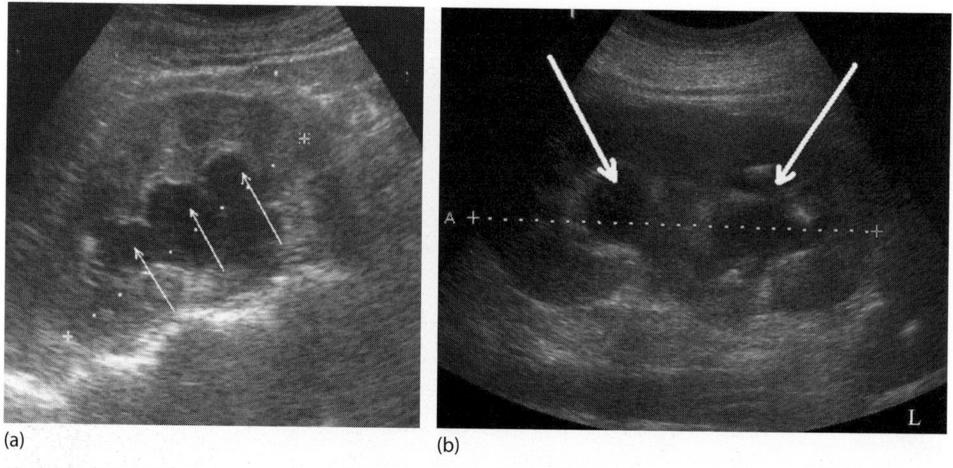

Fig. 4.10. (a) Hydronephrosis. Longitudinal section (LS) US kidney shows dilated renal pelvis and calyces, filled by anechoic fluid (arrows) without internal echoes to suggest infection. (b) Pyonephrosis. LS US of kidney shows dilated renal collecting system with internal echoes seen in calyces, particularly lower pole, consistent with pyonephrosis (arrows).

Technique

3.5–5 MHz curvilinear transducer.

Findings

1. Dilated renal pelvis and calyces (anechoic or containing low-level internal echoes, representing pus).
2. May see gas in emphysematous pyelonephritis (markedly hyperechoic foci with a comet-tail artefact).
3. Normal size or enlarged kidneys.
4. Preserved cortical depth.

Pearls

- Try to visualize proximal and distal ureter as its calibre is helpful in establishing the level of obstruction.

Suggested reading

Refer to Section 4.1.

Laing FC. Renal sonography in the intensive care unit. *J Ultrasound Med* 2002;**21**:493–494.

4.11 Acute renal failure (ARF)

Obstruction presenting as ARF is the single most important indication to perform US. See Fig. 4.11.

Clinical

Oliguria, vomiting, confusion, bruising, GI bleeding, pulmonary edema.

Technique

3.5–5 MHz curvilinear transducer.

Findings

1. Often normal appearance of both kidneys.
2. Dilatation of collecting system in otherwise normal kidneys suggesting it is of recent onset and the likely underlying cause of ARF.
3. Small echogenic kidneys indicate a background of chronic kidney disease.
4. Enlarged kidneys with loss of normal parenchymal structure, replaced by innumerable cysts, in adult polycystic kidney disease.
5. Echogenic material in branches/main trunk of renal vein, with enlarged kidney displaying prominence of pyramids indicating renal edema, points to renal vein thrombosis as cause of ARF.

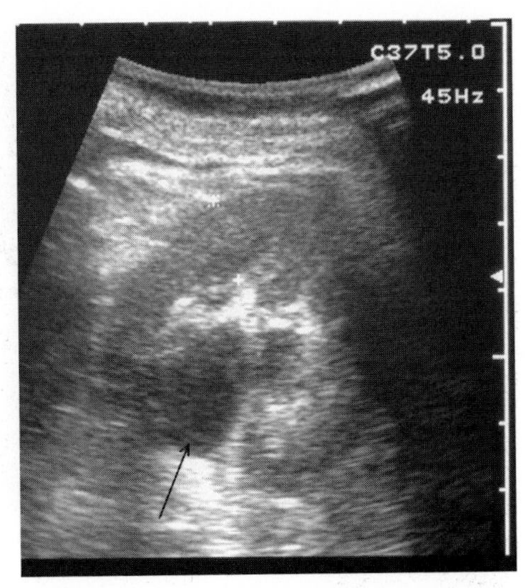

Fig. 4.11. Acute renal failure. US kidney shows hydronephrosis (arrow) presenting as acute renal failure. Normal renal cortical thickness (between calipers) indicating recent onset of renal impairment.

Pearls

- Ultrasound often normal in ARF. Acute obstruction often feared but rarely found.
- Adult polycystic kidney disease may first present with ARF.
- Look for vascular cause for ARF such as renal artery stenosis or thrombosis.

Suggested reading

Platt JF *et al.* Acute renal failure: possible role of duplex Doppler US in distinction between acute prerenal failure and acute tubular necrosis. *Radiology* 1991;**179**(2):419–423.

4.12 Renal vein thrombosis

Occlusive versus non-occlusive thrombus formation within renal vein. There may be bilateral/unilateral/segmental renal vein involvement. See Fig. 4.12.

Clinical

Acute renal failure.
Nephrotic syndrome.

Technique

3.5–5 MHz curvilinear transducer; Doppler US.

Findings

Renal parenchyma

1. Enlarged low-echogenicity (= swollen) kidney(s).

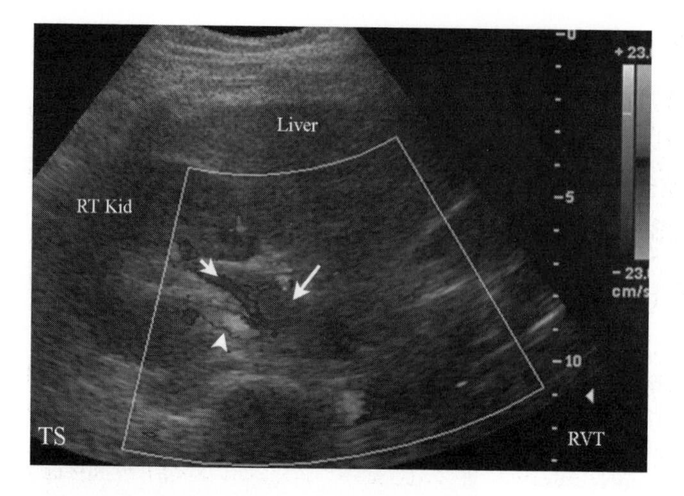

Fig. 4.12. Renal vein thrombosis US abdomen shows edematous right kidney and thrombus (long arrow) within the dilated ipsilateral renal vein. The flow within the renal vein is compromised (short arrow). The Doppler waveforms of the right renal artery (arrowhead) demonstrated reverse diastolic flow (not shown). (Photo courtesy of Drs. Gail Hansen and Mariam Thomas, UCLA-Olive View Medical Center, California.)

2. Loss of corticomedullary differentiation.
3. Eventually shrunken, hyperechoic kidneys.

Renal vein

1. Increased calibre.
2. Echogenic thrombus.
3. Lack of flow.

Renal artery

Increased resistance (decreased diastolic flow).

Pearls

- Renal vein thrombosis starts in small branches and propagates towards main renal vein and IVC.
- Echogenic thrombus only present in the first few days.
- Tumor thrombus usually demonstrates arterial flow whereas bland thrombus is avascular.

Suggested reading

Clark RA *et al.* Renal vein thrombosis: an undiagnosed complication of multiple renal abnormalities. *Radiology* 1979;132:43–50.

4.13 Intra-abdominal collection

Intra-abdominal collections include hematoma, urinoma, biloma, lymphocole, pseudocyst and abscess. Intra-abdominal abscess is an emergency. See Fig. 4.13.

Clinical

Pyrexia, abdominal pain, often following intra-abdominal surgical intervention.

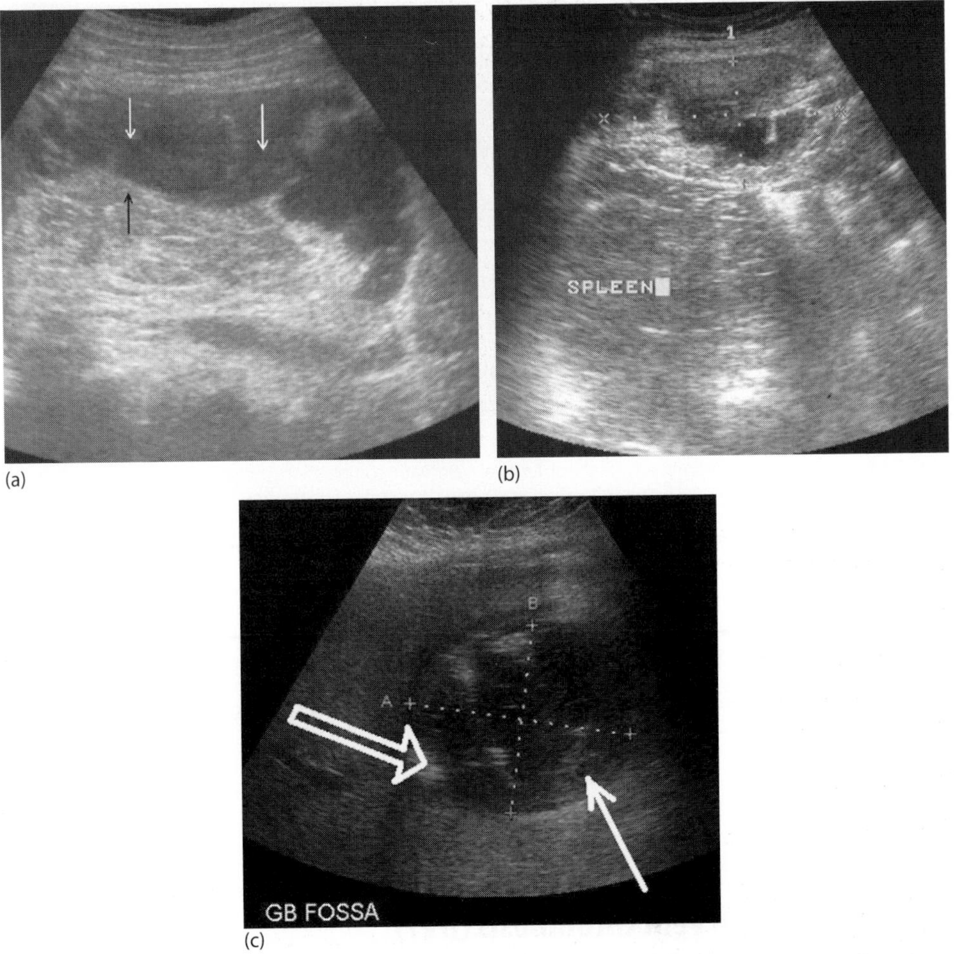

Fig. 4.13. (a, b) Subphrenic collection. (a) US abdomen in a post-operative patient with persistent fever shows loculated fluid with internal septations (white arrows) superior to liver (black arrow), consistent with subphrenic abscess/collection. (b) Mixed echogenicity collection (between calipers) anterior to spleen noted in the same patient. (c) Collection in the GB bed. US abdomen following laparoscopic cholecystectomy shows echogenic areas in the surgical bed (between calipers) representing solid material (white arrow) and gas (open arrow; note posterior shadowing), consistent with an abscess.

Technique

3.5–5 MHz curvilinear transducer.

Findings

1. Depending on the content of the collection; from clear fluid to mixed echogenicity, partially solid/partially cystic structure.
2. Low-echogenic walled-off collection with internal debris and high echogenicity foci (gas) is consistent with a gas-forming abscess.
3. Hematoma in the acute stage appears as an echogenic collection with no definite wall.

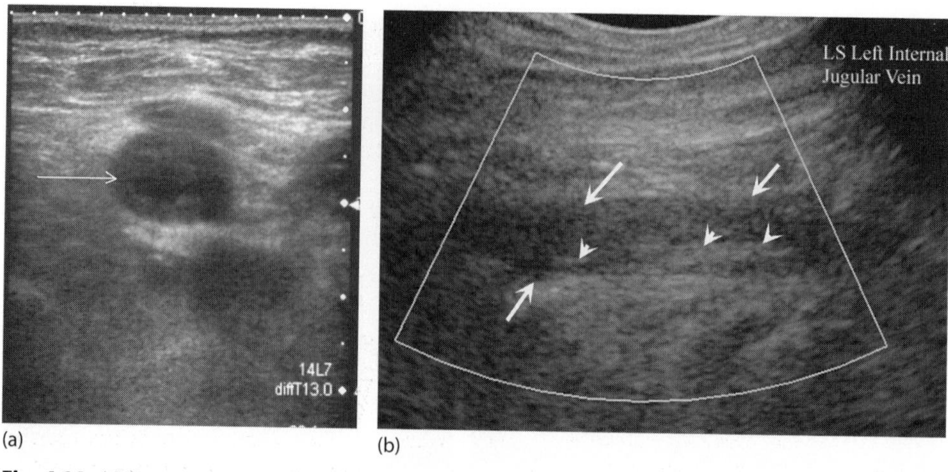

Fig. 4.14. (a) Deep vein thrombosis. TS US of femoral vein with compression shows lack of compressibility of dilated femoral vein and near occlusive echogenic intraluminal thrombus (white arrow). The femoral vein lies deep to femoral artery (which has compressed, indicating adequate pressure has been applied). (b) Left internal jugular vein thrombosis. LS US shows echogenic thrombus (arrowheads) within the dilated left internal jugular vein (arrows).

Pearls

- If the collection is well visualized on ultrasound and a safe route can be established, a US-guided drainage is indicated; otherwise use CT-guided drainage.

Suggested reading

Halber MD. Intra-abdominal abscess. *Am J Roentgenol* 1979;**133**(1):9–13.

4.14 Acute deep vein thrombosis (DVT)

Presence of thrombus in a deep vein; of recent origin (vs chronic DVT). Majority occur in deep leg veins. 1–2% of DVT affect upper limb veins (often following repeated catheterization). See Fig. 4.14.

Clinical

Unilateral limb swelling, redness, increased temperature, tenderness. Above-knee DVT is a strong risk factor for pulmonary embolism.

Technique

7.5 MHz linear probe; gray scale and color Doppler.

Leg veins

Compression: Compress with the probe every 1–2 cm, starting at the common femoral vein in the groin (lying medial to common femoral artery), along the femoral vein in the thigh down to the level of adductor canal. Continue over the popliteal vein in the popliteal fossa down to its trifurcation. Gentle hand pressure along the distal lateral thigh above the knee joint may help to assess the compressibility of distal femoral vein at adductor canal.

Depending on local practice and expertise: Scan the calf veins (two veins accompanying each of the calf arteries – posterior tibial, peroneal and anterior tibial, as well as intramuscular veins in gastro-cnemius and soleus; however, isolated anterior tibial vein thrombosis does not happen so no need to scan).

Make sure that transducer is in true transverse orientation in relation to the vein when performing compression.

Flow: Demonstrate flow with color and spectral Doppler if compression inadequate/inconclusive (use power Doppler if available).

Phasicity: Demonstrate phasicity of the flow in common femoral vein with respiratory cycle/during Valsalva maneuver (decrease in flow in inspiration, increase in expiration).

May need augmentation (by squeezing the calf) to demonstrate flow, particularly in calf veins. The patient may produce calf vein compression during dorsiflexion of the foot. It is essential to have optimal settings on for detecting potentially slow flow (velocity setting at 3–6 cm/s).

Upper limb veins

Axillary and subclavian veins accessible; brachiocephalic vein and superior vena cava – inaccessible to ultrasound (require contrast venogram). Demonstrate flow with color and spectral Doppler (more pulsatile than leg veins).

Findings

1. Vein does not compress completely on firm pressure with the transducer.
2. Vein distension.
3. Intraluminal echoes representing thrombus.
4. No flow demonstrable on color, spectral or power Doppler, or with augmentation.
5. Collaterals may be seen.
6. Lack of phasicity of flow in common femoral vein indicative of more proximal obstruction.

Pearls

- In large leg, 3.5–5 MHz curvilinear transducer necessary to improve deep resolution.
- Use very light pressure at first to identify the vein, without effacing it.
- Echogenicity of thrombus changes with its age – fresh may be hypoechoic, therefore difficult to see.
- Enquire about previous DVT – expect narrow vein with echogenic walls and presence of collaterals in up to 50% of patients with previous DVT; however, chronic DVT may be indistinguishable from acute DVT.
- Use augmentation sparingly – fresh thrombus may be displaced during compression of the calf and may result in pulmonary embolism.
- Try to demonstrate the proximal extent of thrombus as this may influence the treatment (e.g. suitability of IVC filter), but beware that pelvic veins are difficult to visualize.
- Remember that the femoral vein may be duplicated in the thigh.
- Suspect superficial or deep venous thrombosis in a pregnant patient with calf tenderness and edema.

Suggested reading

Polak F. Doppler ultrasound of the deep leg veins. A revolution in the diagnosis of deep vein thrombosis and monitoring of thrombolysis. *Chest* 1999;**99**:165s–172s.

4.15 Femoral artery pseudoaneurysm

Extravasation of blood through a defect in the vessel wall (e.g. due to arterial puncture, trauma, necrosis), contained by a pseudo-capsule. See Fig. 4.15.

Up to 2.2% of patients present following arterial puncture during a diagnostic/interventional procedure.

Clinical

Large or progressive groin swelling, extensive skin bruising, and rarely hypotension (with associated pelvic hematoma) and anterior abdominal wall swelling. Mostly due to inadequate groin compression following femoral artery puncture.

Indications

Confirmation of diagnosis in a patient with suggestive history and finding of a groin swelling, prior to treatment (ultrasound compression of pseudoaneurysm neck; injection of thrombin; surgery), aimed at prevention of pseudoaneurysm rupture, compression of vital structures or peripheral embolization.

Technique

7.5 MHz linear transducer.
Identify normal vascular anatomy in the groin and its relationship to the pseudoaneurysm.

Findings

1. Anechoic/hypoechoic mass adjacent to the common/superficial femoral or profunda artery, often with identifiable neck connecting it to the artery.

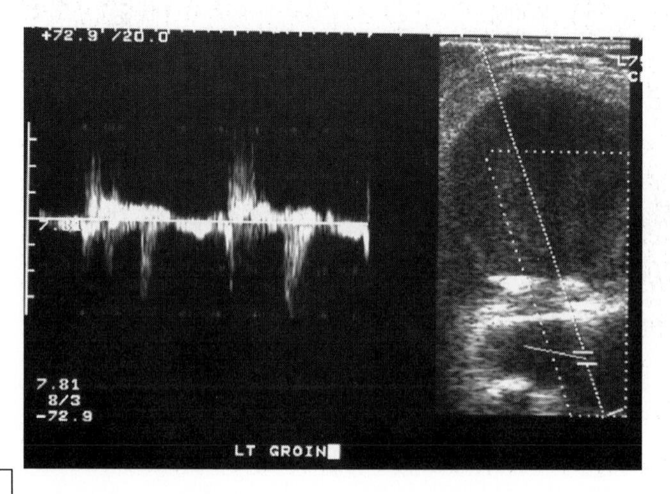

Fig. 4.15. Femoral artery pseudoaneurysm. US groin in a patient with progressive swelling at the femoral puncture site following an interventional procedure shows characteristic bidirectional flow (registered both above and below baseline) in the neck of a femoral artery pseudoaneurysm.

2. Turbulent (swirling) flow in the mass (blood enters during systole, exits during diastole), giving yin-yang symbol-like appearance.
3. May contain echogenic material representing thrombus.

Pearls

- A significant proportion of femoral pseudoaneurysms will undergo spontaneous thrombosis, so follow-up scanning to assess natural progress is useful.
- Beware of possibility of concomitant arteriovenous fistula (communication between the artery and accompanying vein, resulting in high flow velocities in both vessels, leading to vibration of perivascular soft tissues – "color cloud").
- Look for pelvic hematoma.

Suggested reading

Mitchell DG *et al.* Femoral artery pseudo-aneurysm: diagnosis with conventional duplex and colour Doppler US. *Radiology* 1987;**165**:687–690.

Stone PA *et al.* Femoral pseudoaneurysms. *Vasc Endovasc Surg* 2006;**40**:109–117.

4.16 Abdominal aortic aneurysm

Localized dilatation of the aorta > 50% of normal diameter (≥ 3 cm). See Fig. 4.16.

Clinical

Presentation varies from incidental finding on lumbar spine X-ray (or other imaging) to rupture with 90% mortality.

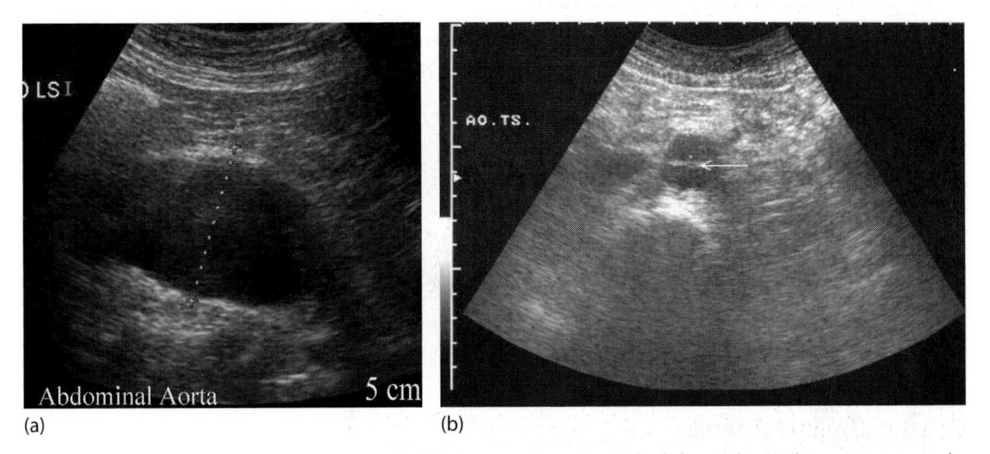

Fig. 4.16. (a) Abdominal aortic aneurysm. US of abdomen in a patient with abdominal pain demonstrates saccular dilatation of abdominal aorta (between calipers). No intraluminal echogenic intimal flap is seen to suggest dissection. (b) Aortic dissection. US of aorta shows an echogenic intraluminal septum (arrow) separating true and false lumen consistent with aortic dissection. The caliber of abdominal aorta is normal (between calipers).

Technique

5 MHz curvilinear probe.

Position the probe just to the left of the umbilicus to start with; scan upwards to the diaphragm and downwards to the bifurcation.

If abdomen is too gassy to find the aorta at the umbilicus, try to follow it down from its upper aspect in the abdomen, at the level of pancreas/celiac axis and superior mesenteric artery.

Findings

Sonographic predictors of rupture:

1. Size > 5.5 cm.
2. Rapid expansion > 1 cm/year or > 6–7 mm/6 months.
3. Saccular shape.

Pearls

- Leak cannot be reliably detected on US.
- If presence of AAA known about and rupture suspected, US is not indicated.
- CTA is a better modality than US to evaluate complications of AAA.
- Aortic aneurysm usually enlarges several mm per year.
- AAA > 5.5 cm is an indication for a repair.

Suggested reading

Jaakkola P *et al.* Interobserver variability in measuring the dimensions of the abdominal aorta: comparison of ultrasound and computed tomography. *Eur J Vasc Endovasc Surg* 1996;**12**(2):230–237.

Kent KC *et al.* Screening for abdominal aortic aneurysms – a consensus statement. *Eur J Vasc Endovasc Surg* 2002;23:55–60.

4.17 Carotid artery dissection

Presence of intimal flap leading to formation of two lumens in common/internal carotid artery (but any neck artery can be involved, e.g. vertebral). See Fig. 4.17.

Clinical

Refer to Section 1.15.

Technique

7.5 MHz linear probe.
B-mode and color/spectral Doppler of common carotid/extracranial internal carotid artery.

Findings

Extracranial carotid dissection

1. Intimal flap (echogenic intraluminal septum oscillating with each cardiac cycle), separating the two lumens (false lumen usually with slower flow than the true lumen); although a classic finding, this is actually rarely seen.

2. Tapering occlusion of internal carotid artery 2–4 cm distal to carotid bifurcation (string sign) or high-grade stenosis (increased systolic flow to > 230 cm/s and diastolic flow > 40 cm/s) of internal carotid artery, in the absence of atheromatous plaque.

Intracranial dissection

1. High-resistance flow in ipsilateral common carotid artery.
2. To-and-fro flow in ipsilateral internal carotid artery (with sharp systolic upstroke and no diastolic flow).
3. Compensatory increased velocity in contralateral common/internal carotid artery.

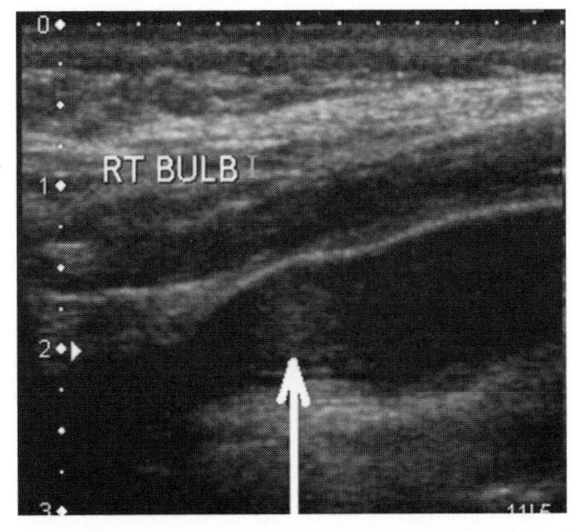

Fig. 4.17. Internal carotid artery dissection. LS US of carotid bifurcation in a young patient with stroke shows occlusion of the internal carotid artery by fresh echogenic thrombus (arrow) due to dissection. The classic double lumen separated by dissection flap is rarely seen.

Pearls

- US can offer reliable exclusion of dissection if examination is entirely normal, but occlusion/high-grade stenosis, although suggestive in the absence of atheromatous plaque, has to be confirmed with MRA or CTA.

Suggested reading

Caplan R. Dissections of brain supplying arteries. *Nat Clinical Pract Neurol* 2008;**4**(1):34–42.

Krishnam M *et al.* Non-occlusive intracranial carotid artery dissection: transcervical carotid Doppler findings. *Clin Radiol* 2005;**60**:512–514.

4.18 Normal pregnancy

Presence of an embryo in endometrial cavity. See Fig. 4.18.

Clinical

The woman may or may not be aware that she is pregnant.

Technique

Transabdominal (TA) scanning should be done initially; transvaginal (TV) if TA is inconclusive.
TA:
3.5–5 MHz curvilinear transducer.

Full urinary bladder (1 litre of fluid 1 hour prior to the scan).
TV:
Needs patient's consent.
5–10 MHz transducer.
Empty urinary bladder.
Necessary if retroverted uterus is present or fine detail of endometrium and ovaries is needed. Always have a chaperone during scanning.

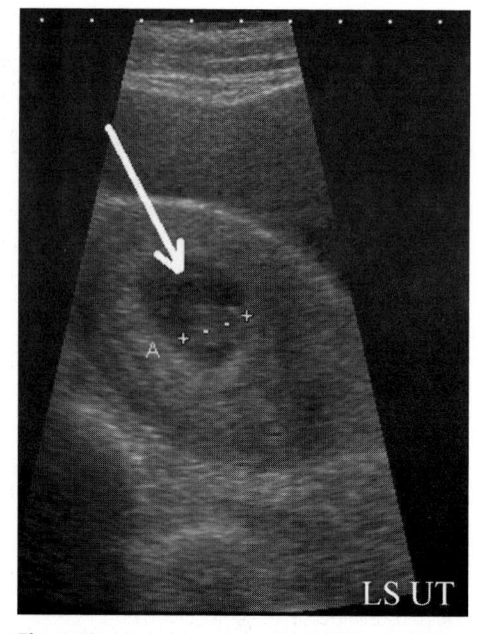

Fig. 4.18. Normal pregnancy. LS US (5,52) pelvis shows a gestation sac – seen as a cystic structure (arrow) surrounded by echogenic ring within the endometrium and embryo (between calipers) within the gestational sac.

Findings

1. Gestation sac (5/52 gestation) – 5 mm cystic structure within the endometrium, surrounded by two echogenic rings ("double decidual" sign) in TS.
2. Yolk sac (between 5/52 and 12/52 gestation) – a thin ring-like structure within the gestation sac.
3. Embryo, with heart beat (6/52 gestation on TV, 8–10/52 on TA; mean HR 175 bpm at 9/52).

Pearls

- Establish the date of LMP.
- Beware of very early US findings of pregnancy including echogenic endometrial thickening in a female of child-bearing age.

Suggested reading

Refer to Section 4.1.

AIUM Practice Guideline for the Performance of Obstetric ultrasound Examinations. www.aium.org/publications/clinical/obstetrics.

4.19 Emergencies in pregnancy

Multiple conditions in pregnancy can present as bleeding per vaginam e.g. ectopic pregnancy, abortion, abnormal placental position, placental abruption, post-partum retained products of conception. Some conditions can complicate normal pregnancy, such as large fibroids, urinary tract calculi and appendicitis. See Fig. 4.19.

Clinical

History of amenorrhea.
Acute abdominal/pelvic pain with bleeding per vaginam.
Positive urinary pregnancy test.

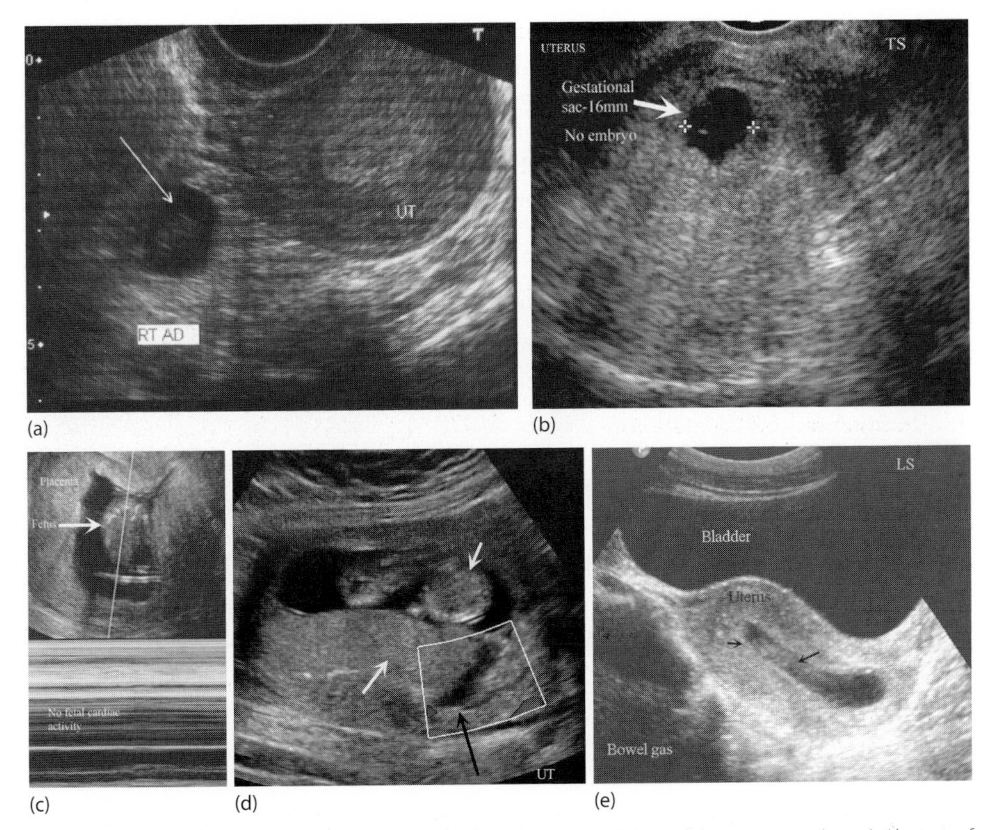

Fig. 4.19. (a) Ectopic pregnancy. TV scan shows an adnexal mass containing solid components (arrow). Absence of intrauterine pregnancy is noted, which supports diagnosis of an ectopic pregnancy. (b) Anembryonic pregnancy/ missed abortion. Endovaginal scan showing an irregular gestational sac in the lower uterine segment measuring 16 mm (between calipers) without any embryo, suggestive of anembryonic pregnancy/missed abortion. (c) Missed abortion. M mode scan of fetus of 12 weeks showing absent cardiac activity. Color Doppler showed no flow within the fetal heart or great vessels. The internal os was closed. (d) Subchorionic bleed. TS US of 13 weeks gestation (arrow) with posteriorly located placenta (long white arrow) and a small hypoechoic lesion (black arrow) separating chorion from inner aspect of uterus without any flow on color Doppler. (e) Retained products of conception. LS of US uterus in an 8 weeks' pregnant woman with bleeding PV shows a bulky uterus with thickened endometrium and split endometrial cavity containing anechoic fluid/ blood and echogenic products of conception (arrows).

Technique

TA scan with full urinary bladder.

TV scan with empty bladder – whenever fine detail is needed or diagnosis is not obvious (patient consent required).

Ectopic pregnancy

Presence of an embryo in location other than endometrium.

$>$ 95% – Fallopian tube; 3.2% – ovary, 2.4% – interstitial, 1.3% – abdominal.

Findings

1. History suggestive of a first-trimester pregnancy.
2. Raised β hCG.

3. Absence of normal intrauterine pregnancy.
4. Intrauterine pseudosac – small fluid collection in endometrium, but without yolk sac or thick ring of decidual reaction being present.
5. Extrauterine non-cystic mass, separate from the normal ovary.
6. Tubal ring – highly echogenic ring with cystic center in Fallopian tube.
7. Free fluid in the pelvis, flank and upper abdomen (often highly echogenic due to presence of blood).

Pearls

- Presence of intrauterine pregnancy excludes ectopic pregnancy for all practical purposes.
- Sometimes serial scanning necessary to make definitive diagnosis.
- Serum β hCG is an important correlate.

Bleeding in first trimester pregnancy: Findings

1. Bulky uterus.
2. Gestational sac at unusually low location.
3. Irregular gestational sac.
4. Cervical canal open (if abortion is incomplete).
5. No fetal cardiac activity in a previously documented live intrauterine pregnancy.

Pearls

- Compare with previous scan for the cardiac activity and location of gestational sac.
- Absence of fetal cardiac activity in a gestation with 15–18 mm mean gestational sac diameter is most suggestive of fetal demise.

Bleeding in late pregnancy: Findings

Abnormal placental position

1. Placenta either reaching the internal os (incomplete placenta previa) or completely covering internal os (complete placenta previa).
2. Abnormal vessel traversing the internal os (vasa previa).
3. Placenta is directly adherent to uterine myometrium without intervening hypoechoic decidual stroma (placenta accreta).
4. Deeper penetration of placenta into the uterine myometrium (placenta increta).
5. Placenta extends up to the uterine serosa in placenta percreta.

Placental abruption

6. Bleeding can be retroplacental, subchorionic or preplacental in location.
7. Well-marginated anechoic or mixed echogenic lesion within the placenta.
8. Localized bulging of the placenta at the site of bleeding.
9. Internal echoes within the amniotic fluid due to intra-amniotic extension of the bleed.

Pearls

- If placenta is low-lying in early pregnancy, rescan after 28 weeks gestation and again in third trimester. Placenta can either migrate into the upper segment or become placenta previa.
- Try to locate a hypoechoic rim between placenta and myometrium.
- Placental lakes are normally present after 20 weeks of pregnancy and are smaller than retroplacental clots and show multiple septations.
- Braxton Hicks (also called "practice") contraction can appear as echogenic area but it disappears after 30–40 min.
- Risk of fetal demise increases with the increase in the area of placental separation.
- History of previous uterine surgery or cesarian section may be a clue to look for in an adherent placenta at the site of scar.
- MRI can play an important role in diagnosing these cases.

Retained products of conception

Clinical

Patient presents with excessive bleeding per vaginam.
History of abortion or childbirth.

Findings

1. Bulky uterus.
2. Thickened endometrium.
3. Hypervascularity on color Doppler imaging (of arterial origin – with high-velocity low-resistance flow).
4. Mixed echogenic (predominantly echogenic) content can be seen within the endometrium.
5. Low-resistance flow can be noted in the echogenic contents on color Doppler.

Urinary tract calculi in pregnancy

Diagnosis of hydronephrosis caused by renal calculus in a pregnant patient may be difficult as there is physiological dilation of pelvicalyceal system and ureter due to hormonal influence and the gravid uterus.

Clinical

Pregnant patient with pain in renal fossa.

Technique

TA with full urinary bladder.
TV for ureterovesical junction calculus.
Color Doppler.

Findings

1. Presence of echogenic calculus with distal acoustic shadowing.
2. Hydronephrosis and hydroureter down to the level of calculus.
3. Difference of 0.1 between the resistive indices of two kidneys.
4. Absence of ureteric jet on the same side even after change in patient position.

Pearls

- Always check fetal cardiac activity on Doppler to document live pregnancy.

Appendicitis in pregnancy

In pregnant women the gravid uterus can prevent reliable evaluation of right iliac fossa for appendicitis.

Findings

See Section 3.11.

Pearls

- Scan in the left lateral position so that uterus falls away from RIF and cecum/appendix comes closer to anterior abdominal wall.

Suggested reading

Coady AM. Ectopic pregnancy: a review of sonographic diagnosis. *Ultrasound* 2005;**13**:18–29.

Rooholamini SA *et al.* Imaging of pregnancy related complications. *RadioGraphics* 1993; **13**:753–770.

Williams PL *et al.* US of abnormal uterine bleeding. *RadioGraphics* 2003;**23**:703–718.

4.20 Follicular cyst

Failure of a follicle to rupture/shrink following ovulation. See Fig. 4.20.

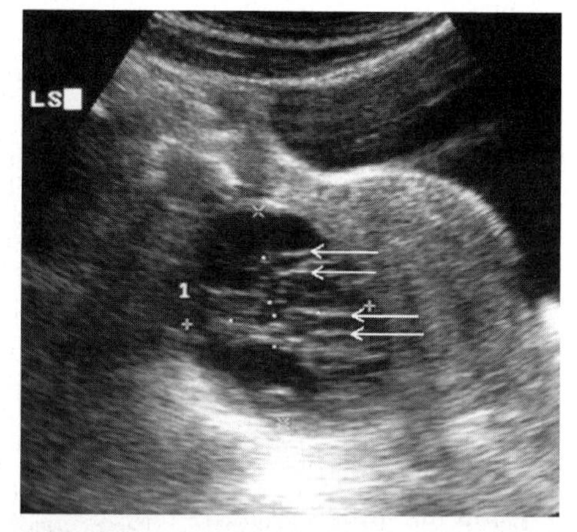

Fig. 4.20. Hemorrhagic ovarian cyst. LS US of pelvis shows a well-defined thin-walled anechoic lesion (between calipers), containing linear internal echoes (arrows) arranged in a layered fashion, suggestive of a hemorrhagic ovarian cyst.

Clinical

Asymptomatic.

Patient can experience unilateral lower abdominal pain if the cyst is large or it undergoes hemorrhage.

Technique

TA and TV.

Findings

1. Thin walled simple ovarian cyst > 2.5 cm.
2. May contain internal echoes representing hemorrhage or infection.

Pearls

- Re-scan after 6–8 weeks to ensure resolution.
- Persistent cyst may need to be punctured to ensure its simple nature. Drainage can be undertaken at the same time.

- Corpus luteum cyst – thicker wall, more often symptomatic.
- Hemorrhagic cyst may mimic ovarian neoplasm, but shows no flow on color Doppler in its solid elements.

Suggested reading

Jain KA. Sonographic spectrum of hemorrhagic ovarian cysts. *J Ultrasound Med* 2002;21:879–886.

4.21 Ovarian torsion

Twisted ovarian vascular pedicle resulting in enlarged ovary with decreased or absent vascularity. Torsion may be persistent or intermittent. See Fig. 4.21.

Clinical

Acute lower abdominal pain – can be intermittent.
Vomiting.
Fever.

Indications

Differentiation from other pathology with similar symptoms.

Technique

TA and TV.

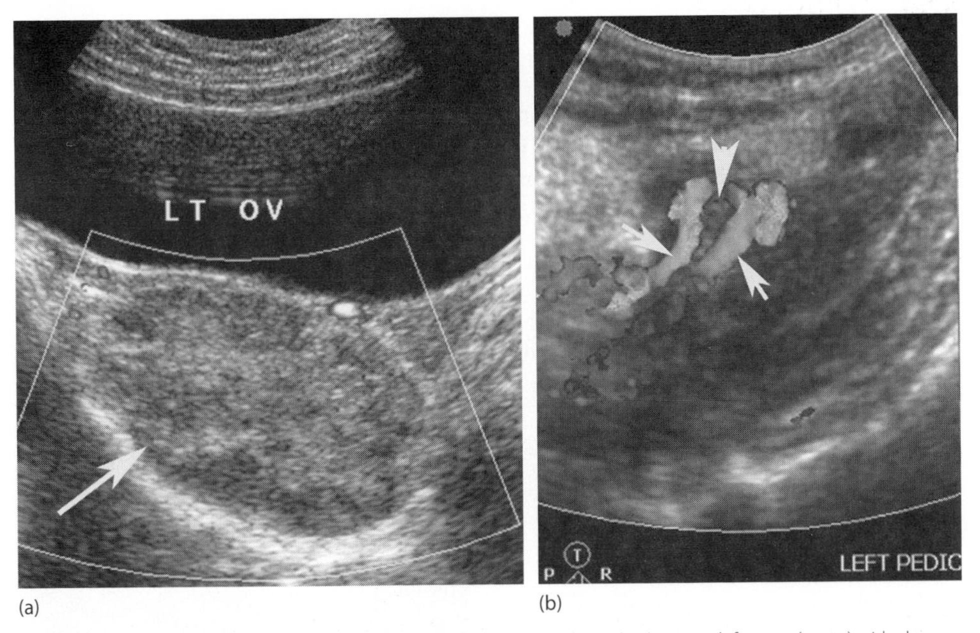

(a) (b)

Fig. 4.21. (a) Ovarian torsion. Power Doppler US of pelvis shows enlarged echogenic left ovary (arrow) with absence of internal flow but presence of pericapsular flow. (Photo courtesy of Dr. Y. Mhashilkar, Wockhardt Hospital, Mumbai.) (b) Twisted ovarian pedicle. US pelvis in a patient with acute abdomen shows circular vascular structures ("whirlpool sign" arrows) within a target-like ovarian mass (arrowhead), consistent with twisted vascular pedicle due to ovarian torsion. (Photo courtesy of Dr. Seema Tardeja, Way 2 Health Diagnostic Centre, Mumbai.)

Findings

Affected ovary

1. Enlargement (volume > 14 ml; calculated as a × b × c × 0.5, where a, b and c are the ovarian dimensions in the orthogonal planes).
2. Low-echogenicity solid structure.
3. Variable position, often in the midline.
4. Decreased/absent vascularity.

Pelvis

Free fluid.

Pearls

- In 70% of cases of torsion of the ovary, there is an underlying lesion present, usually benign (e.g. follicular cyst, dermoid, etc.).
- Peripheral arrangement of follicles often seen in torted ovary.
- Ovarian torsion may be intermittent.

Suggested reading

Andreotti R *et al.* The sonographic diagnosis of ovarian torsion: pearls and pitfalls. *Ultrasound Clin* 2007;2:155–166.

Lee J *et al.* Diagnosis of ovarian torsion with colour Doppler sonography: depiction of twisted vascular pedicle. *J Ultrasound Med* 1998;17(2):83–89.

4.22 Liver transplant

US is a simple, fast and bedside non-invasive imaging modality of choice to identify various complications in the transplanted liver. See Fig. 4.22.

Clinical

Abdominal pain/ tenderness, nausea and vomiting, and deteriorating liver function.

Technique

5–7 MHz curvilinear transducer.
Gray-scale, color and spectral Doppler.

Findings: Post-operative

1. Hepatic artery stenosis: increased velocity (> 200–300 cm/s), turbulence.
2. Hepatic artery occlusion: no detectable flow.
3. Biliary leak or obstruction.

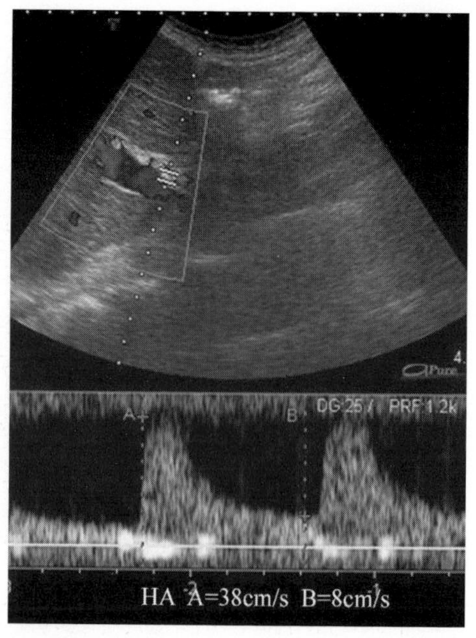

Fig. 4.22. Transplanted liver. Color Doppler and spectral US of transplanted liver shows normal flow in hepatic artery.

4. Fluid collection(s) – bile leakage/abscess.
5. Infarction: wedge-shaped hypoechoic area.

Pearls

- Live donor transplantation is a better option than cadaveric liver transplantation.

Suggested reading

Shaw AS *et al.* Liver transplantation. *Imaging* 2002;**14**:314–328.

Shaw AS *et al.* Ultrasound of non-vascular complications in the post liver transplant patient. *Clin Radiol* 2003;**58**:672–680.

4.23 Kidney transplant

US is a simple, fast and non-invasive imaging modality of choice to identify various complications of renal allograft. See Fig. 4.23.

The transplanted kidney is usually placed in either iliac fossa and the donor renal artery anastomosed to the external or rarely the internal iliac artery. The transplant renal vein is typically anastomosed to the external iliac vein and the donor ureter is plugged into the bladder dome.

Clinical

Deteriorating renal function.

Technique

5–7 MHz curvilinear transducer.
Gray scale, color and spectral Doppler.

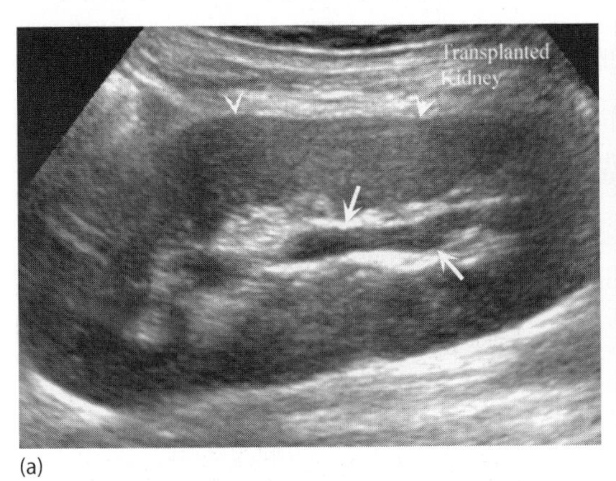

(a)

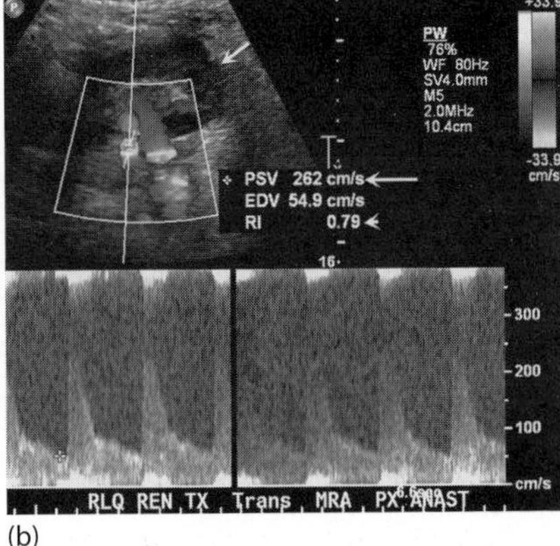

(b)

Fig. 4.23. (a) Transplanted kidney. Gray scale US scan on day 1 after renal transplant (arrowheads) shows physiological mild splitting of pelvicalyceal system (arrows). (b) Transplanted renal artery. Color Doppler scan of renal transplant shows high PSV (long arrow) and resistance to flow (short arrow) proximal to anastomosis. The waveforms of intra-renal arteries were parvus et tardus with delayed systolic peak (not shown), most likely due to renal artery stenosis at the site of anastomosis.

Findings: Normal

1. Parenchymal echogenicity is the same as in a normal native kidney.
2. The transplant renal artery is seen in between the anteriorly placed renal pelvis and posteriorly placed renal vein. In the normal native kidney the renal vein lies anterior to the renal artery and renal pelvis is posterior to the renal artery.
3. Normal allograft kidney may show minimal pelvicalyceal dilatation due to its anterior location, intrarenal edema, transient hydronephrosis, transient edema at the uretero-vesical anastomosis.

Findings: Complications

Obstruction

1. Mild dilatation of the pelvicalyceal system can be seen in up to 30% of non-obstructed transplant kidneys (secondary to post-operative edema at the ureteric anastomosis and decreased ureter peristalsis).
2. True obstruction – individual calyces dilate. This has to be treated promptly with percutaneous nephrostomy and correction of source of extrinsic compression of collecting system.

Perirenal fluid collection

US may not be able to differentiate between causes – lymphocele (most frequent; weeks/months, septated, often recurrent), hematoma (immediately post-operative), urinoma (weeks).

1. Lymphocele: Anechoic perirenal collection with thin wall and no internal echoes.
2. Hematoma: May be seen as a heterogeneous collection with areas of high echoes indicating varying stages of hemorrhage.
3. Urinoma: May be seen as solitary or multiple collections around the transplant kidney. Typically seen as a homogeneous well-defined anechoic collection without internal echoes or septations. Rapid increase in size is a common feature. US may assist in diagnostic tap which characteristically shows a high creatinine level in a urinoma.

Acute tubular necrosis

Commonest cause of primary transplant failure, but no specific US signs.

1. Enlarged kidney.
2. Prominence of renal pyramids.
3. Decreased/reversed diastolic flow.

Rejection

1. May be due to multiple reasons; in cellular, vascular or combined mechanism.
2. No single reliable sign.

Renal parenchyma

1. Decreased cortico-medullary differentiation.
2. Thickened cortex.

3. Enlarged pyramids.
4. Decreased echogenicity of renal sinus fat.

Vessels

1. Increased arterial flow resistance (decreased or reversed diastolic flow, later – decreased systolic flow).
2. Resistance index: RI = peak systole – end diastole/peak systole.
3. Non-perfusion.

Other vascular complications

Renal artery stenosis

Usually at the site of anastomosis with the iliac artery.

1. Turbulent flow.
2. Increased peak systolic velocity (> 300 cm/s) proximal to the stenosis.
3. Tardus parvus waveform of intrarenal arteries – the most important finding.
4. Absent diastolic flow if tight.

Renal vein thrombosis

Rare; see Section 5.12.

Pearls

- Ensure urinary bladder empty before diagnosing renal obstruction.
- Color Doppler alone may appear normal even in severe vascular rejection (use spectral Doppler as well).

Suggested reading

Refer to Section 4.1.

Akbar SA *et al.* Complications of renal transplantation. *RadioGraphics* 2005;25(5):1335–1356.

4.24 Pancreatic transplant

Pancreatic transplant has emerged as an established and most effective alternative treatment option for severe type 1 diabetes mellitus, especially in patients with end-stage diabetic nephropathy. Although the graft survival rate has improved significantly over the years (1 year survival rate is above 70%), complications such as graft rejection, pancreatitis, vascular thrombosis, pseudoaneurysm and peripancreatic collection are common. US plays an important role in post-operative evaluation of normal appearance and various complications of pancreatic transplant. See Fig. 4.24.

Clinical

Raised serum creatinine and abnormal blood biochemistry with or without fever and leukocytosis.

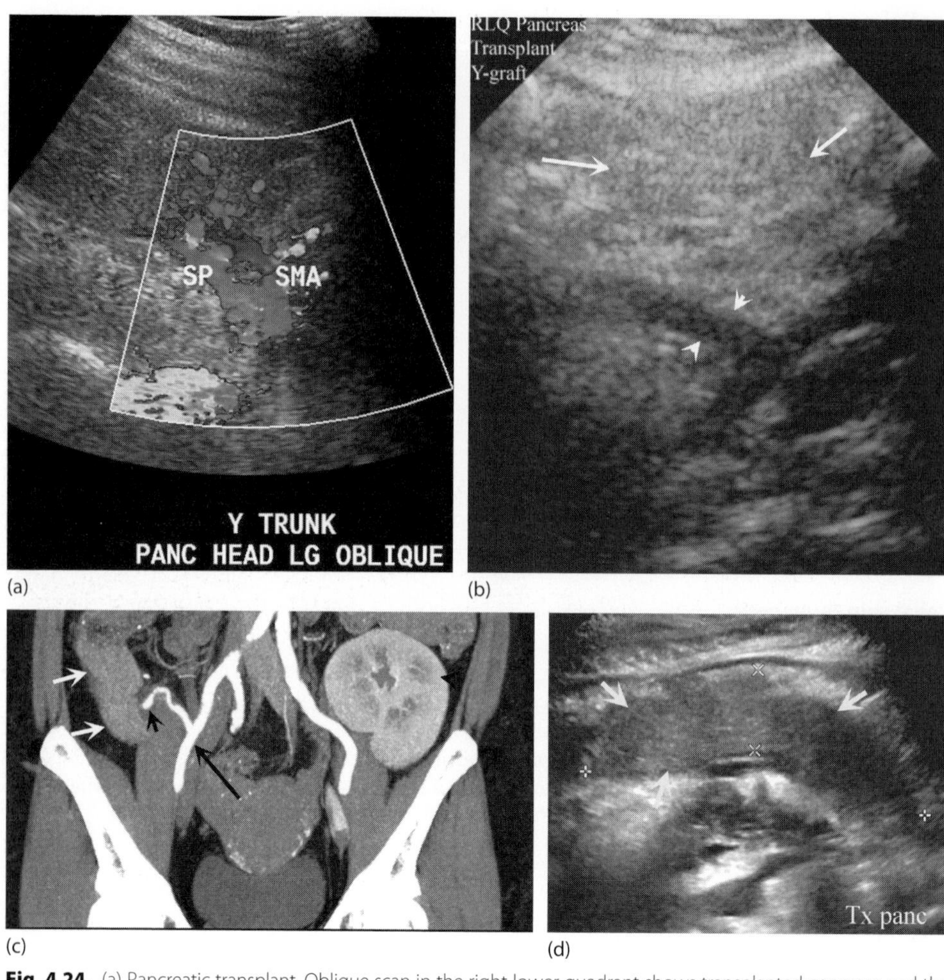

Fig. 4.24. (a) Pancreatic transplant. Oblique scan in the right lower quadrant shows transplanted pancreas and the arterial Y graft formed by superior mesenteric artery and splenic artery. (b, c) Pancreatic and renal transplant. (b) US pelvis shows transplanted pancreas (arrows) and a part of the Y graft (arrowheads). (c) Coronal CECT abdomen shows transplanted pancreas (arrow), kidney (arrowhead) and a patent limb of Y graft (short black arrow). The other limb of Y graft formed by donor superior mesenteric artery is thrombosed. (d) Transplant pancreatitis. US shows diffusely enlarged and hypoechoic transplanted pancreas (arrows) consistent with pancreatitis. Note trace of hypoechoic peripancreatic fluid.

Technique

3.5–5 MHz curvilinear transducer, color and spectral Doppler to assess pancreatic and vascular flow pattern.

Findings

Normal pancreatic graft

1. Typically seen in the right iliac fossa in an intraperitoneal location as homogeneous soft-tissue echo with increased surrounding fat echogenicity (due to omentum).
2. Normal parenchymal color flow is seen within pancreas. Y-shaped vascular graft anastomosis between the recipient common iliac artery and donor vessels (splenic and

superior mesenteric artery). A small portion of donor duodenum is anastomosed to the recipient bladder.

Complications

1. Fluid collection in the surgical bed: Anechoic/hypoechoic with or without internal echoes: anastomotic leak (duodenal–vesical), abscess, hematoma (may be hyperechoic), peripancreatic fluid in graft rejection or pancreatitis.
2. Pancreatitis: Swelling, indistinct pancreatic border, hypoechoic foci, perigraft fluid, foci of air within the graft (infected or emphysematous pancreatitis).
3. Vascular complications: Stenosis (raised peak velocity), thrombosis (echogenic intravascular material, no flow), pseudoaneurysm (color Doppler typically shows swirling blood within the sac).
4. Rejection: No specific signs, may see gland enlargement, focal or diffuse hypoechoic areas, normal pancreatic duct diameter.

Pearls

- Ultrasound findings are non-specific.
- CT or MR angiography can be useful to assess vascular complications.
- Three types of pancreatic transplantation in the order of frequency: simultaneous pancreas and kidney, pancreas after kidney and pancreas transplant alone.

Suggested reading

Nikolaidis P *et al.* Role of sonography in pancreatic transplantation. *RadioGraphics* 2003;23:939–949.

4.25 Pericardial effusion

Accumulation of fluid in the pericardial sac (normally 15–50 ml is present). See Fig. 4.25.

Clinical

Chest pain, palpitations, dyspnea, hiccoughs, syncope.

Technique

5 MHz curvilinear transducer in paraxyphoid or apical region.

Findings

1. Small: Accumulates posteriorly first.
2. Large (> 1 cm depth): May cause tamponade, leading to collapse of the chambers (RA and RV, later LA, rarely LV); pericardiocentesis life saving.
3. Diastolic RA collapse in effusion suggests tamponade: needs immediate pericardiocentesis.

Pearls

- Beware of false positives: pleural effusion, pericardial thickening, epicardial fat pad, mediastinal lesions.

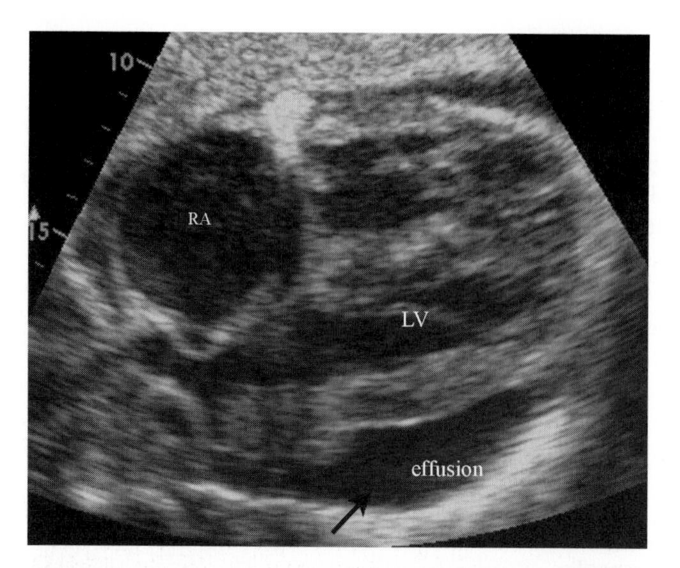

Fig. 4.25. Pericardial effusion. Echocardiogram shows anechoic fluid in the pericardial space (arrow) surrounding the heart, consistent with pericardial effusion. Diastolic right atrial collapse, a sign of cardiac tamponade, was absent (not shown). (Photo courtesy of Dr. Keith Tonkin, UCLA.)

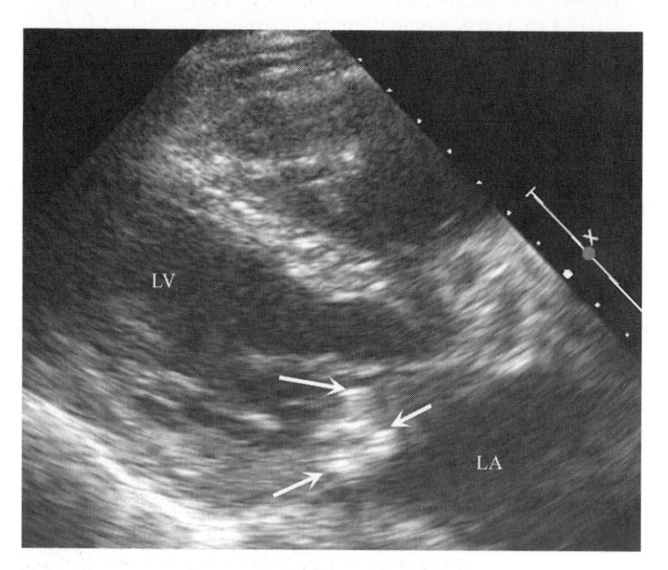

Fig. 4.26. Bacterial endocarditis. Parasternal view of echocardiogram shows nodular echogenic vegetations on the mitral valve (arrows).

Suggested reading

Wann S, Passen E. Echocardiography in pericardial disease. *Am Soc Echocardiogr* 2008;**21**(1):7–13.

4.26 Bacterial endocarditis

Infection involving endocardium, usually valvular. See Fig. 4.26.

Clinical

Fever, weight loss, malaise, night sweats, clubbing.

Technique

5 MHz curvilinear transducer.

Findings

1. Irregular valve thickening.
2. Echogenic irregular mass.
3. Site of vegetations – may be attached to a leaflet or a cusp, in a chamber or in outflow tract of LV.
4. Look for paravalvular leak and focal abscess.

Pearls

- US cannot differentiate between active vs healed lesions in endocarditis. It is difficult to differentiate a vegetation from a thrombus in the right atrium. Cardiac MRI may be indicated to differentiate the two.
- $\leq$ 8 mm size vegetation is better seen on transesophageal echo than MRI.
- Mobile vegetations $\geq$ 10 mm in size are more prone for embolic events.
- Aortic regurgitation due to endocarditis is an indication for surgery.

Suggested reading

Roy P *et al.* Spectrum of echocardiographic findings in bacterial endocarditis. *Circulation* 1976;53:474–482.

4.27 Appendicitis

Inflammation of the appendix. See Fig. 4.27.

Clinical

Refer to Section 3.11.

Technique

7.5 MHz linear or curvilinear transducer.

Start at the point of maximum tenderness and apply gradual compression to displace bowel gas in the cecum and ascending colon ("Gradual compression technique of Puylaert").

Findings

1. Non-compressible, blind ending, immobile.
2. $\geq$ 7 mm in diameter.

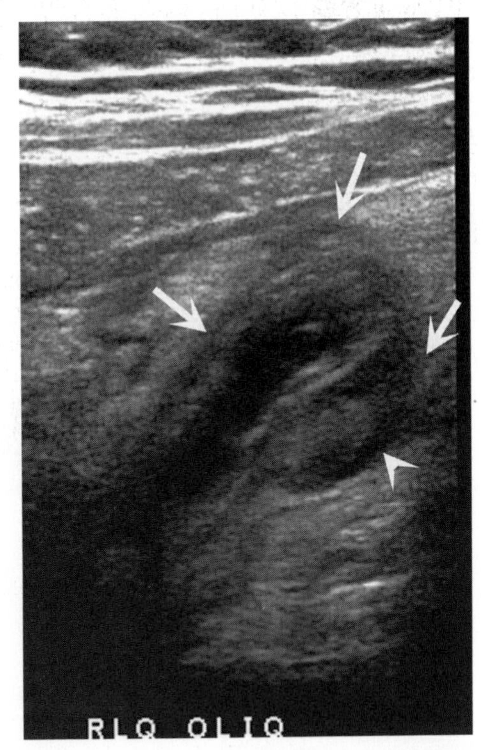

Fig. 4.27. Acute appendicitis. US scan shows dilated, blind ending, tubular structure with wall thickening (arrows) and adjacent peri-appendicial fluid collection (arrowhead) due to acute appendicitis.

3. Irregular outline/loss of layered appearance due to impending perforation.
4. Fecolith obstructing the lumen.
5. Hyperechoic surrounding fat.
6. Enlarged mesenteric lymph nodes.
7. Increased vascularity.
8. Free fluid.
9. Para-appendiceal fluid collection if appendicular abscess develops.

Pearls

- Urinary bladder: Preferably half full (so assessment of pelvic organs possible but not hampering compression).
- If US negative for appendicitis: Perform abdominal and pelvic US scan to look for other causes of symptoms. CT is more sensitive and specific for appendicitis than ultrasound.

Suggested reading

Refer to Section 4.1.

Puylaert JB. Acute appendicitis: US evaluation using graded compression ultrasound. *Radiology* 1986;153:355–360.

4.28 Pancreatitis

Inflammation of pancreatic gland. See Fig. 4.28.

Clinical

Refer to Section 3.12.

Indications

Visualization of biliary stones, especially those responsible for obstruction, as an underlying etiology.
Detection of pseudocysts.

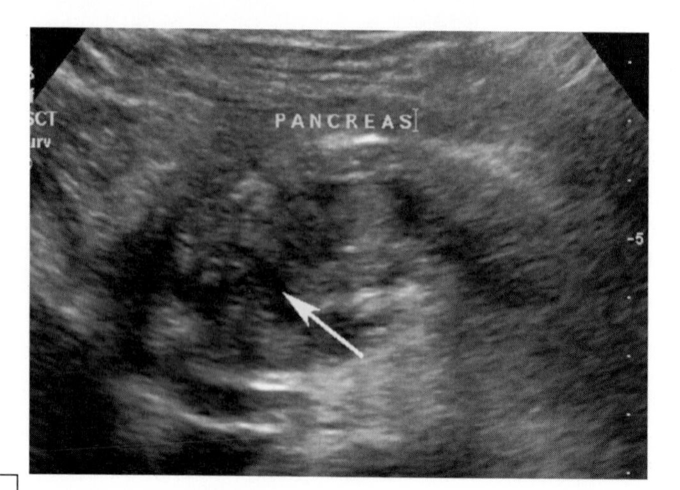

Fig. 4.28. Acute pancreatitis. US abdomen shows diffusely swollen pancreas with a heterogeneous predominantly hypoechoic collection in the head of pancreas (arrow), consistent with acute pancreatitis with necrosis. (Photo courtesy of Dr. S. Maniar, Wockhardt Hospital, Mumbai.)

Technique

3.5–5 MHz transducer; B mode and color Doppler.

Try to overcome commonly troublesome bowel gas, obscuring the pancreas, by scanning through the left lobe of the liver and through stomach after filling it with 500 ml of water (the latter probably impractical in a patient who is vomiting).

Findings

1. Enlarged pancreas of decreased echogenicity (normal pancreas is uniformly hyperechoic).
2. Presence of gallstones/dilatation of biliary tree due to an impacted calculus.
3. A phlegmon may be seen in acute stage as ill-defined peripancreatic heterogeneous fluid.
4. Rounded fluid collection in proximity of the pancreas, representing a pseudocyst; may contain internal echoes.
5. Lack of blood flow in splenic vein on color Doppler with a filling defect, representing thrombosis.
6. Aneurysm of splenic or gastroduodenal artery.
7. Presence of calcification within the pancreas in acute on chronic pancreatitis.

Pearls

- US is not necessary for making the diagnosis, but crucial for excluding biliary stones and obstruction leading to pancreatitis. If the common bile duct is dilated, urgent ERCP and sphincterotomy may be required.
- Pseudocyst(s) and aneurysm formation take 2–3 weeks to develop from the onset of symptoms.
- Use of color Doppler is mandatory to differentiate between pseudocyst and aneurysm as inadvertent puncture of pseudoaneurysm can lead to life-threatening hemorrhage.

Suggested reading

Bollen T *et al.* Update on acute pancreatitis: ultrasound, computed tomography and magnetic resonance imaging features. *Semin Ultrasound CT MRI* 2007;**28**(5):371–383.

4.29 Testicular torsion and acute epididymo-orchitis

Twist in the spermatic cord (when the testis is abnormally mobile e.g. due to bell and clapper configuration), cutting off vascular supply to the testis. See Fig. 4.29.

Clinical

Acute onset severe testicular pain.

Elevation of testis over symphysis pubis results in pain in epididymo-orchitis but relieves pain in testicular torsion.

Indications

If clinically suspected, needs urgent surgery (no place for imaging).

Sometimes, however, the clinical picture is not clear-cut (e.g. epididymitis).

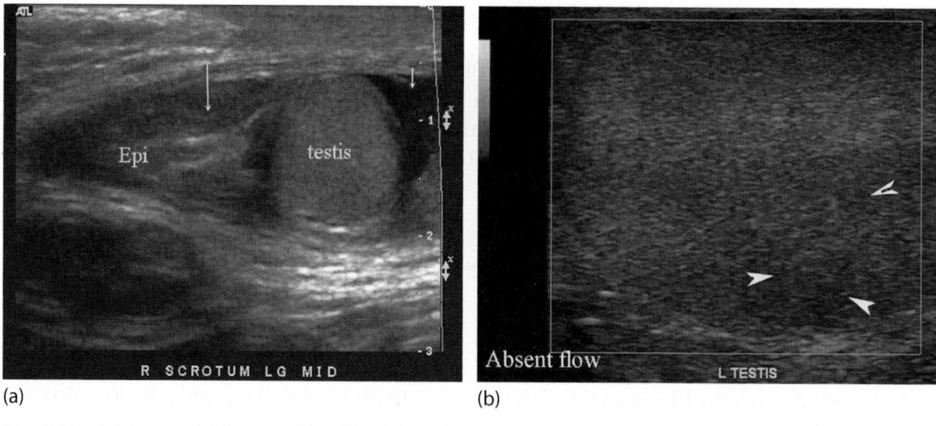

(a) (b)

Fig. 4.29. (a) Acute epididymo-orchitis. US of the right scrotum shows enlarged, swollen epididymis (long arrow) and testis with mild reactive hydrocele (short arrow). Increased vascularity of both the epididymis and testis on color Doppler not shown. (Photo courtesy of Dr. Kiev, UCLA.) (b) Proven left testicular torsion. Power Doppler US of the left testis shows absence of internal flow with an ill-defined hypoechoic lesion (arrowheads) suggestive of infarction. (Photo courtesy of Dr. M. Bapat, Amruta Imaging, Thane, India.)

Technique

7.5–12 MHz probe.
Color Doppler.
Privacy while scanning is important; ideally get a male chaperon.
Use liberal amount of skin gel to avoid artefacts from pubic hair. Start with mid-line view allowing comparison of the two testes; followed by transverse and longitudinal views of each testis, starting with the asymptomatic side to establish the baseline.

Findings

Torsion

1. Enlarged testis, with reduced echogenicity (swollen).
2. Lack of perfusion of testis on color Doppler.
3. Hydrocele may be present.
4. Enlarged epididymis, with reduced echogenicity and no flow.

Epididymo-orchitis

1. Usually unilateral involvement.
2. Enlarged hypoechoic epididymis; hyperechoic if hemorrhage has occurred.
3. Associated reactive fluid in the scrotal sac without internal echoes (hydrocele) or with internal echoes (pyocele).
4. Testicular enlargement (compare the size with contralateral normal testis).
5. Heterogeneous testicular architecture.
6. Increased vascularity of testis and epididymis with decreased vascular resistance (Resistive index < 0.5; peak systolic velocity > 15 cm/s).
7. If flow reversal is noted during diastole it suggests venous infarction.

Pearls

- Do not delay surgery to perform an ultrasound scan for confirmation.
- Scan the normal side first to optimize the vascular settings for detection of flow.
- Complications of untreated epididymo-orchitis include infarction, abscess formation and gangrene.

Suggested reading

Dogra VS *et al.* Sonography of the scrotum. *Radiology* 2003;227:18–36.

4.30 Psoas abscess and hematoma

Focal infection/bleed within the psoas muscle, frequently extending into iliacus muscle. See Fig. 4.30.

Clinical

Flank pain, limited hip movement, thigh swelling.
Pyrexia in case of abscess (often PUO).

Technique

3.5–5 MHz curvilinear transducer.

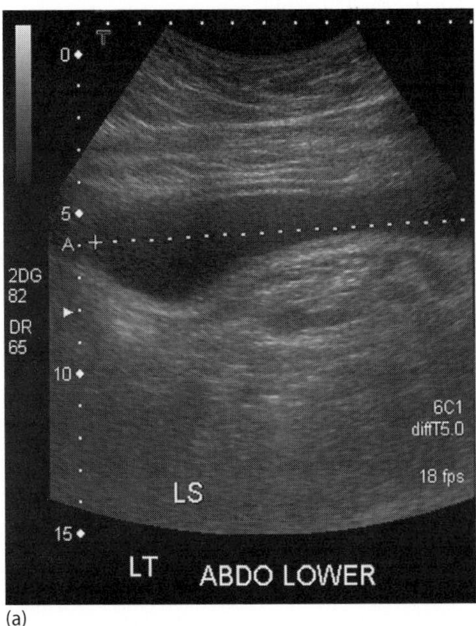

(a)

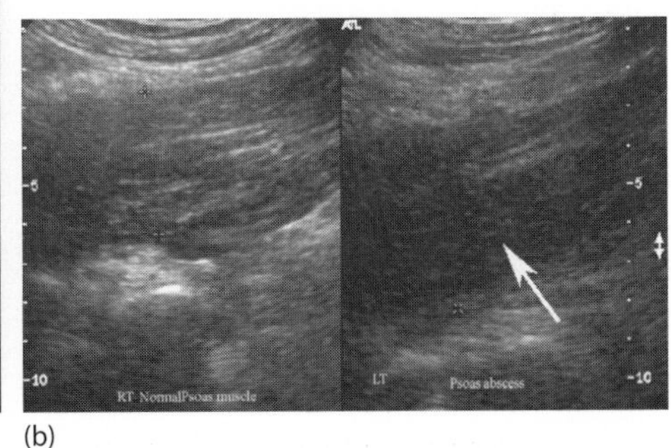

(b)

Fig. 4.30. (a) Psoas muscle hematoma. Anechoic fluid collection (between calipers) representing resolving hematoma in psoas muscle. (b) Psoas abscess. US shows heterogeneous but predominantly hypoechoic collection in left psoas muscle (arrow), consistent with an abscess. Compare the normal striated echotexture of right psoas muscle. (Photo courtesy of Dr. S. Nair, Wockhardt Hospital, Mumbai.)

Findings

Abscess

1. Thick-walled septated lesion in psoas muscle, containing multiple internal echoes.
2. High-echogenicity foci due to presence of gas.

Hematoma

1. The appearance depends on the age of hematoma; a fluid collection containing internal echoes with layering is evident. Gradually it becomes anechoic with age.

Pearls

- Think of an underlying cause for the abscess (i.e. intra-/retroperitoneal or spinal/paraspinal septic process, intravenous drug use) or hemorrhage (coagulopathy/anticoagulants, AAA rupture/repair, trauma).

Suggested reading

Van Dyke JA *et al.* Review of iliopsoas anatomy and pathology. *RadioGraphics* 1987;**17**(1):53–84.

Chapter 5

Fluoroscopy

John Curtis and Mayil S. Krishnam

5.1 General principles

In an emergency setting, non-vascular fluoroscopic studies with contrast are carried out using either barium sulphate or non-ionic water-soluble contrast media (WSCM) media. If esophageal perforation is suspected, WSCM is first administered in concentration of 60% solution of ionic contrast medium (the resultant iodine concentration is 282–292 mg/ml) or non-ionic agents with an iodine concentration 300 mg/ml. Non-ionic contrast medium is preferred to ionic contrast media. If the defect communicates with the mediastinum, pleura or peritoneal cavity, the contrast agent will be re-absorbed. If barium is used, it will spill into the pleural or peritoneal cavity, potentially causing a fibrotic reaction. If no leak is demonstrated by WSCM, a double-contrast barium study can be performed to better delineate the gastrointestinal mucosa in order to demonstrate small tears. See Fig. 5.1.

Ionic contrast media such as sodium and meglumine diatrizoate (Gastrografin) is to be *avoided* if there is a suspected communication with an airway or risk of aspiration, due to its ability to induce a chemical pneumonitis and pulmonary edema.

The ideal barium suspension which can be used in the GI tract without altering its concentration is not yet available. It needs to be altered according to the part of bowel to be imaged.

For lower GI emergencies, non-ionic water-soluble contrast medium or gastrografin is preferred. Barium should be avoided due to the risk of barium peritonitis in the presence of bowel perforation.

Prior to proceeding to CT or emergency fluoroscopy studies, a plain radiograph should be obtained especially in patients with an acute abdomen due to suspected small or large

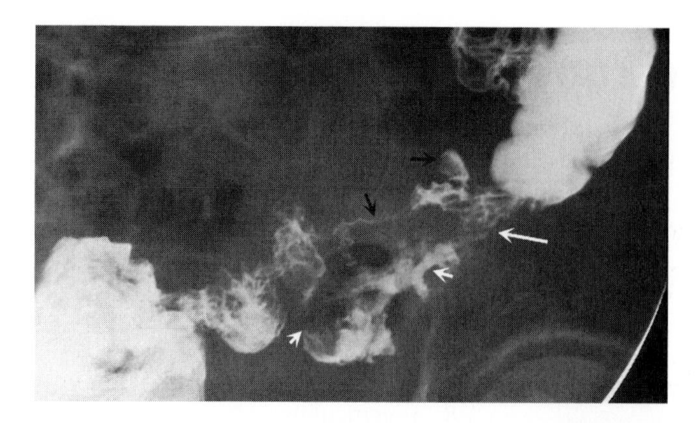

Fig. 5.1. Diverticulitis with pericolonic abscess. Single-contrast enema shows thickening and narrowing of sigmoid colon with associated diverticula (black arrows). There is contrast tracking through the wall (large white arrow) resulting in a large pericolonic collection (short white arrows).

bowel obstruction and colitis. It is also useful in upper GI emergencies such as esophageal perforation, and volvulus.

Proceed to CT or contrast studies, especially when the plain film is discordant with the clinical features. CT is more sensitive than plain radiographs in identifying the transition point in the bowel and to visualize underlying pathology.

Suggested reading

Adam A, Dixon AK. *Grainger and Allison's Diagnostic Radiology. A Textbook of Medical Imaging,* 5th edition, Vol. 1. Churchill Livingstone, 2008.

Gore RM, Levine MS. *Textbook of Gastrointestinal Radiology*, 2nd edition, Vol. 1. Saunders, 2000.

5.2 Spontaneous esophageal perforation

Complete rupture of esophageal wall results in perforation and is a surgical emergency. See Fig. 5.2.

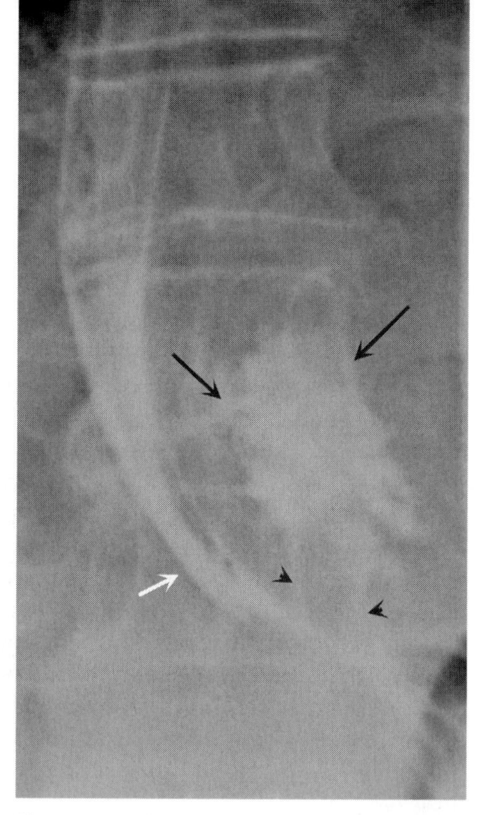

Fig. 5.2. Boerhaave's syndrome. Contrast swallow shows oral contrast filling the mid to distal esophagus (white arrow) and irregular pool of extraluminal contrast (black arrows) adjacent to the site of distal esophageal perforation (arrowheads).

Clinical

In Boerhaave's syndrome, complete perforation can occur spontaneously following retching or vomiting and it usually originates in the distal esophagus. The patient may present with severe constant chest pain and signs of subcutaneous emphysema.

Technique

Frontal chest radiograph.

Findings

1. Pneumomediastinum on a chest radiograph is highly suggestive of the diagnosis in the presence of the appropriate clinical setting.
2. Pneumoperitoneum suggests extension of the tear into the stomach.

Fluoroscopy

1. Table erect, patient in RAO (LPO) position to project the esophagus away from the thoracic spine.
2. A spot control film is to differentiate opacities relevant to the examination from those present before contrast administration.
3. Video facilities are useful for recording the examination.
4. WSCM is swallowed under direct screening/video. If no leak or perforation is demonstrated proceed with a barium swallow.

Findings

1. A focal dynamic extra-luminal contrast leak from the esophagus is seen while doing fluoroscopy screening.
2. The track of contrast leak is ill defined and irregular.
3. The contrast may collect in the mediastinum or pleural cavity.
4. Pneumothorax may be appreciated.
5. The diameter of the contrast track at the esophagus gives approximate estimate of diameter of perforation.

Pearls

- In Boerhaave's syndrome usually the distal esophagus is affected. Sometimes a small early perforation is difficult to see in just one view – screen the patient in all the above views.
- Video fluoroscopy screening may be helpful in reviewing the examination.
- If in doubt, a CT thorax after oral contrast can be performed to exclude perforation.
- Surgical closure of perforation is usually indicated. Follow-up imaging should not demonstrate any residual contrast leak in complete closure.

Suggested reading

Refer to Section 5.1.

Gimenez A *et al.* Thoracic complications of esophageal disorders. *RadioGraphics* 2002;22:S247–S258.

5.3 Esophageal anastomotic leak

Following esophagectomy, the surgically created anastomosis between the residual upper native esophagus and the gastric pull up or small bowel loop such as jejunum or ileum may disrupt, resulting in post-operative anastomotic leak. This can result in serious complications such as mediastinitis and abscess formation, which require immediate and aggressive management. See Fig. 5.3.

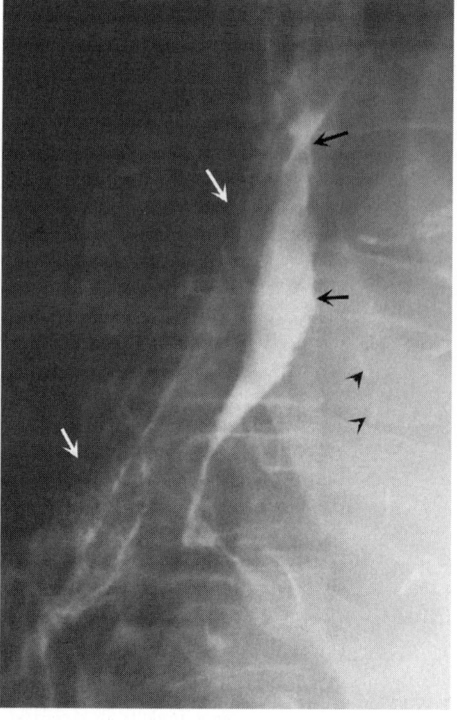

Fig. 5.3. Esophageal anastomotic leak. Contrast swallow in a patient following Ivor Lewis procedure shows contrast leak from the anastomotic site, pooling of contrast in the mediastinum (black arrows), surgical clips (arrowheads), and distal gastric tube (white arrows).

Clinical

The patient may be unwell with or without pneumothorax, surgical emphysema or a pleural collection on the initial post-operative chest radiograph.

Persistent leak can lead to mediastinitis which increases morbidity and mortality.

Technique

Non-ionic water-soluble contrast or gastromiro.

Gastrografin is contraindicated (risk of pulmonary edema and chemical pneumonitis). For ICU patients make sure all tubes, lines and wires are handled safely.

It is more comfortable for the patient to lie supine during the procedure.

Before the procedure make sure you know the location of the proximal and distal anastomotic sites. The leak is usually from the proximal anastomotic site.

Fluoroscopy is centered over the proximal anastomotic site then AP, lateral and opposite oblique views are obtained while swallowing.

If no leak is demonstrated at the proximal anastomotic site then the distal anastomotic site can be studied.

Findings

1. Dynamic contrast leak from the esophageal lumen.
2. Contrast may pool in the mediastinum or pleural space as a collection.

Pearls

- CT thorax with oral non-ionic water-soluble contrast is helpful to identify esophageal leak in very sick patients, and to exclude or confirm any associated collection/abscess.
- Oral contrast should be given just prior to scanning. Do not administer the contrast via NG tube.
- The presence of high-density contrast in the mediastinum or pleural space, with or without the presence of irregular contrast pooling near the surgical anastomotic site on non-contrast CT, is consistent with anastomotic dehiscence.

- Follow-up contrast swallow examinations can be performed until there is resolution of the anastomotic leak. The extraluminal track size and length reduce during healing if conservative management is taken for a small anastomotic leak.
- CT can assist the drainage of a mediastinal abscess.

Suggested reading

Kim TJ *et al.* Postoperative imaging of esophageal cancer: what chest radiologists need to know *Radiographics* 2007;**27**(2):409–429.

Kim SH *et al.* Esophageal resection: indications, techniques, and radiologic assessment. *Radiographics* 2001;**21**(5):1119–1137; discussion 1138–1140.

5.4 Esophageal dissection

Intramural esophageal dissection is a rare emergency in which there is a sudden onset of dissection in the esophageal wall with a false track between the mucosal and muscular layers of the esophagus. See Fig. 5.4.

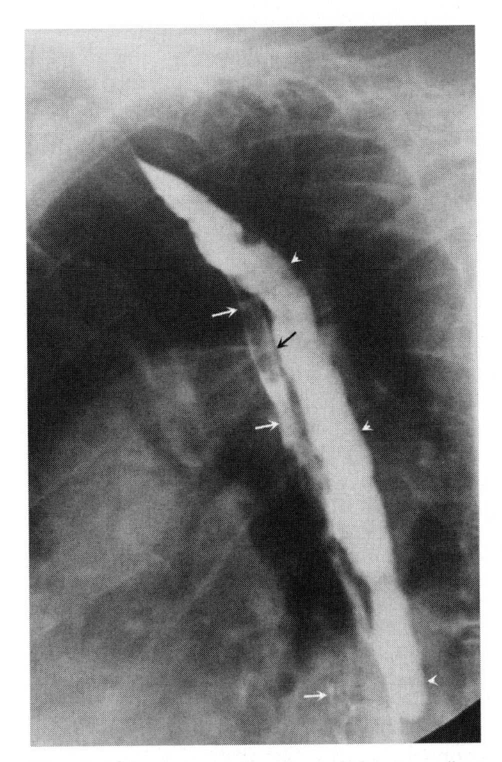

Fig. 5.4. Esophageal dissection. Contrast swallow shows a blind-ending false lumen (arrowheads) originating from upper esophagus. Note the true lumen of the esophagus (white arrows) parallels with the false lumen and extends to stomach. Note "mucosal stripe" sign (black arrow).

Clinical

Esophageal dissection can occur spontaneously or following endoscopy, anticoagulant treatment and forceful swallowing. It presents with severe chest pain and is exacerbated with swallowing.

Technique

See esophageal perforation.

Urgent contrast swallow.

Gastromiro or non-ionic water-soluble contrast.

Both oblique and lateral views.

Findings

1. Extra-luminal contrast in a well-defined false track.
2. The false and true lumina lie parallel to each other and give an appearance of the so-called "double barrelled" esophagus.
3. "Mucosal stripe" sign – a radiolucent thin mucosal stripe between contrast in the true and false lumina.
4. In perforation a contrast leak forms an irregular track dispersing into the mediastinum and/or pleural space.

5. In dissection the false lumen is well defined and usually blind ending and also lies parallel to the native lumen of the esophagus.

Pearls

- CT thorax can be performed immediately after contrast swallow to demonstrate the intramural contrast in dissection and high-density pleural or mediastinal collection in full thickness perforation. See CT esophagus.
- Follow up with upper GI contrast swallow can be performed until the dissection resolves. Typically the false track size and length reduce over time during the healing process if the standard conservative management has been adopted.

Suggested reading

Refer to Section 2.12.

Constantine S. Oesophageal dissection: contrast studies and CT in diagnosis and monitoring. *Australasian Radiol* 2003;47:198–201.

5.5 Gastric volvulus

Gastric volvulus is a rare but potentially life-threatening condition in which the stomach twists on itself. It is thought to be due to laxity or anomaly of the gastric suspensory ligaments. Diaphragmatic defects may predispose to this condition which is rarely encountered before 50 years of age. There are two types of volvulus: organo-axial – twist along its long axis (long axis is a line from the cardia to the pylorus); and mesentero-axial – twist occurs perpendicular to the long axis. See Fig. 5.5.

Clinical

The three clinical features suggestive of *acute gastric volvulus* are:

Abdominal pain.

Retching without vomiting.

Inability to pass a nasogastric tube into the stomach.

The mesentero-axial volvulus is associated with chronic symptoms of abdominal pain and retching.

Technique

Supine abdominal radiograph.

Barium or water-soluble contrast meal.

Findings

1. Massively dilated stomach in LUQ possibly extending into chest.
2. Intrathoracic double air–fluid level on AXR.
3. Air in the gastric wall in cases of vascular compromise.
4. Inability of barium to pass into stomach (when obstructed).
5. The greater curvature of the stomach lies superior to the lesser curvature in an organoaxial twist.
6. In mesentero-axial twist, the gastric antrum lies above the fundus.

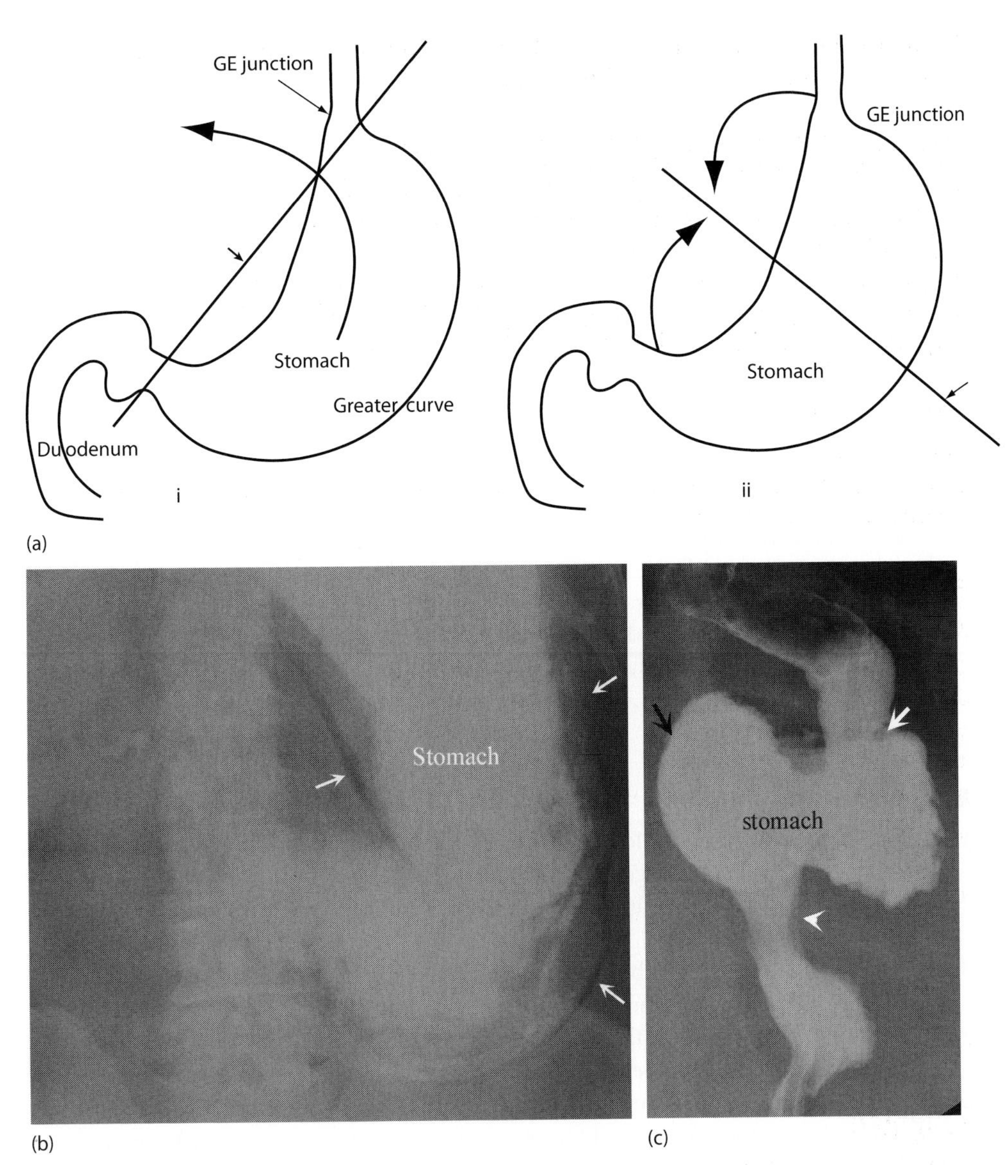

Fig. 5.5. (a) Gastric volvulus. (i) Organo-axial gastric volvulus – twist along the long axis (short arrows) from GE junction to cardia. (ii) Mesentero-axial gastric volvulus – twist perpendicular to the long axis (arrow). (b) Emphysematous gastritis. Contrast meal in a diabetic patient shows a massively dilated stomach with intramural gas (arrows), a sign of ischemia. No evidence of volvulus. (c) Gastric volvulus. Upper GI contrast study shows twisted stomach with resultant superiorly placed greater curvature (black arrow) and inferiorly facing lesser curvature (arrowhead) of the stomach. Also there is herniation of the stomach into the thorax above the gastro-esophageal junction (white arrow).

Pearls

- Volvulus may often be asymptomatic.
- Unless the twist reaches 180 degrees, obstruction tends not to occur.

- When the twist exceeds 180 degrees, obstruction results which may be life threatening unless surgically corrected.
- Vascular compromise is more common with the organo-axial type and there is a strong association with hiatus hernia.
- Gastric wall emphysema may result due to volvulus.

Suggested reading

Refer to Section 5.1.

5.6 Small bowel obstruction

Refer to Section 3.17. See Fig. 5.6.

Technique

Supine abdominal radiograph from the symphysis pubis upwards.

The hernial orifices must be included.

Supplemental films with a horizontal beam are used to detect free peritoneal gas (erect chest radiography and left lateral decubitus films after 10 minutes delay to allow gas to collect between the liver and abdominal wall).

Proceed to CT or contrast studies, especially when the plain film is discordant with the clinical features.

Findings

AXR

1. Central dilated small bowel loops. Mechanical – deflation of colon. Ileus – usually associated with a dilated large bowel.
2. The jejunum > 4 cm diameter and the ileum > 3 cm diameter. Check the level of obstruction.
3. In the erect position small "beads" of air become trapped by the valvulae conniventes resembling the "string of beads" sign – seen in mechanical obstruction rather than ileus.
4. In the erect position an air–fluid level greater than 2.5 cm length is a marker for mechanical obstruction rather than ileus.
5. Look for pneumoperitoneum and associated pathology.
6. Look for pneumatosis in cases of bowel ischemia. Always look for portal venous gas – high of risk mortality.
7. Look for air in the biliary tree and for an ectopic radio-opaque gallstone in cases of gallstone ileus.

Fluoroscopic findings

1. Barium does not inspissate in small bowel obstruction so can be given safely in suspected case of small bowel obstruction (unlike large bowel obstruction). However if urgent laparatomy is indicated as in the case of complete small bowel obstruction neither barium nor WSCM should be used.
2. Site of obstruction – an abrupt change in caliber of lumen from distended to collapsed bowel.
3. Dilatation proximal to the site of obstruction.

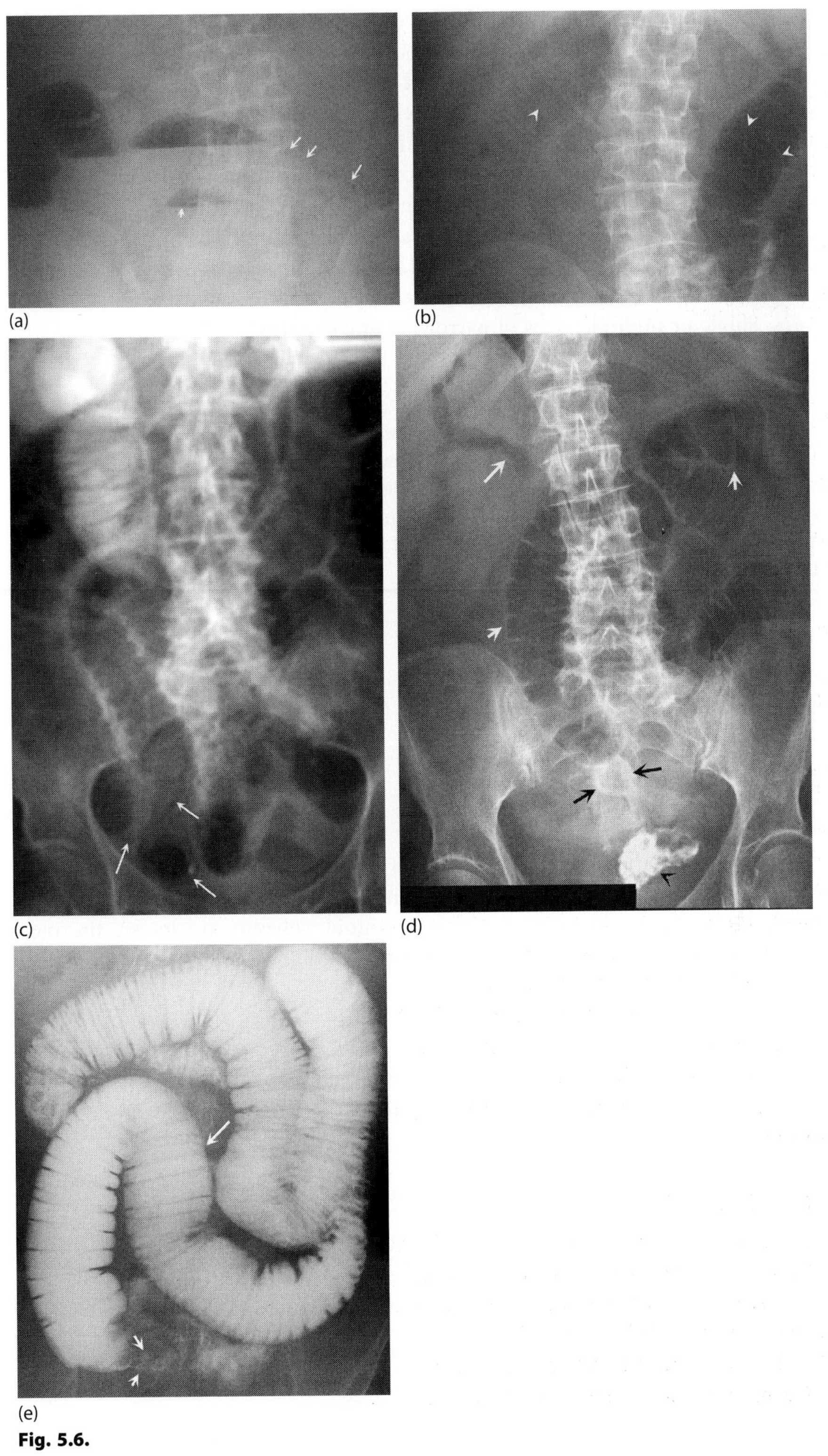

Fig. 5.6.

4. Exaggerated, normal or reduced peristalsis according to the duration of obstruction.
5. Adhesive bands causing the obstruction: A sharp, straight or slightly curved edge of bowel at the site of crossing of adhesion, band of radiolucency across the bowel.
6. Metastatic obstruction: Extrinsic mass effect with tethering of mucosal folds. Rounded and irregular margins at the site of narrowing, long segmental narrowing, annular, tight ring of narrowing, desmoplastic distortion (not seen in primary adenocarcinoma).
7. Internal or external hernias causing SBO: Multiple crowded small bowel loops in an abnormal location enclosed within a hernial sac. Do not change position with time. Delayed barium emptying from the obstructed loops. At the neck of hernia entering and returning loop may show a smooth narrowing.
8. Strictures: Single or multiple areas of narrowing due to varied etiology.

Pearls

- CT of the abdomen should be carried out in all patients who have acute small bowel obstruction.
- Distal small bowel obstruction may be caused by a cecal carcinoma – in such cases a contrast enema may be needed to confirm the diagnosis.
- There may be benefit in contrast studies if the small bowel obstruction is proximal.
- The valvulae conniventes cross the bowel without interruption unlike haustral folds in the colon which are interrupted.

Suggested reading

Refer to Section 5.1.

Silva AC *et al.* Small bowel obstruction: what to look for. *Radiographics* 2009;**29**:423–439.

5.7 Large bowel emergencies

Sigmoid volvulus

Large bowel volvulus comprises 10% of all cases of large bowel obstruction in developed countries. Volvulus occurs where there is a segment of large bowel attached to a mobile mesentery, thus allowing it to twist. Cecal and sigmoid volvulus are by far the most common. Transverse colon volvulus is extremely rare. See Fig. 5.7.

Clinical

75% of all large-bowel volvulus.
It is seen in old-age and institutionalized individuals often on anticholinergic drugs.
Patients often give a chronic history with intermittent acute attacks.
Non-specific abdominal pain, absolute constipation and abdominal distension.

Caption for Fig. 5.6 (a) Small bowel obstruction. Erect AXR shows small bowel obstruction with air–fluid levels (short arrow) and the "string of beads" sign due to small pockets of gas collecting between the valvulae conniventes (arrows). (b) Small bowel obstruction. Supine AXR in mechanical small bowel obstruction demonstrating air-filled small bowel loops. Intraluminal fluid is not better appreciated on this view. Note the valvulae conniventes (arrowheads). (c) Bowel ischemia. Small bowel meal shows dilated small bowel with intramural gas consistent with ischemia (arrows). (Photo courtesy of Dr. Julian Tuson, University Hospital Aintree.) (d) Gallstone ileus. Plain KUB (kidney, urinary tract and bladder) shows air in the biliary tree (long white arrow), small bowel obstruction with collapse of the large bowel and an ectopic gallstone in the distal ileum (black arrows) (Rigler's triad). Note incidental calcified fibroid (black arrowhead). (e) Jejunal obstruction. Small bowel meal demonstrates a shouldered stricture (short arrows) in the jejunum with partial obstruction. Note the grossly dilated small bowel loops (long arrow). The patient was subsequently diagnosed with non-Hodgkin's lymphoma of jejunum.

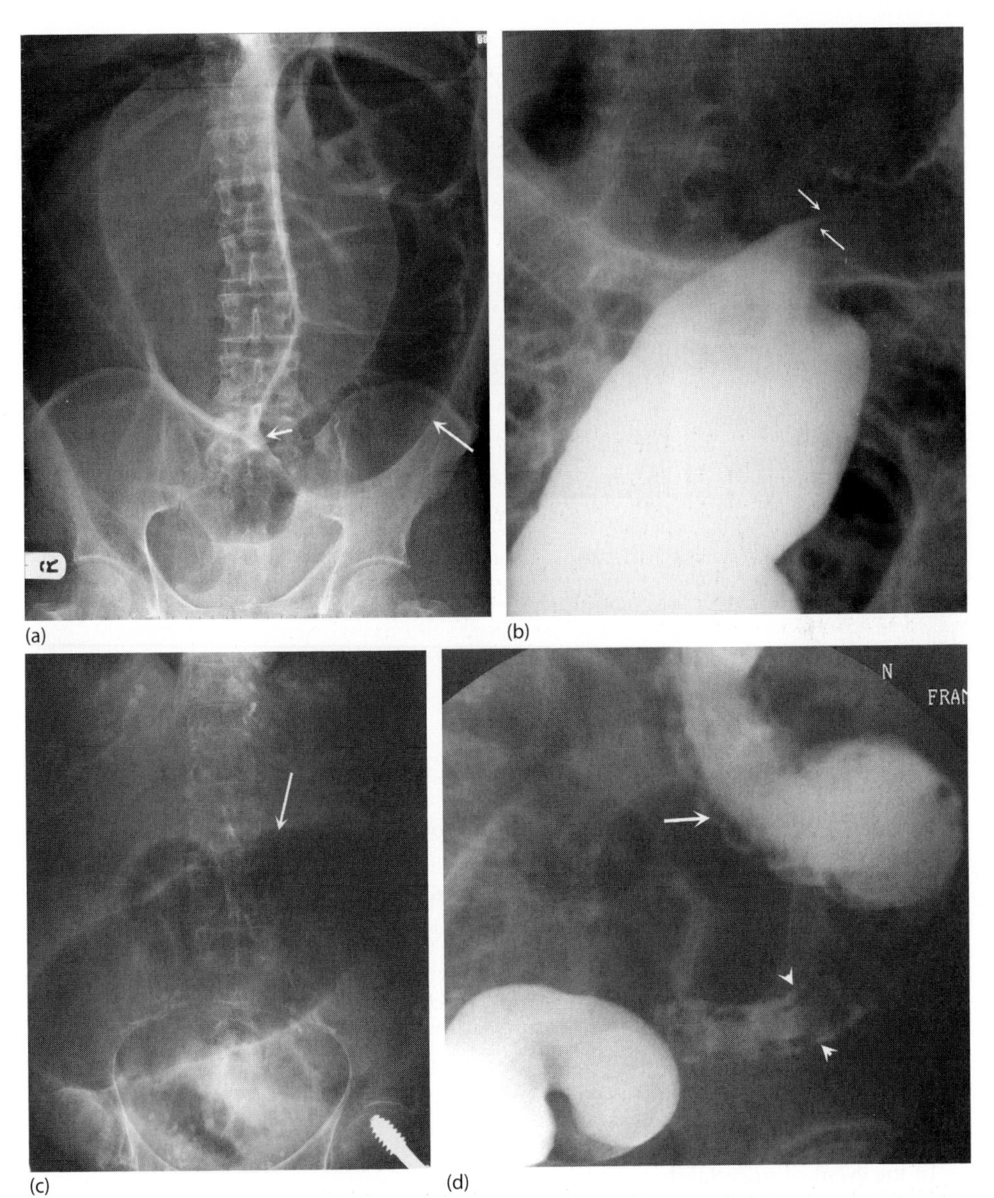

Fig. 5.7. (a) Sigmoid volvulus. Plain AXR shows absence of rectal gas, the left flank overlap sign (long arrow) and "coffee bean" shape to the twisted sigmoid loop. Note the inferior convergence (short arrow) overlying the sacrum. (b) Sigmoid volvulus. Barium enema shows an abrupt caliber change in the sigmoid colon (arrows) resembling the beak of a bird of prey, consistent with sigmoid volvulus. (c) Cecal volvulus. Plain AXR shows dilated cecum lying across the midline and over towards the left upper quadrant (arrow). Note distal small bowel obstruction and deflation of colonic gas distal to the cecum. (d) Active ulcerative colitis. Instant contrast enema shows multiple flask-shaped ulcers with narrow neck (arrow) and broad base (arrowheads), involving entire colon, consistent with collar stud ulcers seen in acute ulcerative colitis.

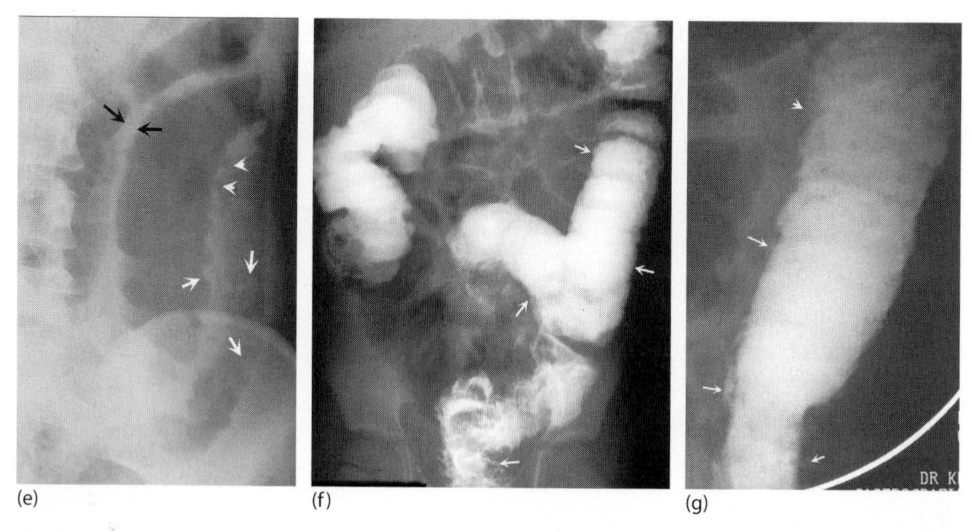

Fig. 5.7. (*cont.*) (e) Ulcerative colitis. Plain AXR shows marked mucosal edema, bowel wall thickening (black arrows) and thumbprinting (arrowheads), pseudopolyp formation involving the transverse colon (white arrows) and splenic flexure. (f) Pseudomembranous colitis. Instant enema shows the diffuse mucosal irregularity and thumbprinting (arrows). (g) Active colitis. Instant contrast enema shows irregular mucosa with multiple mucosal ulcerations (arrows) in descending colon, consistent with active colitis. The patient was subsequently diagnosed with ulcerative colitis.

Findings

AXR

1. Classically the ahaustral sigmoid loop twists around the mesenteric axis giving an "inverted U" or "coffee bean" appearance.
2. The apposing inner walls of the afferent and efferent limbs give a "white stripe" appearance.
3. The three most specific signs are:
   Left flank overlap sign – this is the overlapping of a dilated descending colon by the "coffee bean" loop. This sign is absent in cecal volvulus since the left colon deflates.
   Apex under left hemidiaphragm.
   Inferior convergence on left.

Contrast enema

1. In the event of uncertainty a contrast enema can be carried out with low pressure barium enema without an inflating rectal balloon. This demonstrates the so-called "bird of prey" sign, denoting the point of torsion.
2. Contrast enema can be terminated once the point of torsion has been demonstrated.
3. Once the decompression of the volvulus is done, an underlying colonic neoplasm can also be ruled out by follow-up barium enema.

Cecal volvulus

This is an ascending colon volvulus where the cecum exists on a mesentery. There is congenital failure of attachment of the right hemicolon to the posterior abdominal wall. It requires a degree of malrotation of the proximal colon.

It affects individuals between 30 and 60 years of age and is more likely to occur in conditions that predispose to colonic distension.

Findings

AXR

1. In 50% of cases, the cecum twists so that the pole lies in the midline or left upper quadrant.
2. In 50% of cases the twists occur axially so that the cecum remains in the same position.
3. Haustral folds are usually seen in the dilated, air-filled ectopically located cecum.
4. Ileo-cecal valve indentation on the medial aspect of cecum.
5. Marked small bowel dilatation.
6. Colonic deflation distal to the cecum.
7. Erect abdominal films – single fluid level (unlike multiple levels in sigmoid volvulus).

Fluoroscopic findings (contrast enema)

1. Beaking like appearance of the bowel at the point of volvulus.
2. Bowel dilatation proximal to narrowing.

Colitis

The "instant" enema and CT abdomen examinations are particularly useful in total active colitis to assess the extent of ulcerative colitis without bowel preparation. As the colitic bowel is free of fecal matter, good quality double-contrast images can usually be obtained.

Contraindications to an instant enema are peritonism, toxic megacolon and perforation.

This examination is not usually suitable for Crohn's disease as mucosal ulceration is patchy and discontinuous and does not necessarily involve the distal colon, unlike ulcerative colitis.

Findings

Crohn's disease

1. Can involve any part of bowel from mouth to anus.
2. When confined to colon, Crohn's disease resembles ulcerative colitis on plain radiograph.
3. Changes suggestive of Crohn's disease: Lymphoid hyperplasia, aphthous ulcers in the normal mucosa, cobblestone formation, transverse contrast strips, fissuring deep ulcers ("rose thorn") producing fistulas and sinus tracts strictures, pseudo-sacculations on the antimesenteric border of ileum.
4. Skip, asymmetric lesions.
5. Pseudopolyps appear as islands of intact edematous mucosa in a surrounding area of sloughed-off mucosa.

Ulcerative colitis

1. Granular mucosa, mucosal stippling, collar-stud ulcers, polyps, strictures.
2. Ileitis (backwash ileitis) in case of active pancolitis involving ileum-patulous, ileocecal valve with reflux associated with a dilated terminal ileum.

3. Enlarged presacral space > 1.5 mm with rectal valve > 6.5 mm thick in case of active proctitis.
4. Rectum is usually involved in ulcerative colitis but may appear normal if the patient is on rectal steroid treatment.

Pseudomembranous colitis

It is associated with *Clostridium difficile* infection, antibiotic use and gives a similar pattern to ulcerative colitis. It usually involves whole large bowel and causes marked mucosal thickening.

Ischemic colitis

1. It tends to involve the region of the splenic flexure and can occur anywhere from the mid transverse colon to the distal descending colon.
2. Typically it spares the rectum.
3. Its distribution is variable as it is dependent on the precise anatomy of the arterial blood supply between the superior and inferior mesenteric arteries via the "wandering artery" of Drummond.
4. Ischemia leads to submucosal hemorrhage.

Active colitis

1. Bowel wall thickening – can only be appreciated when there is intraluminal gas (the silhouette sign).
2. Loss of haustral folds.
3. "Featureless abdomen" – there is complete absence of gas and feces, usually seen in total active colitis.
4. If distal extent of formed fecal matter is up to sigmoid colon, proctitis is present.
5. If distal extent of formed fecal matter is up to proximal colon the colitis extends up to it.
6. Granular, indistinct mucosa.
7. Ulcerations in the inflamed mucosa.
8. Intramural gas shadows in case of fulminating colitis with necrosis.
9. In chronic burnt-out ulcerative colitis, if colon measures > 5 cm suggest fulminant colitis causing transmural involvement.
10. Perforation – results from severe transmural inflammation.
11. Marked dilatation of colitic bowel – toxic megacolon. Dilatation of large bowel other than the cecum to a diameter of 5.5 cm. In toxic megacolon the patient is very sick.

Pearls

- The presence of the left flank overlap sign is the most important sign that establishes a diagnosis of sigmoid volvulus.
- Sigmoid volvulus with obstruction causes global large bowel dilatation. Cecal volvulus with obstruction causes the distal colon to deflate.
- Barium enema is useful in establishing sigmoid volvulus where there is doubt. This is usually unnecessary in cecal volvulus.
- Transverse colon and splenic flexure volvulus are both very uncommon.

- Less specific signs of sigmoid volvulus on plain radiograph are: The apex above T10 vertebra; the liver overlap signs; usually absence of rectal gas unless a digital examination has been carried out. Cecum with feces in its normal position in the right flank.
- Presence of formed feces in a given segment of large bowel suggests no active colitis in that segment.
- Complete absence of feces is a good indicator of active colitis.

Suggested reading

Refer to Section 5.1.

Burrell HC *et al.* Significant plain film findings in sigmoid volvulus. *Clin Radiol* 1994;**49**:317–319.

Thoeni RF, Cello JP. CT imaging of colitis. *Radiology* 2006;**240**:623–638.

5.8 Diverticulitis

Refer to Section 3.18. See Fig. 5.8.

Technique

Contrast enema is the optimal test for mucosal disease but does not always reveal the true extent of the intramural pathology. CT is useful for demonstrating this.

Barium is contraindicated in cases of suspected perforation. CT is preferred in this situation as it allows assessment of extraluminal pathology such as associated abdominal or pelvic abscesses.

Findings

1. Diverticula, some with distortion.
2. Stricture formation, narrowing and spasm.
3. Barium "tracking" into intramural abscess sinus tracks.
4. Fistulation with epithelial lined hollow organs or rarely the skin.
5. Pericolic abscess formation.
6. In vesico-colic communication, the fistula is rarely seen.
7. May be frank perforation in severe cases.

Pearls

- Mucosal ulceration, absence of diverticula, "shouldering" of stricture favor carcinoma.
- Co-existing diverticula are present in 30% of patients with carcinoma.
- Mucosal preservation, diverticula with distortion, sinus tracking of contrast into intramural abscesses, absence of shouldering of stricture favor diverticulitis.

Suggested reading

Refer to Section 5.1.

Tack D *et al.* Suspected acute colon diverticulitis: imaging with low-dose unenhanced multi-detector row CT. *Radiology* 2005;**237**:189–196.

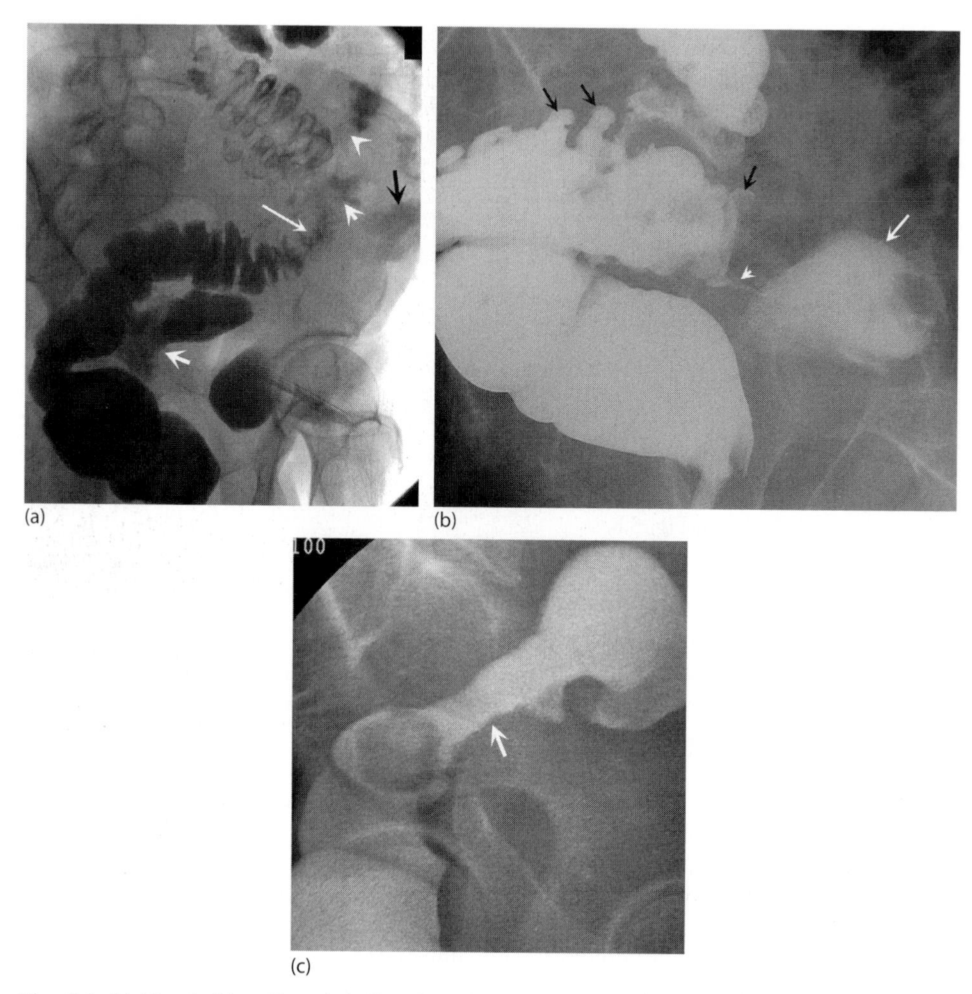

Fig. 5.8. (a) Diverticulitis with sealed-off perforation. Instant contrast enema shows pericolonic thickening, mucosal irregularity and luminal narrowing of the sigmoid colon (white arrow). Note the fistulae (arrowheads) communicating with small bowels (black arrow) and a pericolonic collection (white arrow). (b) Diverticulitis with vesico-colic fistula. Barium is seen entering the bladder (white arrow) through a fistulous communication (arrowhead). Multiple diverticula (black arrows) are seen arising from descending and sigmoid colon. (c) Rectosigmoid carcinoma. Instant-contrast enema in a patient with suspected large bowel obstruction shows irregular narrowing of recto-sigmoid region (arrow) with mild shouldering, suggestive of rectosigmoid carcinoma.

5.9 Bowel perforation

A perforated viscus may lead to free intraperitoneal gas or pneumoperitoneum. See Fig. 5.9.

Technique

Plain film erect or supine – if perforation is present there is no time for further examination. Proceed to surgery.

Contrast examinations have a limited role in emergency. If conservative treatment is planned, there is some merit in assessing the source of perforation e.g. duodenal perforation with water-soluble contrast examinations such as a contrast meal.

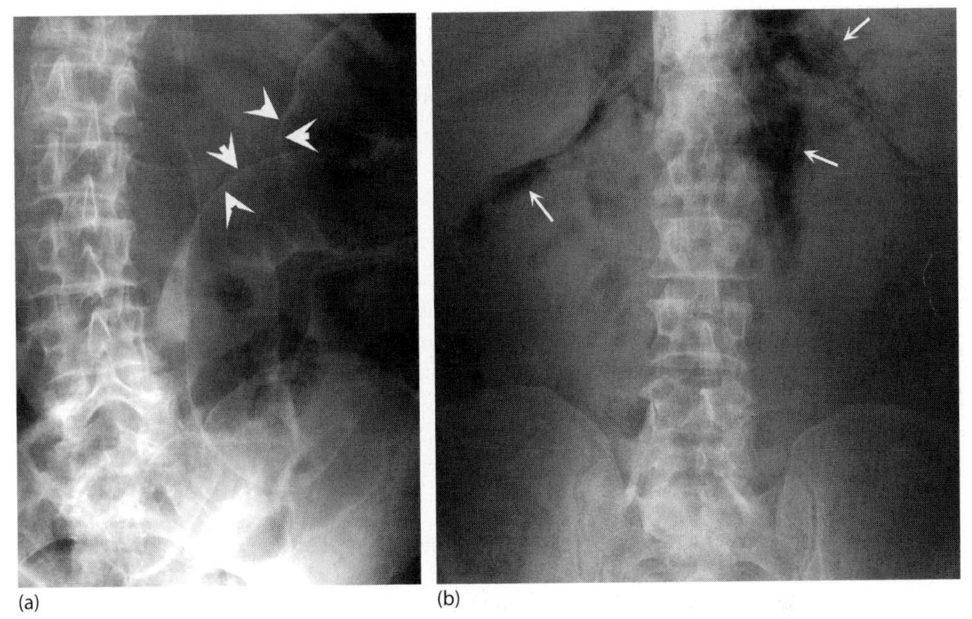

Fig. 5.9. (a) Pneumoperitoneum-Rigler's sign. Gas is present on both sides of the bowel wall (arrowheads) – intraluminal gas and extraluminal gas. This renders the bowel wall visible on both sides, not just the interface of the bowel wall. (b) Pneumoretroperitoneum. Note that the trapped gas is streaky and outlines retroperitoneal structures (arrows). This can occur following perforations of the retroperitoneal colon (ascending and descending) at colonoscopy and the second part of the duodenum at ERCP.

Barium is absolutely contraindicated in suspected perforation because of chemical peritonitis. Prior to laparotomy, CT abdomen and pelvis with oral non-ionic contrast may be performed to identify the site and cause of perforation if needed, although its role is questionable if a decision to undergo laparotomy has been made.

Findings

1. A sliver of gas under the diaphragm on an erect chest radiograph or in the least dependent part on a left lateral decubitus film.
2. Supine AXR film – can detect free intraperitoneal gas in about 60% of patients with pneumoperitoneum.
3. Best detected in the right upper quadrant.
4. Rigler's sign – both sides of bowel wall seen (silhouette sign).
   Cupola sign – gas under mid-diaphragm on a supine abdominal film.
   Subhepatic air – free air under the inferior margin of the liver.
7. Football sign – air lies under the anterior abdominal wall on supine film. The "football" is an American football shape.
8. Falciform ligament sign – air outlines the falciform ligament over the liver.

Pearls

- Pneumoperitoneum on a supine abdominal radiograph is very important to recognize.
- Free gas under the left hemidiaphragm on an erect chest radiograph can be confused with colonic or stomach gas. A left lateral decubitus film may be required but it is important

to allow the patient to settle in this position for 10 minutes before the radiograph is obtained.

- Perforation without free gas can occur in cases where there is very little intraluminal gas.

Suggested reading

Refer to Section 5.1.

5.10 Nephrostogram

Nephrostography is carried out during or after nephrostomy to determine the cause or the progress of an obstruction. On occasions the timing of the nephrostogram is delayed to avoid inducing bacteremia at the time of nephrostomy, especially when there is infection or pyonephrosis. See Fig. 5.10.

Technique

Sterile conditions.

Withdraw urine from the renal pelvis before injecting contrast to avoid dilution.

Half-strength or 150 w/v contrast media is used to avoid obscuring radiolucent calculi.

Gentle introduction of "bubble-free" contrast is essential to avoid mimicking radiolucent ureteric calculi. This can be avoided by priming the extension tubing before injection.

Obtain AP and right and left oblique views. Check the bladder for any contrast before, during and at the end of procedure.

Findings

1. Contrast outlines the point of partial or complete obstruction.
2. If the cause of obstruction is relieved (stone passed) then the contrast easily empties into the bladder.

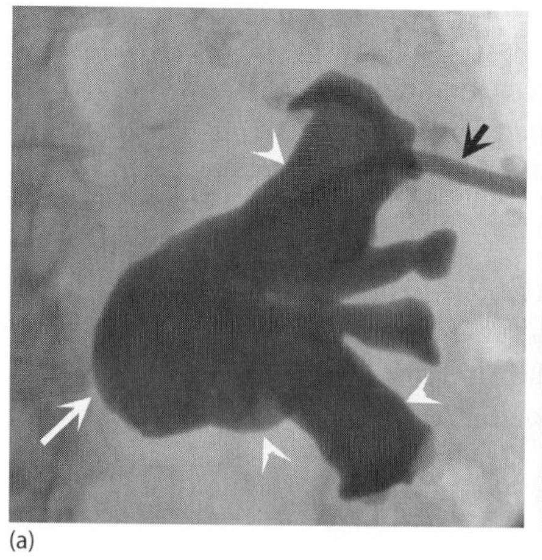

(a)

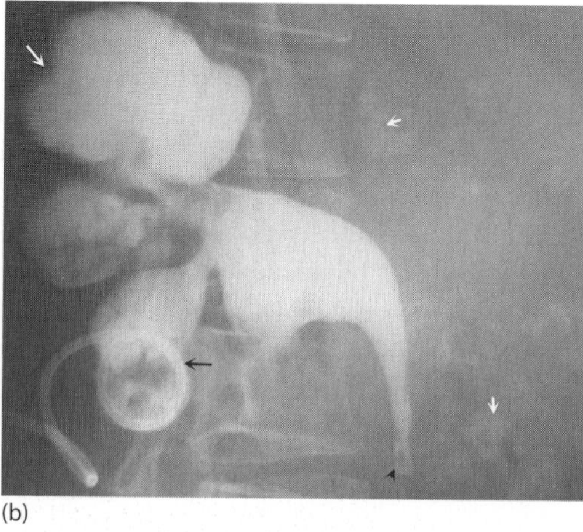

(b)

Fig. 5.10. (a) Nephrostogram. Note grossly dilated and clubbed calyces (arrowheads) and dilated renal pelvis (white arrow), with an abrupt termination at the pelvi-ureteric junction (PUJ); features are consistent with PUJ obstruction. (b) Obstructive hydronephrosis. Right hydronephrosis is due to an impacted calculus in the right upper ureter (arrowhead) in a patient with bilateral medullary sponge kidney. Note papillary calcification in the left kidney (white arrow) and nephrostomy drainage catheter (black arrow).

3. Presence of contrast in the bladder from the ureter on the affected side indicates only partial obstruction.

Pearls

- If there is any suggestion of infection, antibiotic prophylaxis is necessary.

5.11 Ascending urethrogram

Urethral injuries are almost exclusively seen in males owing to the difference in urethral length and also the relative protection of the urethra in women. See Fig. 5.11.

Female urethral injuries are often associated with extraperitoneal bladder injury.

Clinical

Blunt injury mainly affects the posterior urethra and is seen in high-speed impact trauma with pelvic fractures.

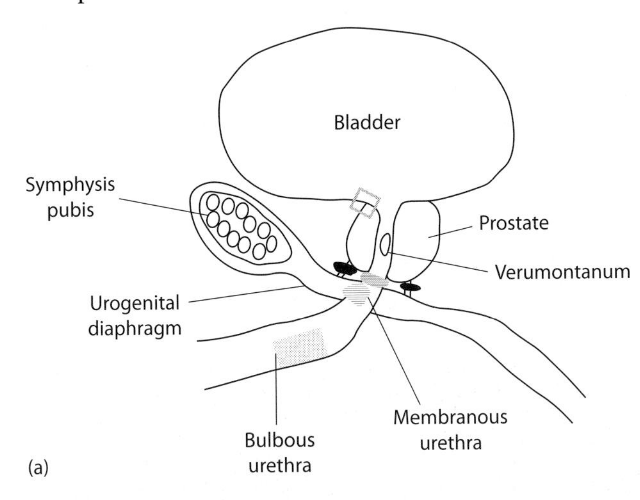

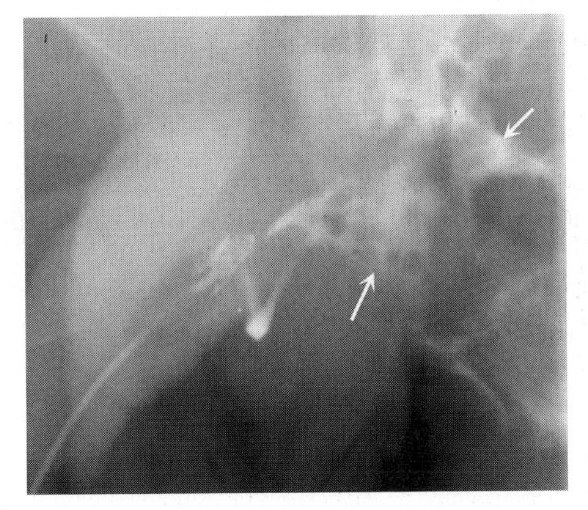

Fig. 5.11. (a) Urethral injuries. Type I (black area), Type II (striped area), Type III urethral injury (hatched area), Type IV urethral injury (gray box) and Type V urethral injury (dotted area). (b) Urethrogram. In a trauma patient an ascending urethrography demonstrates that contrast localizes in the perineum (arrows) and fails to reach the bladder due to mixed bulbous and membranous urethral injury.

Up to 14% of pelvic fractures in males are associated with injury to the posterior urethra. In those with urethral injury there is a 20% incidence of bladder laceration.

Anterior urethral injury is associated with straddle trauma and is usually seen on its own without additional injury.

There are five types of injury.

1. Type I urethral injury: Urethra intact but elongated at the site of disruption due to puboprostatic ligament disruption. No extravasation of contrast at urethrography.
2. Type II urethral injury: Disruption of membranous urethra above an intact urogenital diaphragm. Contrast extravasates into the extraperitoneal space above the urogenital diaphragm but fails to enter the perineum. Associated with incontinence.
3. Type III urethral injury: The membranous urethra is ruptured with laceration of the urogenital diaphragm. Contrast enters both the perineum and extraperitoneal space. Associated with incontinence. This is the most common type of uretheral injury.
4. Type IV urethral injury: Bladder base injuries result in extraperitoneal leak of contrast.
5. Type V urethral injury (Straddle): Contrast collects around the bulbous urethra due to anterior urethral injury.

Technique

Ascending (or retrograde) urethrography is the initial investigation of choice in cases of urethral trauma.

Demonstrates entire urethra, the anatomical site and extent of urethral damage.

The most widely used method is insertion of a Foley catheter into the urethra.

An aseptic technique.

Intravenous antibiotic prophylaxis.

The catheter is held in place by a balloon inflated to 1.5 ml in the navicular fossa of the penis. Use lubricants such as lidocaine jelly to anesthetize urethra prior to catheter placement.

If possible the patient should be placed in a posterior oblique position of 45 degrees with the penis lying laterally. Approximately 20 ml of iodinated contrast media is instilled gently filling the anterior (penile) urethra. Often there is natural sphincter resistance to filling more proximally but this is easily overcome with gentle pressure.

Findings

1. Extraluminal contrast pooling in the perineum or extraperitoneal space.
2. Mucosal irregularity and tracking of contrast into the urethral wall.

Pearls

- Bladder catheterization per urethram is contraindicated in suspected urethral trauma until a urethrogram has been carried out.
- CT also has a role in determining the types of urethral injury.

Suggested reading

Ali M *et al.* CT signs of urethral injury. *Radiographics* 2003;23:951–966.

Kawashim A, Sandle CM. Imaging of urethral disease: a pictorial review. *RadioGraphics* 2004;24: S195–S216.

5.12 Cystogram

Bladder rupture

In adults the bladder is protected within the bony pelvis and is less susceptible to trauma than in infants where the bladder is more prominent, less protected and has a more "intraperitoneal" location. In adults the bladder is primarily an extraperitoneal organ. See Fig. 5.12.

A small volume mobile bladder is less susceptible to trauma than a distended relatively fixed bladder. This is because, when full, the bladder is compressed against the spine.

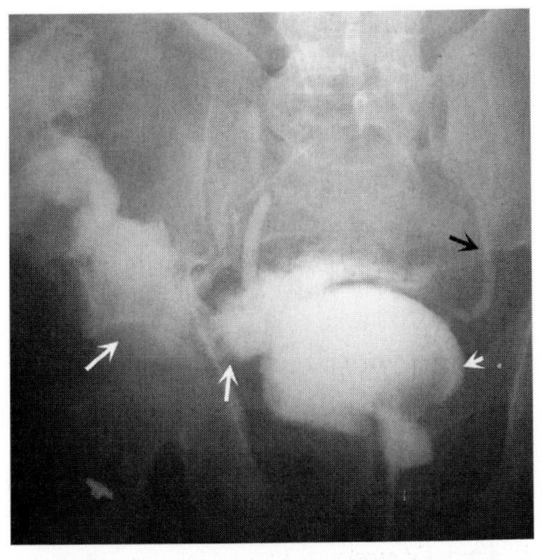

Fig. 5.12. Intraperitoneal bladder rupture. Cystogram demonstrates extraluminal contrast pooling in the right paracolic gutter (white arrows). Urinary bladder (short arrow) and ureter (black arrow).

The base of the bladder is attached to the urogenital diaphragm inferiorly by ligaments and posteriorly by the rectum. Pelvic fractures can easily cause extraperitoneal rupture. The dome of the diaphragm is relatively mobile and it is at this site where penetrating or blunt trauma can lead to intraperitoneal rupture.

Intraperitoneal and extraperitoneal ruptures occur with equal frequency and in approximately 10% of cases they occur simultaneously. Road traffic accidents and sports injuries are the principal causes of injury.

95% of extraperitoneal rupture is due to blunt trauma and pelvic fracture, mainly of the Malgaigne type.

5% of patients with pelvic fracture will have extraperitoneal bladder rupture.

Clinical

Refer to Section 3.7.

Technique

Ensure no urethral injury – if necessary rule out by performing ascending urethrography initially. A 16F urinary catheter is inserted under sterile precautions, ideally into an empty bladder. Residual urine is fully drained via the catheter. Urografin or non-ionic water-soluble contrast media is instilled hung from a drip stand at least 50 cm above the pa[illegible]nt. Spot films in the antero-posterior and oblique positions are obtained when co[illegible] shown to extravasate the bladder. Videofluoroscopy is also useful.

Findings

1. Extraperitoneal bladder rupture: Produces streaky, fixed, linear ar[illegible] [illegible]ere is no perivesical potential space, anterior and lateral to bladder. The [illegible] contrast usually is confined to the lower pelvis below the hi[illegible]
2. Intraperitoneal bladder rupture: contrast extravasation li[illegible] pools into the paracolic gutters and outlines pelvic lo[illegible] "streakiness."

3. Normal appearances are seen in bladder contusion. CT may reveal subtle changes.
4. Perivesical pelvic hematoma causes narrowing of the bladder in the pelvis.

Pearls

- If male urethral injury is suspected a CT scan can be carried out to look for bladder and urethral injury.

Suggested reading

Refer to Section 5.11.

Vaccaro JP, Brody JM. CT cystography in the evaluation of major bladder trauma. *RadioGraphics* 2000;**20**:1373–1381.

Srinivasa RN *et al.* Genitourinary trauma: a pictorial essay. *Emergency Radiology* 2009;**16**:21–33.

5.13 Intravenous urography

Intravenous urography (IVU) is helpful in demonstrating the anatomy in recurrent stone disease, in those patients for whom surgery is planned. It can also determine complete from partial obstruction. See Fig. 5.13.

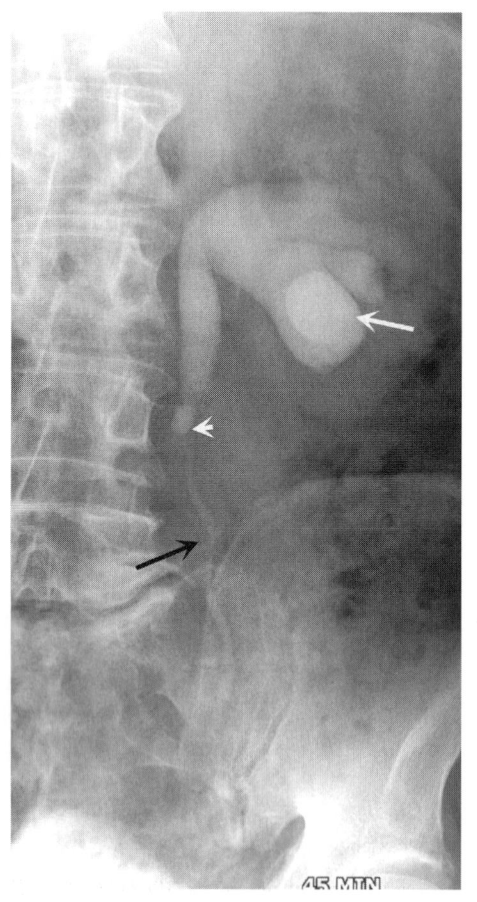

Fig. 5.13. Acute ureteric calculus. Intravenous urogram shows hydronephrosis (white arrow) and abrupt caliber change (arrowhead) of the ureter at the site of the calculus. Contrast is seen distal to the calculus indicating partial obstruction (black arrow).

Clinical

Refer to Section 3.13.

Technique

Plain abdominal film from the symphysis pubis upwards to include the renal areas – demonstrate radiodense opacities along the urinary tract.

Oblique radiographs – to localize the radio-opacities.

IVU.

Compression is withheld in acute renal and ureteric colic to avoid peripelvic contrast extravasation and also avoid a further reduction in the glomerular filtration rate that is p[illegible]valent in patients with acute obstruction.

[illegible]avenous contrast (300 mg I per kg [illegible]ht) is given.

[illegible]gth film immediately and at [illegible]ken.

[illegible]nters the calyces, serial [illegible] find the point of [illegible]s up to 24 hours

It is usual to combine the IVU with ultrasound to search for hydronephrosis.
Prone films may assist ureteric filling.

Findings

1. Increasingly dense nephrogram.
2. Hydronephrosis may be surprisingly minimal especially in the first 48 hours of obstruction.
3. The time delay in the appearance of the nephrogram and pyelogram depends on the degree of obstruction. The nephrogram intensification peaks at about 60 minutes following injection.
4. "Standing" column of contrast terminating at the site of obstruction which, in the case of ureteric stones, is usually at the pelvi-ureteric junction, the pelvic brim and the vesico-ureteric junction.
5. In severe obstruction peripelvic contrast extravasation may be seen suggesting a high obstructing pressure.

Pearls

- Phleboliths in the pelvis can cause confusion until contrast has outlined the ureters.
- CT – can detect stones greater than 2 mm in diameter and those stones that are radiolucent on radiographs and hence can be superior to IVU.

Suggested reading

Refer to Section 5.1.

5.14 Pegogram

Percutaneous endoscopic gastrostomy (PEG) or radiologically inserted gastrostomy (RIG) tubes are placed percutaneously into the body of the stomach. See Fig. 5.14.

They are used for short- or long-term feeding in patients who are unable to take food orally. An external tube provides the conduit for feeding.

Pegograms or tubography via the PEG tube can be very useful in assessing the patency of a tube, searching for leaks and for misplaced tubes.

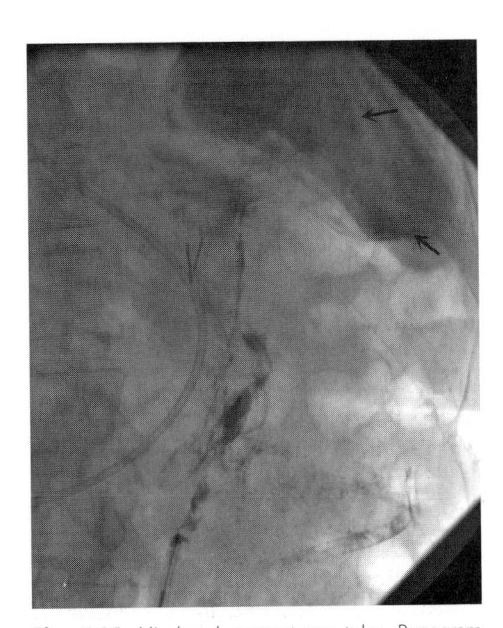

Fig. 5.14. Misplaced gastrostomy tube. Pegogram demonstrates intraperitoneal pooling of contrast around the spleen in the left upper quadrant (black arrows) due to misplaced PEG.

Technique and possible findings

Control film.

Inject contrast slowly via the tube looking for the position of the tube, peritoneal leak and reflux into the esophagus.

Be familiar with types of gastrostomy or jejunostomy tubes and their ports.

Findings

1. Normal: Contrast easily passes through the tube and fills the stomach. No hold up. No intraperitoneal contrast pooling.
2. Abnormal: Contrast leaks outside the stomach and into the peritoneal cavity. Absent or inadequate contrast opacification of small bowel and stomach.

Pearls

- A malpositioned gastrotomy tube should prompt immediate notification of the referring clinicians.

Suggested reading

Levine CD *et al.* Imaging of percutaneous tube gastrostomies: spectrum of normal and abnormal findings. *Am J Roentgenol* 1995;**164**(2):347–351.

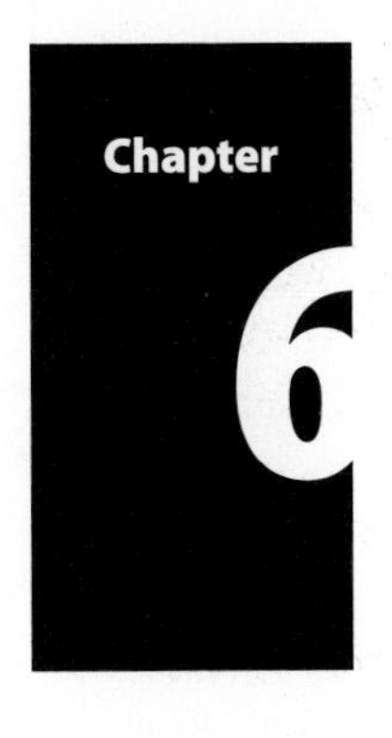

Magnetic resonance imaging

Sacha Niven and Mayil S. Krishnam

6.1 General principles

The patient may be critically ill and require monitoring, or even artificial ventilation; MR-compatible equipment will therefore be required for these cases. See Fig. 6.1.

T2-weighted sequences usually show pathology, but fat-suppressed T2 sequences (STIR) are much more sensitive for cases such as marrow replacement and edema in bone; they are also useful for the orbits.

Examples of imaging protocols

Routine brain:	T1 sagittal, T2 axial, FLAIR coronal.
Ischemic brain:	Add in DWI and ADC.
Intracranial hemorrhage:	Add Gradient-recalled-echo T2*.
Routine spine:	T1 sagittal, T2 sagittal, T1 and T2 axials through relevant levels.
Trauma spine:	Add in STIR sagittals.
Metastasis/infection spine:	Add in STIR sagittal, T1 sagittal post-gadolinium, T1 axials post-gadolinium through relevant levels.

Signal characteristics relative to brain/spinal cord signal

Tissue/Sequence	T1	T2	FLAIR
Fat	High signal ++	High signal+	High signal+
Water/CSF	Low signal	High signal++	Low signal
Air/gas	Low signal++	Low signal++	Low signal++
Dense calcium	Low signal+	Low signal+	Low signal+
Punctate calcium	Variable, often High signal	Low signal	Low signal
Proteinaceous fluid	Variable, often High signal	High signal	High signal
Blood < 5 hours	Low signal	High signal	High signal
Blood 5 hours–4 days	Isointense	Low signal	Low signal
4–7 days	High signal	Low signal	
>1 week	High signal	High signal	High signal
>2 months	Low signal	Low signal+	Low signal+

Pearls

- MRI can be an unsafe environment for some patients. Put safety first.
- A single sequence in a single plane will often not answer the question. A subtle change in the temporal lobes will be easier to see on coronal than axial imaging.
- Gadolinium-enhanced images can be very helpful in the correct setting.

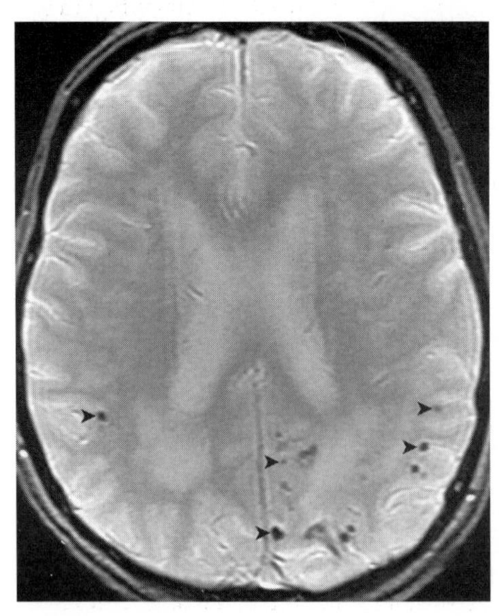

Fig. 6.1. Intracranial microhemorrhage. Gradient echo T2 axial image of brain in a patient with amyloid angiopathy shows multiple dark signal microhemorrhages (arrowheads) at the gray–white matter junction.

Suggested reading

www.mrisafety.com.

www.emedicine.com.

Atlas SW. *Magnetic Resonance Imaging of the Brain and Spine* Lippincott Williams and Wilkins, 2008.

6.2 Spinal cord compression

Spinal cord compression is a radiological emergency and MRI is the investigation of choice to assess the cause and degree of compression. See Fig. 6.2.

Clinical

Symptoms and signs include localized back or limb pain/tenderness, weakness, paresthesia, sensory level, pyramidal signs, and sphincter disturbance. Note reflexes may be absent in coexisting cauda equina compression.

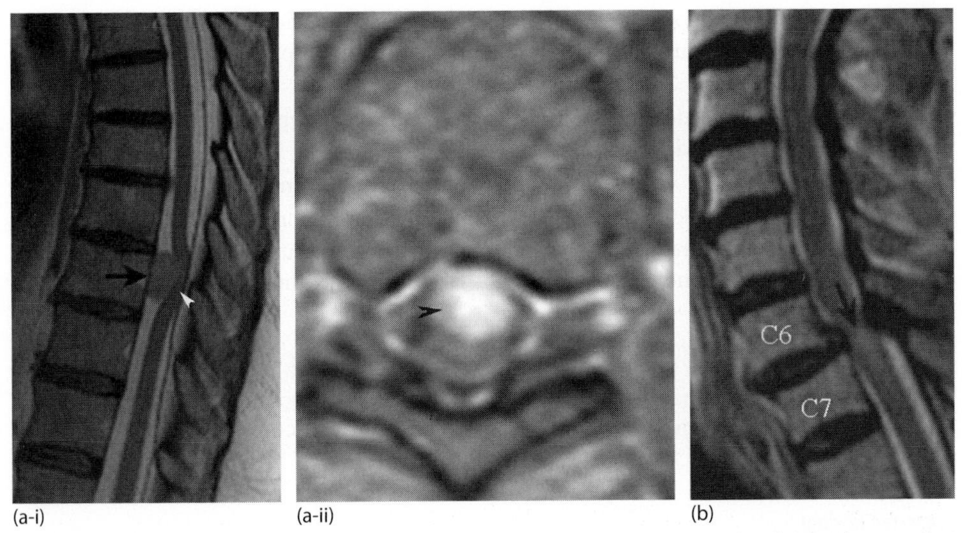

Fig. 6.2. (a) Spinal cord compression. T2 sagittal (i) spine shows an intradural extra-axial well-defined intermediate signal mass (arrowhead) compressing the thoracic spinal cord. Post-gadolinium T1 axial image (ii) shows vivid enhancement of the mass (arrowhead). (b) Spinal cord compression T2 sagittal C-spine shows an acute disc prolapse at the C6/C7 level and resultant significant compression of spinal cord and high-signal cord edema (arrow).

Causes

Infective: Discitis. Epidural abscess.
Degenerative: Disc prolapse (usually cervical region). Presents with radicular symptoms.
Tumor: Bone metastases (bronchus, breast, prostate, renal). Neurofibroma/meningioma.
Hemorrhage: Spontaneous epidural hematoma.

Technique

T1- and T2-weighted sagittal MRI with axial slices through an area of interest. Fat-suppressed T2 (STIR) sequences are more sensitive to marrow edema or replacement (metastases). Gadolinium may be required if infection, malignancy, or an arteriovenous fistula are suspected.

Findings

1. Compression of the spinal cord which will often have abnormal high signal within it at, or adjacent to, the level of compression.
2. Discitis and epidural abscess are often found together. The disc space is often narrowed and there will be abnormal high signal in the disc on T2 (much more obvious on STIR). There will be enhancement of both the disc and epidural collection.
3. Disc prolapse is usually seen to be contiguous with an intervertebral disc and have similar signal on T1. T2 signal can be variable. Sequestered fragments can be seen separated from a disc in some cases; the signals from these can be very variable but they usually do not enhance much and if they do, it is usually rim-like.

4. Metastases usually involve a vertebral body. The posterior elements of the vertebrae, especially the pedicle, are often involved and there may be a paravertebral mass. Look at the entire field of view for the primary.
5. Neurofibromas: Well-defined, multiple, dumb-bell shape (when it extends through a root exit foramen), vivid enhancement.
6. Meningiomas: Usually well defined, and enhances vividly, and may have a dural tail.
7. An arteriovenous fistula: Increased signal in the conus which may extend upwards to the cervical level. The spinal venous plexus is distended with multiple vessels seen on the surface of the conus and cord; this may be best seen following gadolinium.

Pearls

- Multiple metastases may be missed on T2, low signal areas in bone marrow on T1 indicate replacement of fatty marrow; STIR is most sensitive to detect other lesions.

Suggested reading

Cole JS, Patchell RA. Metastatic epidural spinal cord compression. *Lancet Neurol* 2008;7(5):459–466.

6.3 Acute ischemic stroke

Ischemic injury to the brain secondary to occlusion of a vessel. See Fig. 6.3.

Clinical

Refer to Section 1.8.

Technique

FLAIR, T2, DWI, ADC, Gradient echo T2* and MRA should be performed.

The sensitivity and specificity of MR in early acute stroke is far superior to that of CT. Diffusion-weighted imaging sequences (DWI) will show restricted diffusion in ischemic brain; this occurs because the dying cells swell and restrict the movement of extracellular

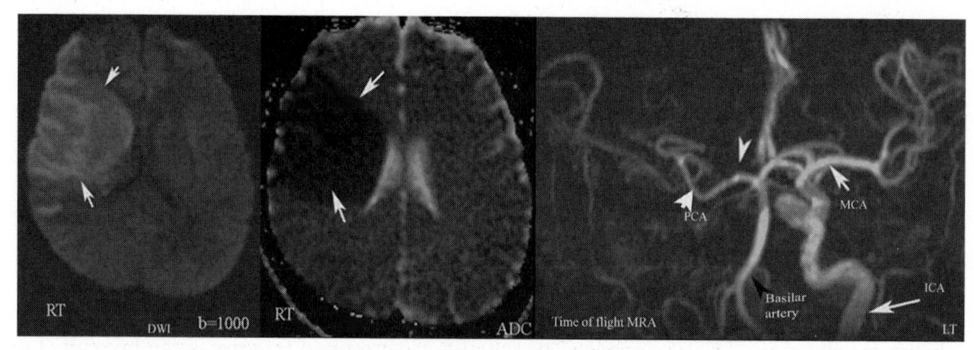

Fig. 6.3. Acute MCA infarction axial DWI image of brain (i) shows high signal (short arrows) and corresponding axial ADC (ii, arrows) shows low signal within the right temporal and frontal cerebral cortex, consistent with acute stroke. MRA TOF image (iii) shows occlusion of entire intracranial ICA and markedly attenuated right MI and A1 (arrowheads).

fluid. This restriction of diffusion can be detected within minutes of onset (at which time the CT will almost certainly be normal). Perfusion MR shows the area of abnormal perfusion, the infarcted brain will have the poorest perfusion and this usually corresponds with the restricted diffusion. In some patients the perfusion defect is seen to extend beyond the area of restricted diffusion; this is likely to be a brain that can be "salvaged" if perfusion can be improved by some form of intervention (e.g. thrombolysis, embolectomy).

Findings

1. In the hyperacute phase (within minutes), DWI shows restricted diffusion (high signal), and perfusion imaging will show decreased perfusion. T1 and T2 will be normal initially, showing sulcal effacement after 2–3 hours (can be subtle). Abnormally increased signal on T2 and FLAIR will develop after approximately 8 hours. On T2 there may be increased signal within the occluded blood vessel (loss of flow void). On MRA, a flow signal in the vessel may be "missing."
2. In the days following a stroke, hyperintensity may be seen on T1-weighted imaging in the damaged cortex. This represents laminar necrosis and is thought to represent lipid-laden macrophage or cholesterol accumulation. It is not a contraindication to anticoagulation. There will be swelling of the infarcted brain; the restricted diffusion will persist for up to about 8 days.
3. If gadolinium is given in the days following stroke there will be enhancement because the blood–brain barrier is broken down. This does not mean that there is an underlying lesion.
4. Old ischemia will be hyperintense on T2, with low signal on T1 (like CSF) and there is loss of brain volume, dependent upon the size of the infarcted area.
5. In the context of new symptoms in a patient with previous ischemia, DWI will identify the acute lesions (hyperintense on DWI and hypointense on ADC).
6. Occlusion of perforating vessels causes infarction of deep structures, e.g. basilar tip occlusion will result in bilateral thalamic and midbrain ischemia. There may or may not be posterior cerebral artery occlusion depending upon the completeness of the circle of Willis.

Pearls

- Acute ischemia will be high signal on DWI and low signal on ADC.
- Always perform both DWI and ADC to evaluate ischemic patients.
- FLAIR imaging is not an ideal sequence to look at old infarcts as they have similar signal to CSF and may suppress on FLAIR.
- Generally gadolinium is not required, it can cause confusing appearances.
- T2 shine through artefact appears as high signal on DWI and ADC.
- Hemorrhages can be seen on gradient echo images.

Suggested reading

Sheerin F, Pretorius PM, Briley D, Meagher T. Differential diagnosis of restricted diffusion confined to the cerebral cortex. *Clin Radiol* 2008;**63**(11):1245–1253.

Wintermark M *et al.* Acute stroke imaging research roadmap. *Stroke* 2008;**39**:1621–1628.

6.4 Intracranial hemorrhage

MRI is very sensitive in identifying microbleeds and small subdural or subtle traumatic subarachnoid hemorrhage. See Fig. 6.4.

Clinical

Refer to Section 1.6.

Technique

Gradient echo sequences (T2*) are more sensitive to susceptibility artefact; this can be used to more readily identify hemosiderin staining from microhemorrhage. MRA may demonstrate a vascular abnormality, phase contrast MRA may be more useful than time-of-flight MRA in the presence of a hematoma, which is not affected by T1 shine-through. Post-contrast imaging may demonstrate an enhancing tumor or small vascular malformation. MRV may demonstrate venous occlusion.

Findings

1. Hemorrhage can have variable signal characteristics depending on how old it is (see Section 7.1). Blood products can sediment within hematomas or the ventricular system, forming layers of differing signal.
2. Several conditions are associated with multiple areas of hemorrhage which may not be seen on CT. Multiple cavernomas, and amyloid angiopathy (15% of spontaneous ICH in over 60s age group). Gradient-echo sequences should be used to identify microhemorrhage.
3. Spontaneous hemorrhage within the cerebellum can have a very distinct margin and appear very rounded. This does not necessarily indicate a bleed in the underlying lesion.

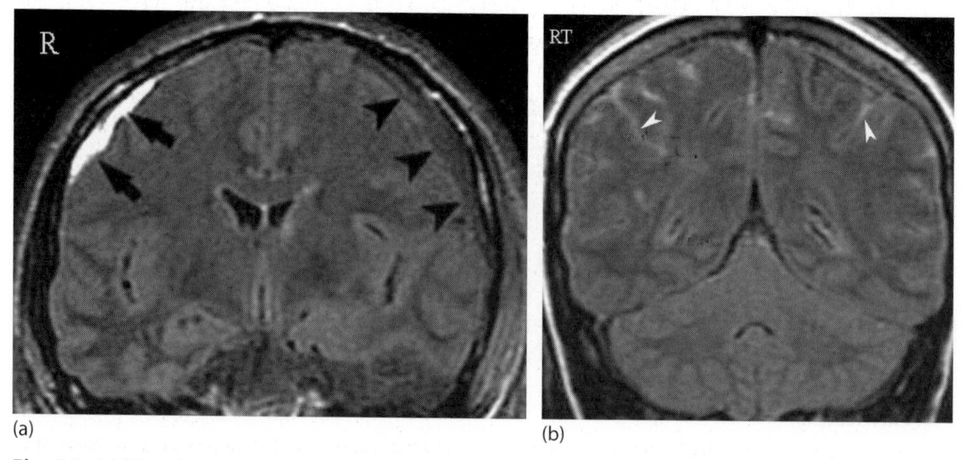

Fig. 6.4. (a) Bilateral subdural hemorrhage. Coronal FLAIR image shows high-signal acute blood (arrows) and low- to intermediate-signal chronic blood (arrowhead) in the right and left subdural space respectively. (b) Traumatic SAH Coronal FLAIR image shows high-signal acute blood in bilateral sulci (arrowheads) with adjacent gyral effacement.

Pearls

- A hematoma may take several months to resolve and artefact from it can mask an underlying lesion for this time. Delayed imaging can be helpful.
- The T1 "shine through" on time-of-flight MRA can obscure an underlying lesion such as an aneurysm or AVM.

Suggested reading

Blitstein MK, Tung GA. MRI of cerebral microhemorrhages. *Am J Roentgenol* 2007;**189**(3):720.

Dainer HM, Smirniotopoulos JG. Neuroimaging of hemorrhage and vascular malformations. *Semin Neurol* 2008;**28**(4):533–547.

6.5 Epidural abscess and discitis

Infection of an intervertebral disc usually involving adjacent bone; the epidural space may also be involved. The epidural space can be seeded with infection without discitis or osteomyelitis. See Fig. 6.5.

Clinical

Discitis: Back pain which may be severe, radicular symptoms, fever, weight loss.

Epidural abscess: Occurs without discitis in approximately 60% of cases. It usually involves the posterior epidural space in the thoracic region. Back pain (chest pain) is usually present, and radicular symptoms are common.

Systemic symptoms are less common than in discitis. Vascular compromise can result in sudden deterioration.

Staphylococcus aureus is the commonest organism. Generally thought to be hematogeneous spread.

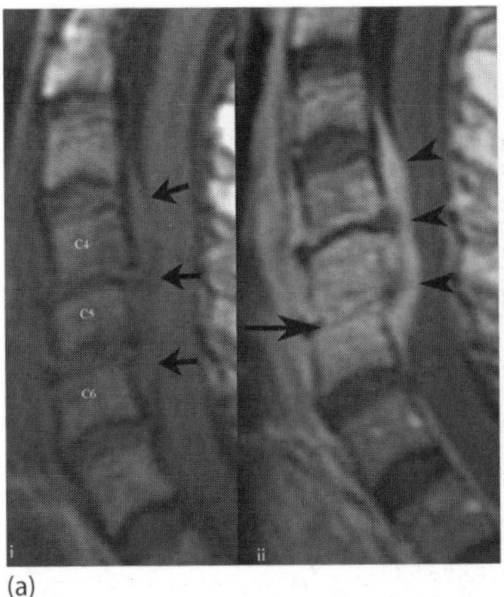

(a)

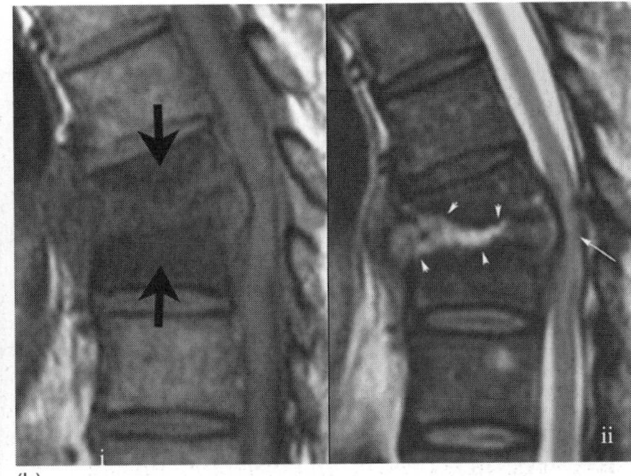

(b)

Fig. 6.5. (a) Discitis with epidural abscess. Sagittal T1 C-spine MRI (i) shows intermediate signal disc space at C4–5, C5–6 and an epidural mass (black arrow) which enhances on post-contrast T1 GRE (ii, arrowheads, arrow indicates disc enhancement). (b) Mid-thoracic discitis. Sagittal MRI of thoracic spine shows increased signal within the disc space on T2 (ii, arrowheads). The adjacent vertebral bodies have a lower signal than normal because of marrow edema (i, arrows) on T1-weighted images.

Technique

T1 and T2 sagittal and axial images. STIR images will show fluid in discs, bone and the epidural space more clearly. Post-gadolinium T1 sagittal and axial images (can use fat-suppression).

Findings

Discitis

1. High signal fluid in the disc space on T2 and STIR.
2. The disc may have lost considerable height.
3. Paraspinal collections are common (often psoas abscess).
4. Enhancement of the disc with contrast. Meningeal enhancement is common.
5. Vertebral body involvement can result in endplate collapse and vertebral body collapse.
6. Occasionally bone fragments are displaced into the epidural space – this can cause cord compression.
7. Associated epidural abscess – usually in the anterior, or lateral epidural space, and limited to the levels above and below the infected disc (tight dural attachments to the bones anteriorly).

Epidural abscess

1. Displacement of the dura may be seen on T1 and T2.
2. Precontrast STIR images will demonstrate a high-signal epidural collection.
3. Low or heterogeneous on T1, difficult to see on T2 (due to high-signal fat).
4. Fat-saturated T1 will show enhancement.

Pearls

- Patients can be remarkably well with back pain alone.
- Always consider in patients who develop recurrent back pain a few weeks after back surgery.
- Look for associated collections.
- A tissue sample, and blood cultures, should be taken prior to antibiotics if at all possible.
- The posterior epidural space is quite large and collections here can extend for a long distance up and down the spine.

Suggested reading

An HS, Seldomridge JA. Spinal infections: diagnostic tests and imaging studies. *Clin Orthop Relat Res* 2006;**444**:27–33.

Cottle L, Riordan T. Infectious spondylodiscitis. *J Infect* 2008;**56**(6):401–412.

Tali ET. Spinal infections. *Eur J Radiol* 2004;**50**(2):120–133.

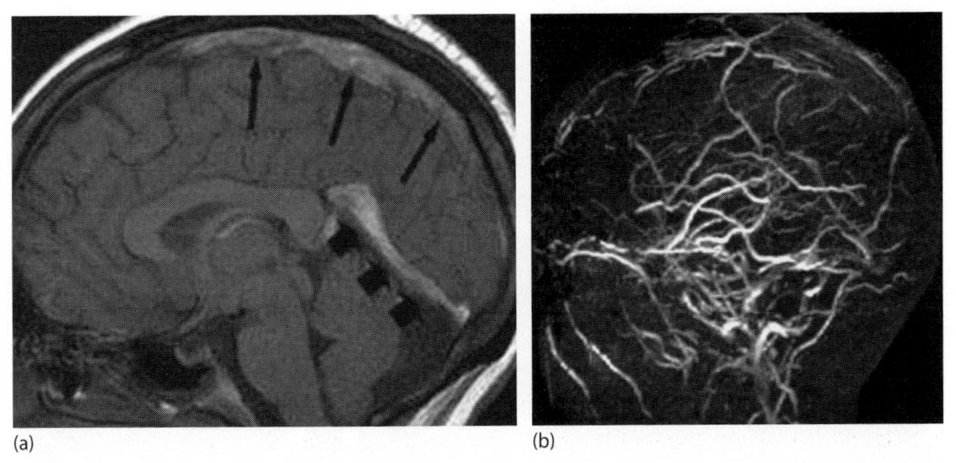

Fig. 6.6. Venous sinus thrombosis. (a) T1 sagittal image of brain without contrast shows hyperintense clot in the straight sinus (short arrows) and the superior sagittal sinus (long arrows). (b) MIP image from a time-of-flight MR venogram showing absence of the large sinuses.

6.6 Cerebral vein or sinus thrombosis

Occlusion of either a superficial or deep cerebral vein/sinus with thrombus. See Fig. 6.6.

Clinical

Refer to Section 1.7.

Technique

T1 sagittal, T2/FLAIR axial/coronal, MR venogram.

Findings

1. High signal-intensity thrombus within cerebral veins on T1 (subacute clot).
2. Absence of flow voids in the cerebral veins.
3. Areas of peripheral hemorrhage often at the gray-white junction.
4. Patchy areas of high signal in the brain parenchyma.
5. Absence of flow in venous structures on the MR venogram.
6. Look for causative factors such as sinusitis, meningiomas, etc.

Pearls

- Clinical presentation is non-specific; the diagnosis is often made by the radiologist.
- Deep venous occlusion is less common and easier to miss if not specifically looked for.
- The transverse sinuses are often asymmetrical. If there is doubt about whether a sinus is partly occluded or just small, CT to look at the jugular foramina can be helpful to see if they are asymmetrical.

Suggested reading

Refer to Section 1.7.

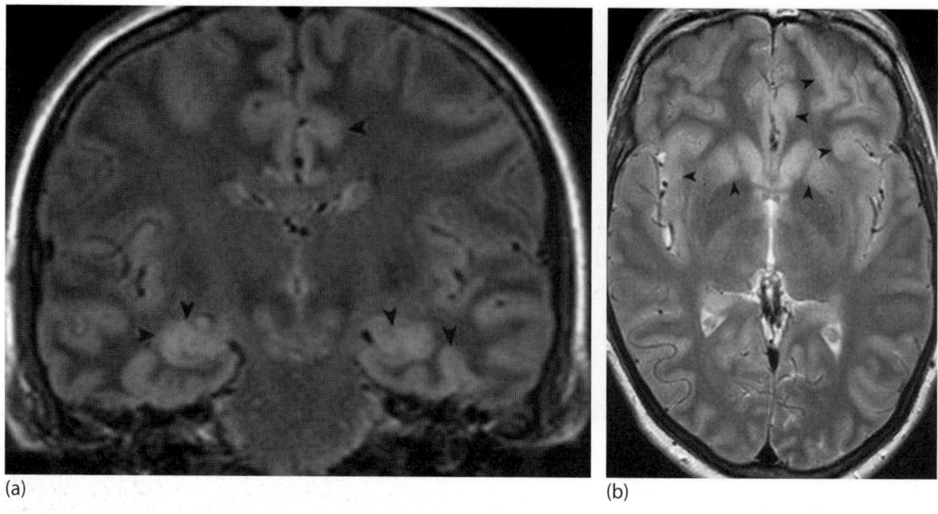

Fig. 6.7. (a) Herpes simplex encephalitis. Coronal T2 FLAIR image of brain shows typical bilateral temporal lobe hyperintensity (arrowheads). (b) Encephalitis. Axial T2 image of brain in a patient with rabies encephalitis shows widespread bilateral gray matter hyperintensity (arrowheads) including basal ganglia.

6.7 Encephalitis

Infection of the brain parenchyma, usually viral. See Fig. 6.7.

Clinical

Refer to Section 1.10.

Technique

CT may appear normal.
T1, T2 and T2 FLAIR.
Coronal FLAIR is the best sequence for the temporal lobes.

Findings

1. The process is usually multifocal with scattered hyperintensity that may become confluent.
2. The temporal lobes are most commonly involved.
3. Affects both gray and white matter.
4. Small areas of acute hemorrhage may be seen in very aggressive disease
5. If gadolinium is given, enhancement may be seen in both the brain parenchyma and in the meninges.

Pearls

- *Herpes* is the most common pathogen.
- The imaging findings are non-specific to the pathogen.
- Inflammation of the medial temporal lobe only (limbic encephalitis) can be seen as a paraneoplastic condition.
- Infiltrative glioma can simulate encephalitis.

Suggested reading

Refer to Section 1.10.

Shankar SK. Neuropathology of viral infections of the central nervous system. *Neuroimaging Clin N Am* 2008;**18**(1):19–39.

6.8 Cauda equina syndrome

The spinal cord usually terminates above the L2 level. The descending nerve roots form the cauda equina. The most common cause of cauda equina compression is a prolapsed intervertebral disc, followed by malignant disease, rarely trauma and epidural abscess. See Fig. 6.8.

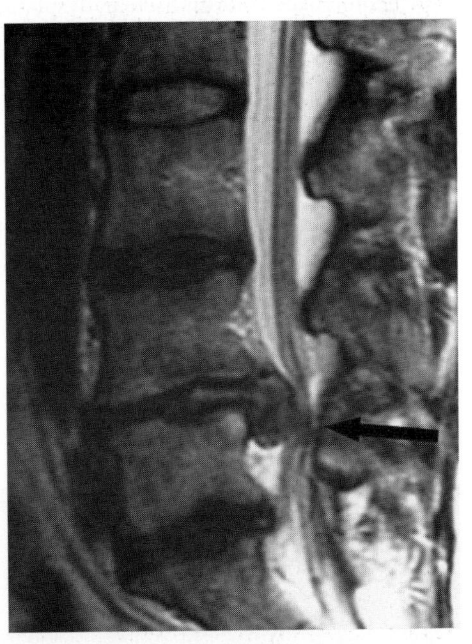

Fig. 6.8. Cauda equina syndrome. T2 sagittal image of lumbar spine demonstrates a large prolapsed L4/L5 disc (arrow) with significant compression of thecal sac by the large disc prolapse.

Clinical

Sciatica (often bilateral), leg weakness, saddle paresthesia and sphincter disturbance.

Technique

T1 and T2 sagittal and axial sequences will demonstrate most pathology. Post-gadolinium and STIR if tumor or infection are present, or in patients with prior spine surgery.

Findings

1. Usually extradural compression of the thecal sac and cauda equina.
2. Prolapsed intervertebral disc with or without sequestered segment most commonly.
3. Malignant disease may replace fatty marrow making the vertebral body lower in signal than normal on T1. It will usually enhance post-contrast, as will epidural collections.

Pearls

- Cauda equina syndrome with loss of bladder/sphincter function is a surgical emergency.
- If compression is not relieved within 48 hours of symptom onset, permanent deficit commonly results. Rapid decompression (< 48 hours) results in a much better prognosis.
- Many patients with a clinical cauda equina syndrome will not have significant cauda equina compression on MR.
- Myelography can be used if MRI is contraindicated.

Suggested reading

Mauffrwey C *et al.* Cauda Equina syndrome: an anatomically driven review. *Br J Hosp Med (Lond)* 2008;**69**(6):344–347.

Winters ME, Kluetz P, Zilberstein J. Back pain emergencies. *Med Clin North Am* 2006;**90**(3):505–523.

6.9 Vessel dissection

Intramural hematoma due to an intimal tear in an artery wall. Dissection is the cause of up to 20% of TIA and stroke in young adults (< 30 years). Carotid dissection accounts for 75%, vertebral for 15%. Intracranial dissection accounts for 10% and may present as subarachnoid hemorrhage. Fibromuscular dysplasia is seen in 15% and is associated with multi-vessel dissection. See Fig. 6.9.

Clinical

Refer to Section 1.15

Technique

T2 axial, FLAIR coronal, and diffusion-weighted imaging of the brain. MRA of the Circle of Willis. MRA of the carotid and vertebral arteries. Pre-contrast T1 fat-saturation axial images of the neck and skull base.

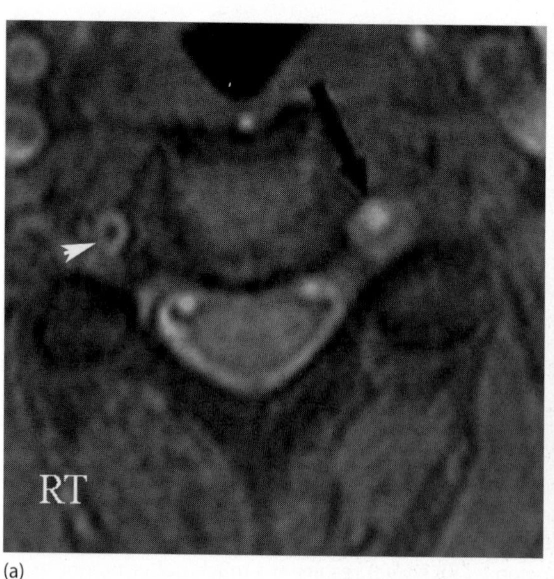

(a)

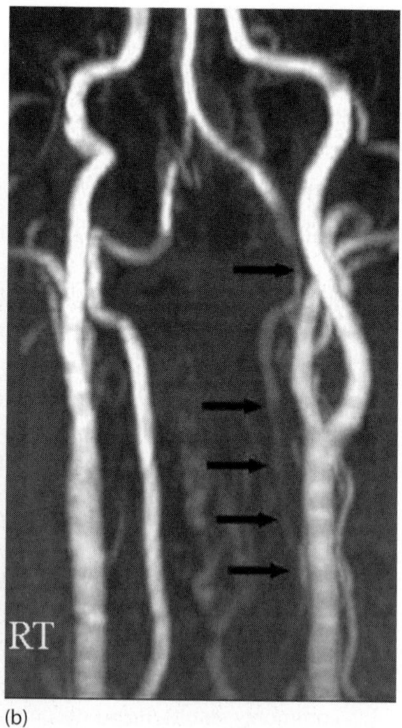

(b)

Fig. 6.9. Vertebral artery dissection. (a) Axial T1 fat-saturation TSE sequence shows semilunar mural high signal in the dilated left vertebral artery (arrow) due to acute intramural hematoma. Also note the normal flow void in the right vertebral artery (arrow). (b) An MIP image from a TOF MRA showing very poor flow in the lower part of the left vertebral artery (arrows) due to dissection.

Findings

1. Brain imaging may show evidence of acute ischemia, even if clinically silent, with restricted diffusion, and possibly increased signal on T2.
2. The normal flow voids seen in the vertebral or carotid arteries may be filled in with clot.
3. Most carotid dissections are just below the skull base, but do extend into the carotid canal.
4. Intracranial MRA may show reduced flow in a carotid siphon or vertebral artery. It may show irregularity of an intracranial vessel if this is involved.
5. Cervical MRA may show irregularity, stenosis, occlusion or dilatation of vessels.
6. The T1 fat-saturation axial images may show crescent-shaped high signal in the vessel wall representing the intramural clot. Alternatively the whole vessel may be high signal if occluded.

Pearls

- On time-of-flight MRA, T1 high signal will shine through – this can mask stenosis in a vessel so the T1 imaging is mandatory.
- Ensure that the fat saturation has been effective.
- Look for an intracranial dissection.
- Posterior inferior cerebellar territory infarcts are often associated with vertebral artery dissection.

Suggested reading

Refer to Section 1.15.

6.10 Central pontine myelinolysis

Non-inflammatory demyelination within the central pons usually secondary to rapid correction of hyponatremia. See Fig. 6.10.

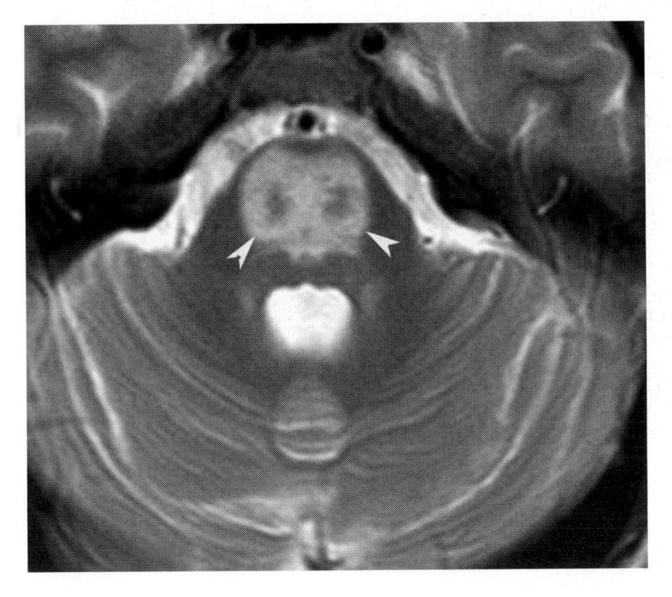

Fig. 6.10. Central pontine myelinolysis. Axial FLAIR image of the brain in an elderly patient with decreased consciousness following rehydration shows central high signal within the pons (arrows). No mass effect is seen.

Clinical

Decreased consciousness levels, brainstem signs (gaze paresis, dysarthria, dysphagia etc.), weakness and paralysis may develop. The patient may become "locked in." Patients may improve over weeks and months but mortality and morbidity are high.

Technique

T1 sagittal, T2 axial and T2 FLAIR coronal imaging.

Findings

1. High signal lesion, on T2-weighted images, within the central pons, there may be some heterogenicity of the signal which represents increased water.
2. There may be swelling of the pons.
3. Hypointense to adjacent brain on T1-weighted images.
4. No contrast enhancement.
5. Extrapontine involvement in 10% (basal ganglia, thalamus, midbrain and cerebellum).
6. In the late stage there may be a CSF signal defect within the pons which can be variable in size.

Pearls

- Usually these patients have been in hospital unwell, or have had a preceding illness.
- Onset of symptoms usually 48–72 hours after IV fluid therapy.
- CT scan is usually normal.
- Prognosis is poor; there is no treatment other than supportive.
- The size of the lesion on MRI does not appear to predict prognosis.

Suggested reading

Kumar S, Fowler M, Gonzalez-Toledo E, Jaffe SL. Central pontine myelinolysis, an update. *Neurol Res* 2006;**28**(3):360–366.

6.11 Pituitary apoplexy

Acute hemorrhage or infarction of the pituitary gland. There is usually a pre-existing adenoma. See Fig. 6.11.

Clinical

Headache, diplopia, nausea and vomiting, field defect, decreased visual acuity. May have pre-existing pituitary dysfunction but often the adenoma will be clinically silent. Sheehan's syndrome is a special case where the pituitary is normal but undergoes infarction post-partum.

Technique

T1 and T2 sagittal and coronal of the pituitary, T2 axial of the brain.

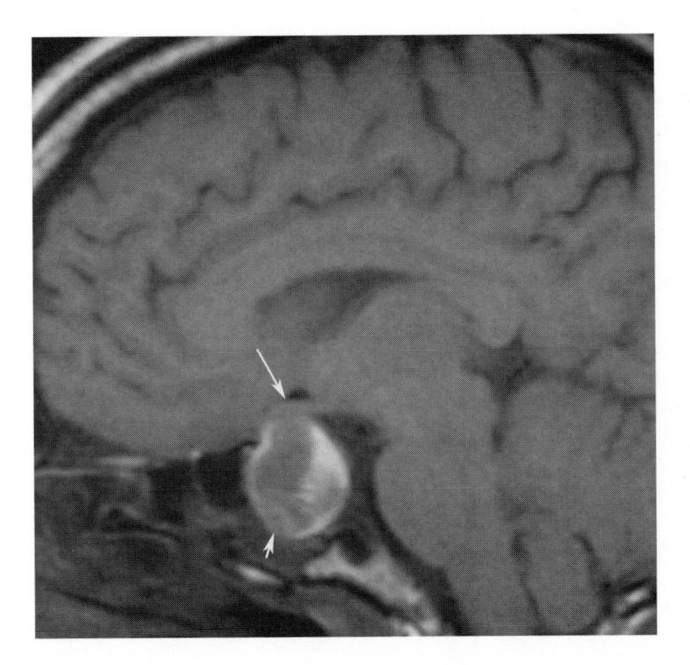

Fig. 6.11. Pituitary apoplexy. T1 sagittal image of the brain shows mixed signal hemorrhage within the pituitary macroadenoma (short arrow). Note an expanded pituitary fossa causing compression, elevation and displacement of the optic chiasm (long arrow).

Findings

1. Increased signal in the pituitary gland on T1 which may be somewhat heterogeneous, representing blood.
2. The pituitary gland is usually enlarged and the pituitary fossa is usually expanded. The pituitary may not be enlarged.
3. There may be only a small area of hemorrhage, or infarction alone with increased T2 signal.
4. In cystic pituitary tumors, blood may be contained within the cyst – this can be mistaken for proteinaceous fluid.
5. The optic chiasm may or may not be compressed.

Pearls

- The clinical diagnosis can be difficult if the only symptom is headache – always review the pituitary gland.
- The presence of visual failure makes this a neurosurgical emergency: Failure to decompress the optic nerves rapidly may result in permanent vision loss.
- The posterior part of the pituitary is normally high signal on T1 due to the presence of neuropeptides.

6.12 Spinal trauma

Traumatic injury to the spinal column and/or the spinal cord. The role of MRI is to identify the cause of neurological deficit in the absence of significant bony injury and prognostically to predict if neurological recovery is likely. See Fig. 6.12.

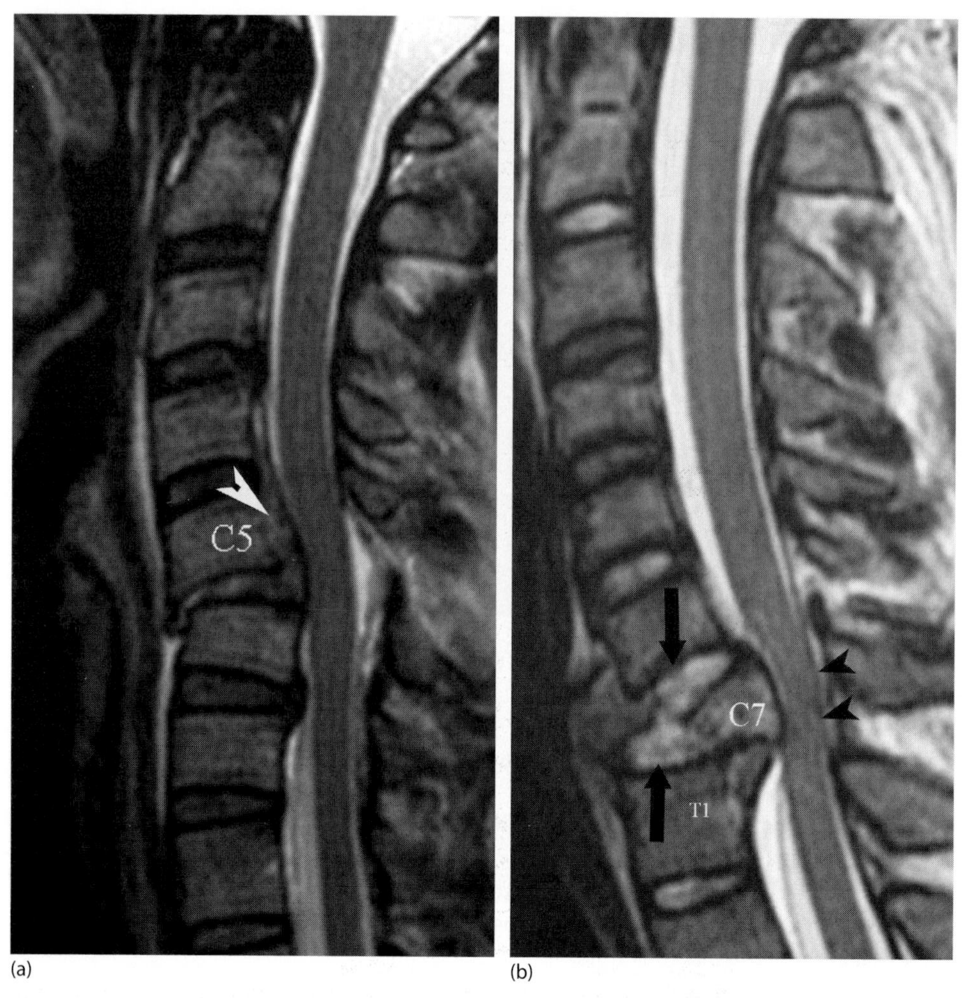

Fig. 6.12. (a) Spinal trauma. Sagittal STIR image of cervical spine in a patient with C5/C6 fracture demonstrates high-signal hemorrhage within the intervertebral disc and a small epidural hematoma (arrowhead), which is causing mild cord compression. Note high-signal prevertebral hematoma along the anterior longitudinal ligament. (b) C-spine burst fracture. Sagittal T2 image of the cervical spine in a patient with a C7 burst fracture shows hemorrhage (large arrows) and cord compression with subtle increase in cord signal due to edema/hematoma (arrowheads).

Clinical

Very dependent on the type and severity of the injury. Cord injury can result from direct contusion, but can also result from vascular compromise.

Technique

Sagittal T1, T2, and STIR and axial T2 through any abnormality.

Findings

1. Bone marrow edema is bright on STIR (the most sensitive sequence for bone injury).
2. Associated epidural hematoma visible as high signal on STIR and T1.

3. High signal anterior and posterior spinal ligaments (normally low signal). This finding alone is a sign of unstable spinal injury.
4. Associated traumatic disc herniation, particularly in the cervical segment, which can compromise the cord.
5. If there has been vascular compromise, the appearances can be normal in the acute stage. Within 24 hours there will usually be high signal in the cord with associated swelling. Typically cord edema (bright on T2 and STIR) is said to have "flame" shaped edges.
6. At areas of focal cord compression there will be increased signal in the cord with swelling of the cord.

Pearls

- Neurological deficit may be very transient but needs to be investigated.
- Minor trauma to pathological bone can result in significant injury.
- Look for ligamentous injury.
- Whole spine STIR sagittal images are an effective screen for associated spine injury elsewhere.

Suggested reading

Kaji A, Hockberger R. Imaging of spinal cord injuries. *Emerg Med Clin N Am* 2007;**25**(3):735–50, ix.

Yucesoy K, Yuksel KZ. SCIWORA in MRI era. *Clin Neurol Neurosurg* 2008;**110**(5):429–433.

6.13 Aortic dissection

MRI has very high sensitivity and specificity for detecting dissection and intramural hematoma. MRI is very useful in order to differentiate an intramural hematoma from an atherosclerotic plaque. See Fig. 6.13.

Indication

Contraindications to contrast CTA due to history of iodinated contrast reaction and renal failure. To further establish the diagnosis of intramural hematoma (if non-contrast CT was not helpful).

Technique

Multiplanar steady-state free-precession (SSFP), pre-contrast fat-saturated T1 GRE. Contrast-enhanced MRA (CE-MRA) × 2 passes, and post-contrast GRE. Dynamic time resolved MRA (TR-MRA, if available.) Cine imaging of the aorta with SSFP, if needed.

SSFP is an ultrafast single-shot bright-blood technique in which blood appears high signal. HASTE is a fast turbo-spin echo used for black blood-imaging of aorta and cardiac chambers. Fast-flowing blood appears black and slow flow blood may appear intermediate signal. Pre-contrast T1 GRE depicts intramural blood as high signal.

TR MRA: High temporal resolution dynamic MRA which requires only 3–5 ml of contrast to assess sequential filling of false and true lumens in communicating dissection, end organ perfusion especially bilateral renals, and contrast filling of branch vessels.

However, small vascular details are better depicted on conventional CE-MRA.

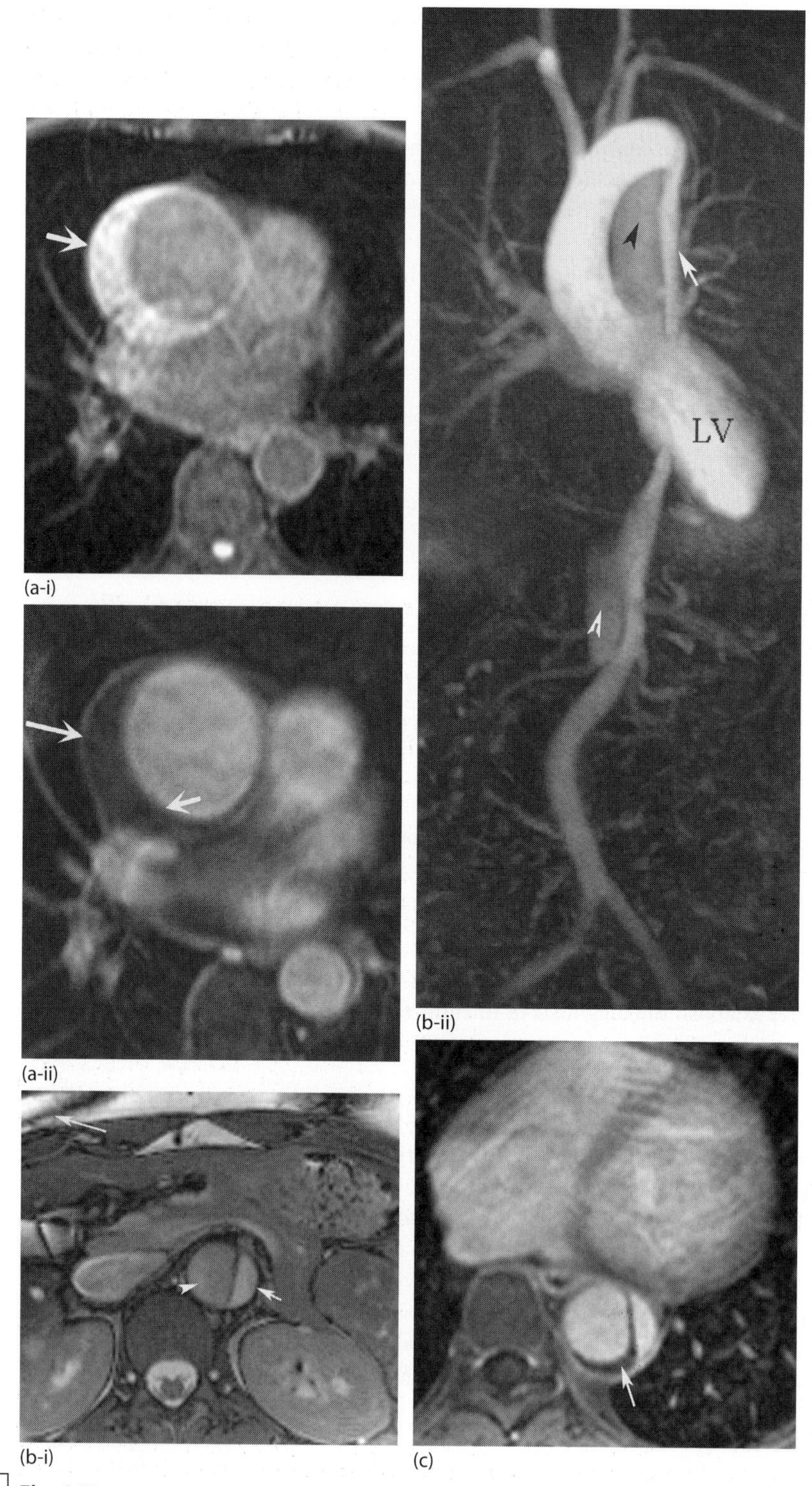

Fig. 6.13.

For rapid detection of aortic dissection, SSFP (axial, sagittal, coronal), HASTE (axial), pre-contrast T1 GRE (axial) are sufficient. If there is an aortic dissection flap on the pre-contrast images, then CE-MRA and post-contrast axial T1 GRE images may be performed.

For non-contrast MRA of aorta (due to risk of NSF or prior allergy to gadolinium), apart from SSFP, HASTE and T1 GRE, SSFP cine images of the aorta in sagittal plane (candy cane views with no more than 4–5 slices), can be performed.

Free breathing 3D SSFP MRA can be performed to assess thoracic aorta in patients where administration of intravenous contrast is not desirable.

Findings

1. Dissection flap is seen as a low-signal linear structure.
2. True and false lumen (early and late filling lumen).
3. Fenestrations.
4. Aneurysm.
5. Entry and exit points.
6. Branch vessels origin and involvement.
7. Extension of the dissection flap.
8. End organ ischemia: Renal infarction, bowel ischemia.
9. Intramural hematoma (IMH): High signal on pre-contrast fat-saturated T1 GRE sequence. No communicating dissection flap.

Pearls

- True and false lumens are easily differentiated on the timing sequence and dynamic time-resolved contrast MRA.
- IMH appears as low signal (no perfusion) on CE-MRA and post-contrast T1 GRE images due to absence of communication with true lumen; junior radiologists can potentially miss this important finding. Non-contrast CT may be complementary and it may show displacement of intimal calcification and mural high density.
- Atherosclerotic thrombus is low density, and margins are irregular with or without associated aneurysm.
- Signal changes of thrombosed clot within the false lumen can simulate as IMH, but should be differentiated by the appearance of differential enhancement/filling of two lumens and the presence of dissection flap in communicating dissection.
- Extravasation of contrast is consistent with rupture – it is important to obtain at least 2–3 passes of contrast MRA and followed by post-contrast 2D or 3D T1 GRE images.
- SSFP sequence will show dissection flap within a few seconds of scan. Gated SSFP may be helpful to assess the aortic root without motion artefacts.
- Traumatic pseudoaneurysm is well appreciated on the sagittal images. It has an irregular margin, and acute angle to aorta, and is usually associated with mediastinal hematoma.

Caption for Fig. 6.13 (a) Intramural hematoma. (i) Axial precontrast TI GRE image shows a thick crescentic mural high signal within the ascending aortic wall. (ii) Axial post-contrast T1 GRE shows the hematoma as low signal and note the typical smooth margin of the opacified aortic lumen. (b) Type B aortic dissection image. (i) Axial SSFP image shows a low-signal intimal flap in the descending aorta separating the true lumen (small arrow) from false lumen (arrowhead). (ii) Single frame of TE MRA shows early opacification of the true lumen (arrow). Prompt enhancement of the false lumen in the proximal descending (black arrowhead) and upper abdominal aorta (arrowhead) is due to fenestrations. (c) Aortic dissection. Post-contrast T1 fat-saturated GRE in a different patient with type B dissection shows a low signal intimal flap separating the perfused false and true lumina. Note the dark signal thrombus (arrow) in the false lumen.

Suggested reading

Krishnam MS *et al.* Noncontrast 3D SSFP MRA of the whole chest: comparison with contrast-enhanced MRA. *Invest Radiol* 2008;**43**(6):411–420.

Lohan DG *et al.* MR imaging of the thoracic aorta. *Magn Reson Imaging Clin N Am* 2008;**16**(2): 213–234.

Roberts DA. Magnetic resonance imaging of thoracic aortic aneurysm and dissection. *Semin Roentgenol* 2001;**36**(4):295–308.

6.14 Acute pulmonary embolism

CT angiography is the investigation of choice but MRA may be indicated in certain patients with suspected pulmonary thromboembolism. MRA has high sensitivity and specificity for detecting PE especially up to segmental pulmonary branch arteries. See Fig. 6.14.

Clinical

Refer to Section 2.7.

Indications

Pregnant women, history of allergic reaction to iodinated contrast, and high serum creatinine. MRI/A is a great tool in the follow-up of patients with chronic PE including in the assessment of right heart function.

Technique

MRI and MRA chest.
Essential sequences:

Multiplanar SSFP–axial, sagittal and coronal planes.
Coronal CE-MRA timed at main pulmonary artery × 2 passes.
Axial and coronal high-resolution post-contrast 3D GRE.

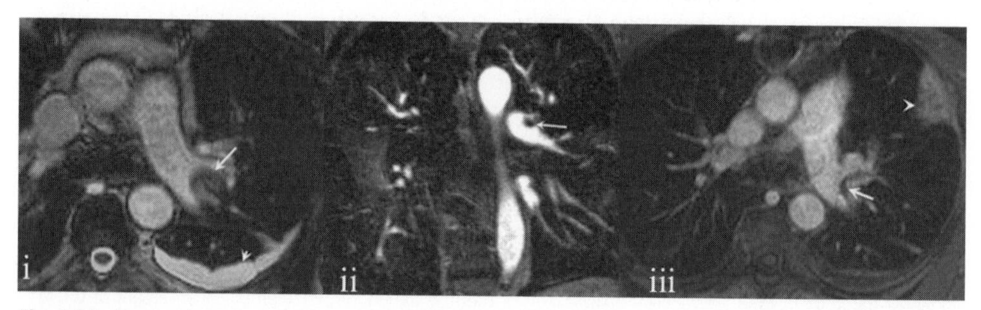

Fig. 6.14. Acute pulmonary embolism. Axial SSFP (i) CEMRA (ii) and post-contrast T1 GRE (iii) images show a low-signal embolus in the distal left main pulmonary artery. Note peripheral wedge shaped consolidation (iii, arrowhead) in the left upper lobe.

Optional sequences:

Axial pre-contrast T1 GRE: Important to have in patients with an atypical chest pain to detect IMH.

Coronal time-resolved MRA.

Limited SSFP cine imaging of heart: 3 short axis and 1 horizontal long axis (4 chamber) views (optional).

Findings

1. Near-occlusive low-signal filling defect within the dilated pulmonary artery – acute thrombus.
2. Enlarged main PA.
3. Sudden cut-off of affected pulmonary arteries.
4. Wall adherent thrombus in chronic PE (arterial diameter may be reduced).
5. Decreased/delayed or absent segmental perfusion of lung parenchyma on dynamic time resolved MRA. CE-MRA shows decreased segmental enhancement of lung parenchyma (mosaicism).
6. Pleural effusion: High signal on SSFP and low signal on contrast MRA and GRE images.
7. Peripheral consolidation.
8. Right heart enlargement (>45 mm measured transversely at end diastole near the basal RV cavity or greater than LV diameter at corresponding level).

Pearls

- Contrast MRA should be performed if there is a clinical indication. Time-resolved MRA may demonstrate dynamic perfusion of the lungs and it may be sufficient to exclude central and proximal PE.
- In pregnant women, the total dose of contrast should be kept minimum (low-dose contrast MRA can be performed).
- Post-contrast images are useful to see low-signal thrombus. Enhancing peri-thrombotic inflammatory soft tissue can be seen rarely.
- Wall adherent thrombus, web, calcification along the wall (low signal) are suggestive of post-thrombotic changes, and with enlarged main PA and segmental perfusion defects, represent chronic PE.
- Post-contrast 3D T1 GRE images of the pelvis and lower extremity can be performed at the same sitting to evaluate for deep vein thrombosis.
- Cine imaging of the heart can be performed to assess right ventricular strain, dilatation and intracardiac thrombus.

Suggested reading

Kluge A *et al.* Real-time MR with TrueFISP for the detection of acute pulmonary embolism: initial clinical experience. *Eur Radiol* 2004;**14**(4):709–718.

Krishnam MS *et al.* Low-dose, time-resolved, contrast-enhanced 3D MR angiography in cardiac and vascular diseases: correlation to high spatial resolution 3D contrast-enhanced MRA. *Clin Radiol* 2008;**63**(7):744–755.

Pedersen MR, Fisher MT, van Beek EJ. MR imaging of pulmonary vasculature – an update. *Eur Radiol* 2006;**16**(6):1374–1386.

6.15 Myocardial viability

In non-viable myocardium (chronic infarction), the myocytes are dead and there is decreased or no chance of recovery after revascularization. In hibernating (chronic ischemia) or stunned (acute stress) myocardium, the LV myocardial function may be decreased but myocytes are viable, therefore, the cardiac function is potentially recoverable after revascularization. See Fig. 6.15.

Contrast-enhanced MRI is the current gold standard technique to assess for myocardial viability.

Clinical

Indications: Myocarditis, atypical chest pain, acute coronary syndrome (ideally after 24–48 hours of onset), prior to revascularization in a known ischemic heart-disease patient, with or without infarction, and cardiomyopathy.

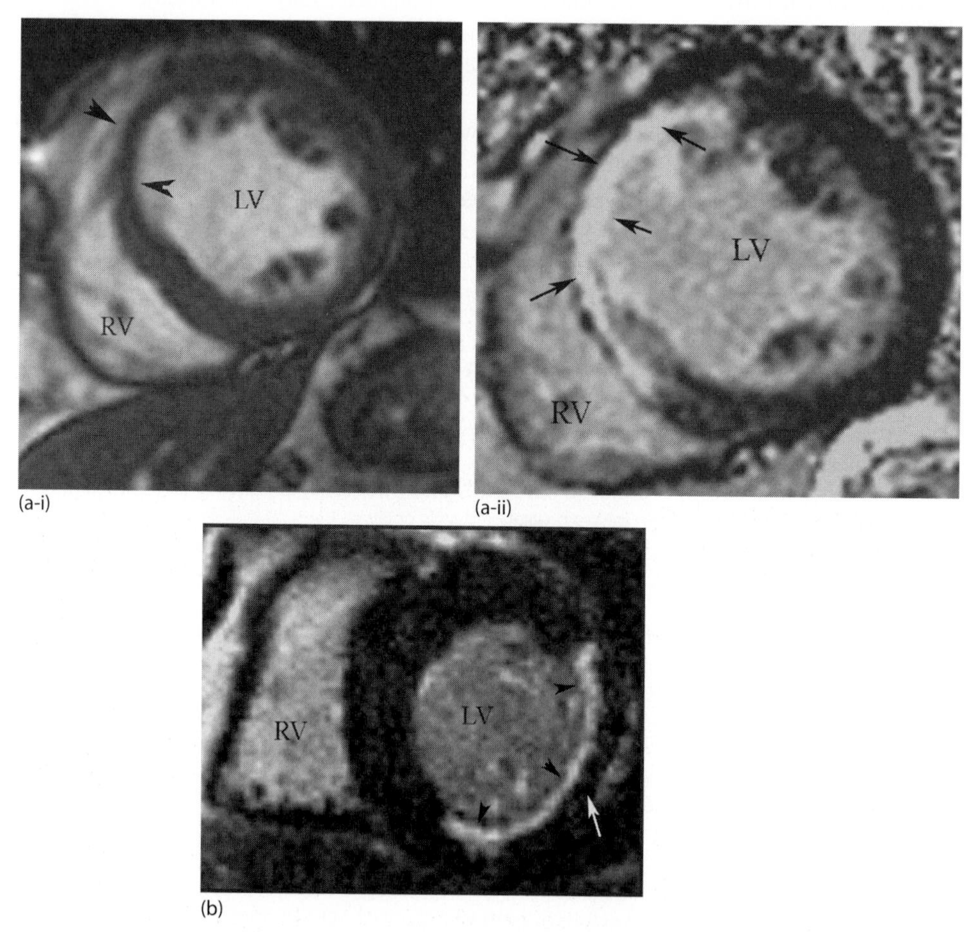

Fig. 6.15. (a) Transmural myocardial infarction. (i) Single frame of short-axis cine MRI shows marked segmental thinning of anterioseptal wall of mid LV. (ii) Delayed post-contrast phase sensitive T1 inversion recovery (IR) image at the corresponding level shows near transmural hyperenhancement of anteroseptal myocardium. (b) Subendocardial LV infarction. Delayed post-contrast T1 IR magnitude image shows segmental linear subendocardial hyperenhancement in the inferolateral LV myocardium with less than 50% transmural extent.

Technique

SSFP cine imaging of the heart, and T1 post-contrast delayed enhancement imaging.

For delayed enhancement, T1 scout images should be performed to decide accurate time to null the myocardium (usually 230–260 ms). Single or double dose of gadolinium (0.1–0.2 mmol/kg) can be given, imaging is usually performed after 10 minutes. Minimum of three short axis slices through the ventricles (3 slices: base, mid and apical), one vertical long axis (2-chamber view showing LA, mitral valve, LV) and one horizontal long axis view of heart (4-chamber view showing RV, LV, RA, LA and AV valves) should be obtained.

Findings

1. Decreased segmental wall motion and thinning of myocardium on cine images.
2. High signal (delayed or late hyperenhancement) in the myocardium on the delayed post-contrast images.
3. Subendocardial pattern of myocardial hyperenhancement.
4. No reflow zone is seen as linear low signal within the subendocardium of delayed myocardial hyperenhancement.
5. Intra-cardiac low signal along the enhancing myocardium indicates thrombus. May be appreciated on cine images but it is better seen on first-pass perfusion and post-contrast delayed images. Mostly it appears as low signal due to hypovascularity.

Pearls

- Segmental linear subendocardial pattern of delayed myocardial enhancement along the coronary arterial distribution is consistent with infarction.
- Less than 50% transmural enhancement of LV myocardium indicates that the adjacent non-enhancing myocardium is viable and adequate and would benefit from revascularization therapy (bypass surgery or angioplasty/stent) to improve cardiac function.
- $>$75% of transmural delayed enhancement indicates that there is negligible recoverable (viable) myocardium and therefore revascularization would not be beneficial in improving the overall ejection fraction.
- Non-subendocardial, patchy, ovoid myocardial enhancement (epicardial or mid-wall) in a non-arterial distribution is suggestive of inflammation/infiltration or scar due to a non-ischemic etiology. The differential diagnosis includes myocarditis, infiltrative disease (sarcoid, amyloid), and rarely, multiple embolic infarction. Mid-wall enhancement is seen in non-ischemic idiopathic dilated cardiomyopathy. Diffuse subendocardial pattern of enhancement may be seen in amyloid and endomyocardial fibroelastosis.
- Ischemia alone does not produce delayed hyperenhancement. It is diagnosed by detecting segmental subendocardial reversible perfusion defect (low signal) on adenosine stress and rest MR imaging. Stress adenosine is usually not performed in the acute setting. Rest perfusion may be helpful in acute setting.
- T2 edema sequence may show myocardial edema in acute infarction.
- Linear low signal within the delayed hyperenhancement denotes microvascular obstruction resulting in the no-reflow phenomenon. Marker of poor prognosis as it forms a substrate for malignant re-entry tachyarrhythymias.
- Segmental hyperenhancement in multiple territories indicates poor outcome.
- LV myocardial segments: Base (Mitral valve to tip of papillary muscle): 6 segments – anterior, anteroseptal, anterolateral, inferior, inferolateral and inferoseptal. Middle

(tip of papillary muscles to its insertion): 6 segments as basal. Apical (distal to insertion of papillary muscles): 4 segments – anterior, inferior, lateral, septal.

- Left anterior descending artery supplies anterior, anteroseptal and apex.
- Right coronary artery supplies inferior, and inferoseptal walls.
- Left circumflex coronary artery supplies lateral wall.

Suggested reading

Vogel-Claussen J *et al.* Delayed enhancement MR imaging: utility in myocardial assessment. *RadioGraphics* 2006;**26**(3):795–810.

6.16 Acute deep vein thrombosis

Intraluminal clot formation within the major draining veins. See Fig. 6.16.

Clinical

SVC obstruction can result in facial and upper extremity edema, engorged veins in the neck, face and arm, and breathlessness.

Indication

Ultrasound is technically difficult for reliable assessment of pelvic veins, IVC and central chest veins like SVC.

Technique

MRI axial and coronal SSSP; pre-contrast axial and coronal GRE (optional in tumor thrombus); coronal MRA, 2–3 passes (40 s delay between 2nd and 3rd passes); and axial and coronal post-contrast GRE (must).
Timing of chest and upper extremity MRV: Pulmonary artery and then 2 passes.
For abdominal, pelvis and lower extremity MRV: Aorta and then 2 passes.

Findings

1. Thrombus is low signal on SSFP.
2. Acute clot may be high signal on T1w GRE.
3. Clot is avascular and shows no enhancement on post-contrast sequences.
4. Post-contrast GRE images better define venous wall and useful to assess post-thrombotic stricture.
5. Dilated and tortuous collaterals. Clot may extend to collaterals.

Pearls

- Acute clot is usually near-occlusive and results in dilated vein and "tram line" sign.
- In chronic DVT, there is non-occlusive and wall-adherent low-signal thrombus. The affected veins may be decreased in caliber. Post-thrombotic venous strictures may be seen. Extensive collateral veins are common.

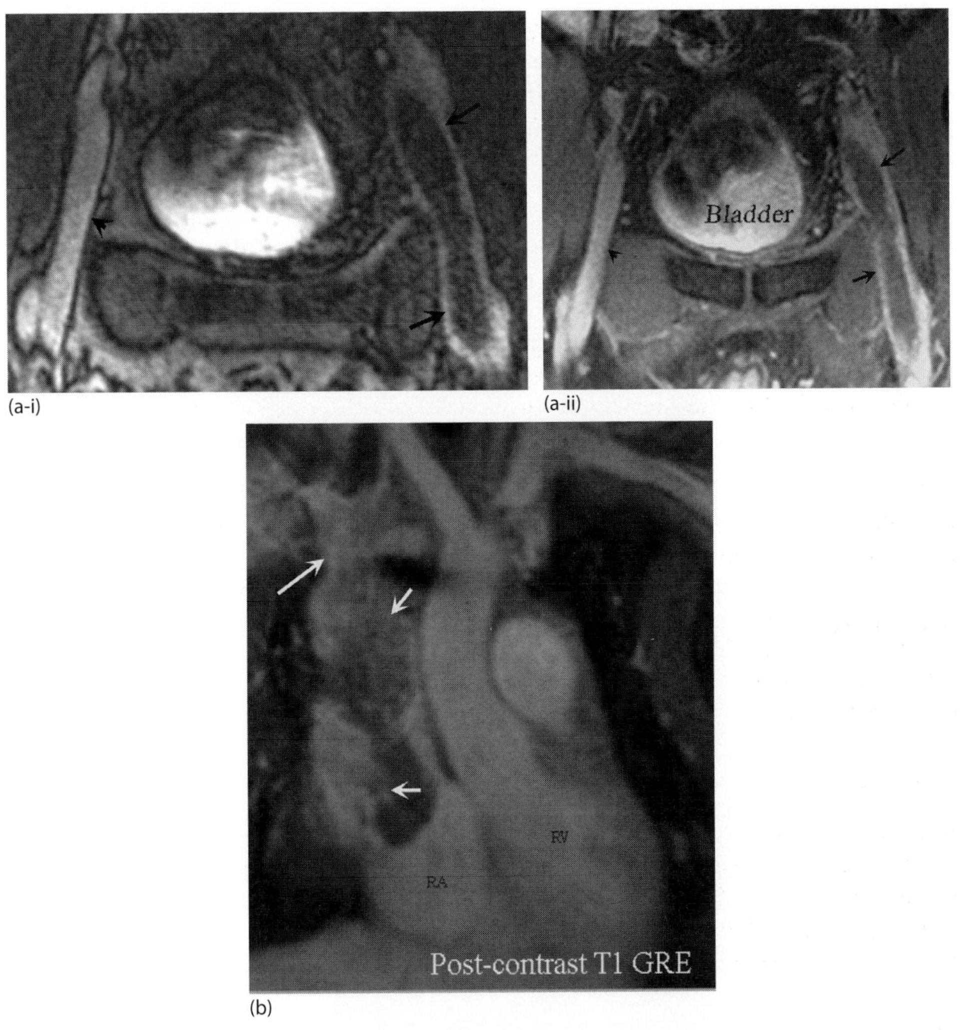

Fig. 6.16. (a) Acute deep vein thrombosis. Contrast-enhanced MRV (i) and post-contrast 3D GRE (ii) images show a near-occlusive low-signal thrombus (arrows) within the dilated left distal external iliac and proximal common femoral veins. Normal right external and common femoral veins (arrowheads). (b) Tumor thrombus. Post-contrast T1 GRE image shows heterogeneously enhancing mass within the dilated SVC (arrow) and right brachiocephalic vein (long arrow), consistent with tumor thrombus which extends to the right atrium and lower neck.

- Time-resolved MRA is helpful to show dynamic flow obstruction in the chest and abdominal veins and resultant collateral drainage pathway.
- Tumor thrombus may show partial internal or heterogeneous enhancement.
- Always check for pulmonary embolus in chest or upper extremity MRV. If indicated, post-contrast GRE images of the chest may be performed while the patient is on the table with lower or abdominal DVT.
- Perivenous enhancing soft tissue may be seen rarely, and it is better appreciated on post-contrast T1 GRE sequence. This likely represents perivenous inflammation due to acute DVT.

Suggested reading

Cantwell CP *et al.* MR venography with true fast imaging with steady-state precession for suspected lower-limb deep vein thrombosis. *J Vasc Interv Radiol* 2006;17:1763–1769.

Polak JF, Fox LA. MR assessment of the extremity veins. *Semin US CT MR* 1999;20:36–46.

6.17 Critical limb ischemia

Occlusive peripheral arterial disease resulting in sudden onset of decreased perfusion to limbs. The affected limb may become non-viable if appropriate measures are not taken immediately. MRA lower extremity of high quality is useful to provide a road map to intervention and to plan treatment. Calcification of arteries does not affect the image quality on MR. See Fig. 6.17.

Clinical

Lower limb claudication, rest pain, skin discoloration, diminished peripheral pulses, gangrene toes and paralysis. Low less than 0.1 Ankle–brachial index.

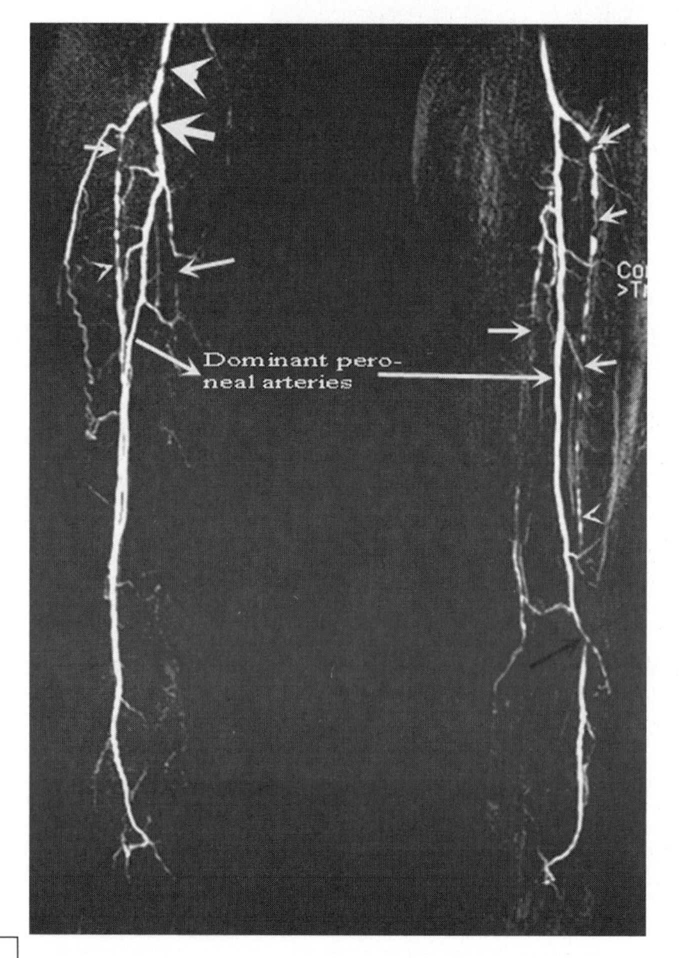

Fig. 6.17. Critical limb ischemia. Coronal thin MIP MRA shows multiple focal occlusions (white arrows) and high-grade stenoses (arrowheads) in the bilateral anterior tibial, and posterior tibial arteries, moderate stenosis in the right tibioperoneal trunk (thick arrow) and a high-grade stenosis in the right popliteal artery (thick arrowhead). The dominant peroneal artery forms the dorsalis pedis artery (black arrow) in both feet.

Technique

Sequences

SSFP scout views of abdomen, thighs and legs; 2 ml of gadolinium test injection to assess the time of contrast arrival in calves and abdominal aorta to plan high resolution MRA.

High-resolution contrast-enhanced MRA of calves – 2 passes.

With another separate contrast bolus injection, CE-MRA of abdomen (only arterial pass) and thighs (2 passes – table is moved immediately to thighs after the abdominal acquisition).

Axial post-contrast T1 GRE (abdomen, thighs, calves); useful to assess any enhancing lesion such as abscess in the context of sepsis or osteomyelitis etc. (pre-contrast T1 STIR is also useful to assess marrow edema of feet bones), graft infection, and thromboemboli within the arteries or grafts.

Findings

1. Total occlusion of arteries due to low-signal thrombus.
2. "Meniscus" sign – near-occlusive intraluminal low-signal embolus.
3. Focal significant obstructive stenosis or multifocal tandem stenoses.
4. Central filling defect in the arteries is consistent with thromboemboli.
5. Chronic thromboemboli may cause multiple eccentric wall-adherent filling defects and irregularity.
6. Popliteal, femoral or aortic aneurysm.
7. Bilateral peripheral arterial irregularities and narrowing with beading may suggest vasculitis.
8. Collaterals.

Pearls

- Systematically check aorta and bilateral common iliac, external iliac, common femoral, superficial femoral, popliteal, anterior tibial, tibioperoneal trunk, posterior tibial, peroneal and dorsalis pedis arteries.
- Stenosis can be graded as mild (less than 50% narrowing), moderate (50–70%), severe (> 70–99%), and total occlusion.
- MRA can overestimate; MIP (maximum intensity projection) can overestimate stenosis. Check both source and MIP images to judge the degree of luminal stenosis.
- Assess any enhancing lesion such as abscess in the context of sepsis or osteomyelitis etc. (precontrast T1 STIR is also useful to assess marrow edema of feet bones).
- Recommend cardiac echocardiogram or MRI to search for the source of thromboemboli.
- Floating thrombus (irregular low-signal mass attached to aorta but protruding into aortic lumen (low density on CTA)) may also be seen in the thoracic or abdominal aorta.
- Mural thrombus within the aneurysm (aortic or popliteal artery) may cause distal thromboembolism.
- Major limitations of MRA are motion artefacts and venous contamination of below-knee trifurcation arteries.

Suggested reading

Ersoy H. MR angiography of the lower extremities. *Am J Roentgenol* 2008;**190**(6):1675–1684. Review.

Habibi R *et al.* High-spatial-resolution lower extremity MR angiography at 3.0 T: contrast agent dose comparison study. *Radiology* 2008; **248**(2):680–692.

Lapeyre M. Assessment of critical limb ischemia in patients with diabetes: comparison of MR angiography and digital subtraction angiography. *Am J Roentgenol* 2005;**185**(6):1641–1650.

Stepansky F. Dynamic MR angiography of upper extremity vascular disease: pictorial review. *RadioGraphics* 2008;**28**(1):e28.

Interventional procedures – basics

Michael Murphy

7.1 General principles

Indications

Ensure there is a true indication for the procedure to be done as an emergency rather than electively.

Imaging

Review imaging prior to decision on intervention, and carry out any additional appropriate imaging.

Patient

Personally review the patient's clinical status including any contraindications, co-existent medical morbidity, stability of patient and any additional factors which may be relevant such as coagulation status.

Consent

Informed consent ideally taken by radiologist performing the procedure.

Monitoring

This will include nursing and anesthetic staff as well as relevant monitoring equipment.

Analgesia

The operating radiologist must be familiar with appropriate peri-procedural use of local anesthesia, opiate analgesia and sedation to minimize patient discomfort.

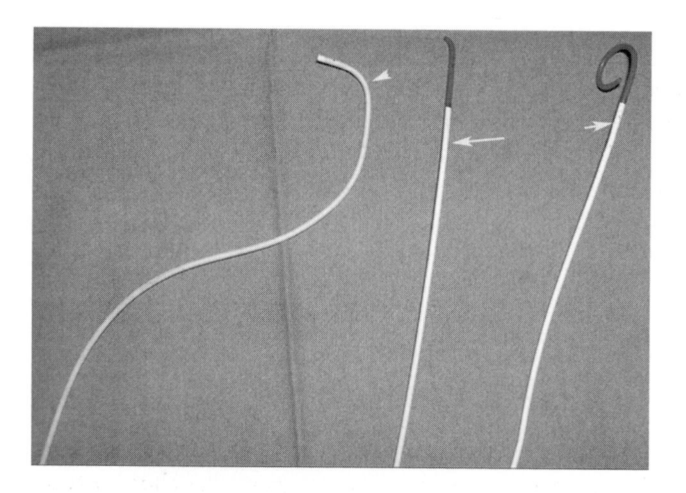

Fig. 7.1. Interventional catheters. Image shows Cobra (arrowhead), Vanschie (long arrow) and pigtail (short arrow) catheters.

Review

The radiologist should review patient and ensure that appropriate monitoring and any subsequent imaging/treatment is organized.

Support staff

Appropriate levels of support for the procedure including radiographic, nursing, medical and anesthetic staff as required for local policies.

Monitoring

Monitoring equipment includes pulse oximetry, ECG, blood pressure monitoring and also potentially an anesthetic machine for more complex cases. A resuscitation trolley with defibrillator should also be available in the room.

Drugs

Be familiar with use and doses of drugs which could potentially be used including:

1. Local anesthetics: Lidocaine, bupivocaine, prilocaine.
2. Analgesics: Opiates such as pethidine and morphine and reversal agent naloxone.
3. Sedatives: Midazolam and reversal agent flumazenil.
4. Anticoagulants: Heparin and reversal agent protamine, use of vitamin K, fresh frozen plasma and platelets for correction of coagulopathies.
5. Thrombolytic agents: Streptokinase, tissue plasminogen activator and urokinase.
6. Antibiotics: According to local guidelines.
7. Vasodilators: Glyceryl trinitrate, for example.
8. Vasoconstrictors: Vasopressin, for example.
9. Resuscitation medications.
10. Iodinated contrast media and medications used to treat anaphylaxis.

Guidewires

There are guidewires of varying sizes from 0.014 to 0.038 inch. Lengths are chosen according to the procedure and may be up to 300 cm long. Wire stiffness varies from floppy tip, e.g. Bentson wire to super-stiff, e.g. Lunderquist (stiff guidewires are not intended for manipulation through vessels, rather to be exchanged/placed through a catheter prior to use). The standard wires used are a straight or J-tipped 0.035 inch wire. Hydrophilic coated guidewires e.g. Terumo are immensely useful for manipulation into hard-to-reach places.

Catheters

Angiographic catheters (see Fig. 7.1) generally used are 4–5 French size, length varies according to intended use. These may be non-selective, e.g. straight/pigtail or selective curved catheters, e.g. Cobra, Sos Omni, Sidewinder, Headhunter, Berenstein, and Vanschie. For super-selection of the arterial tree microcatheters are indispensable. These can pass through the lumen of a selective catheter to pass into smaller more peripheral arterial branches e.g. hydrophilic Progreat catheter or Tracker system.

Sheaths

These have a hemostatic valve to allow multiple catheter wire exchanges.

Needles

18 gauge needles of varying length can take up to 0.038 guidewires; 21 gauge needles take 0.018 guidewires.

Micropuncture

System which allows initial puncture with 21/22 gauge needle and uses an 0.018 wire, over which a dilator is placed. A larger wire can then be passed for more stable access. Useful for gaining access safely to small vessels and renal/biliary systems, e.g. AccuStick system.

Drains

Generally 6–14 French, although larger drains are available. The size used depends on type of fluid/pus being drained. Commonest are pigtail-type drains which may be locking, non-locking or sump type drains.

Other

Angioplasty balloons, vascular and non-vascular stents, vena caval filters, embolization materials and coils, thrombectomy/embolectomy catheters, mechanical thrombectomy devices and arterial closure devices.

Pearls

- You must review the patient, indication and any prior imaging, and obtain consent for all procedures.
- Prepare/drape the patient appropriately and use local anesthetic as needed for all procedures.

Suggested reading

Baum A, ed. *Abrams' Angiography: Vascular and Interventional Radiology, 4th edition*. Little, Browne, 1997.

Beard J, Gaines PA, eds. *A Companion to Specialist Surgical Practice – Vascular and Endovascular Surgery, 3rd edition*. Elsevier Ltd., 2006.

Kadir S, ed. *Current Practice of Interventional Radiology*. BC Decker, 1991.

Kandarpa K, Aruny JE, eds. *Handbook of Interventional Radiologic Procedures, 3rd edition*. Livingstone, 2000.

Kessel D, Robertson I, eds. *Interventional Radiology. A Survival Guide, 2nd edition*. Elsevier Churchill Livingstone, 2005.

Whitehouse GH, Worthington BS, eds. *Techniques in Diagnostic Imaging, 3rd edition*. Blackwell Science, 1996.

Wyatt MG, Watkinson AF, eds. *Endovascular Intervention – Current Controversies*. tfm Publishing Limited, 2004.

7.2 Pigtail drainage of abscess

The majority of abscesses can be drained percutaneously with appropriately sized catheters as long as there is a safe access route to the collection. See Fig. 7.2.

Methods: Drainages may be carried out under ultrasound, fluoroscopy or CT guidance, or a combination of these. There are essentially two methods of placing the drainage catheter in the collection.

The *trocar technique* can be used for large, easily accessible collections. This is a one-step procedure where the catheter, which is mounted on a stiffener and central needle, is passed directly in the collection under image guidance (after making a small incision with a scalpel in the skin and subcutaneous tissues). The central needle is removed and fluid aspirated to confirm correct location after which the catheter is advanced over the stiffener into the collection with the stiffener remaining in a stable position.

A *Seldinger type technique* can be used for smaller or more remote collections; here a small needle (21G or 18G) is passed into the collection through which a guidewire is passed.

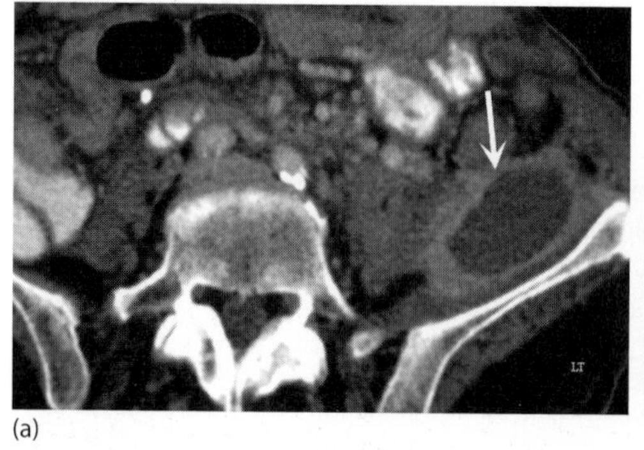

(a)

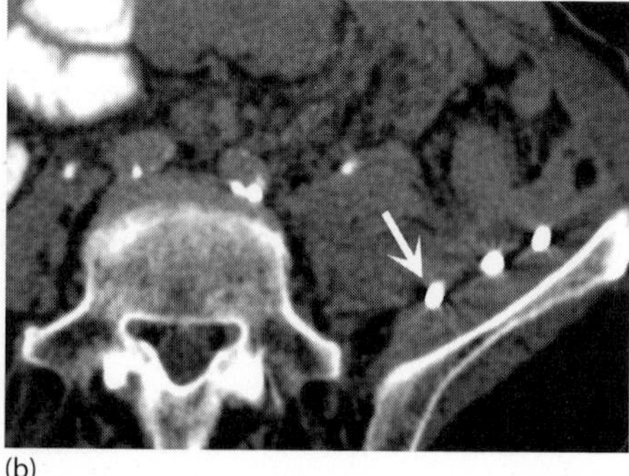

(b)

Fig. 7.2. (a, b) Pelvic abscess and pigtail drainage. (a) Axial CT scan of pelvis shows left iliacus muscle abscess (arrow). (b) Axial CT following insertion of pigtail drainage catheter and aspiration of pus shows near complete drainage of the abscess. The tip of the pigtail catheter is visible in the residual cavity (arrow).

Once guidewire access has been obtained, the tract can be dilated using fascial/vascular dilators or the cathether can be advanced directly over the guidewire into the collection. Once the system reaches the collection the catheter is advanced over the stiffener as above and stiffener and guidewire removed.

The size of drainage catheter used will need to increase with the thickness/viscosity of the fluid/pus aspirated.

Indications

1. Sepsis.
2. Relief of symptoms such as pain.

Contraindications

1. Absolute: Absence of safe route for drain passage.
2. Relative: Coagulopathy (often can be corrected).

Equipment

Selection of needles of varying lengths.
Guidewires (commonly 80 cm, 0.035 inch J wire).
Selection of drainage catheters (commonly 8–14 French locking pigtail).
Fascial/vascular dilators.
Connectors and drainage bags.
Sterile probe covers if using ultrasound.
Surgical blade or scalpel.

Procedure

Position patient appropriately for expected route of access and imaging modality chosen (under ultrasound, fluoroscopy or CT guidance or a combination of these).

Choose Trocar or Seldinger type technique as described above. Secure catheter by locking the pigtail and suturing catheter to skin surface, or by using one of the many patented skin fixation devices. Aspirate the collection using 50 ml syringe. Attach catheter to the drainage bag with appropriate connectors. Send sample of fluid to laboratory and leave catheter on free drainage.

Follow-up

1. Ensure the catheter is aspirated and irrigated with 5–10 ml sterile saline *twice daily.*
2. If fluid does not drain the catheter may have to be exchanged for a larger bore catheter over a guidewire.
3. Catheter should be removed once the drainage is minimal e.g. 5–10 ml/day, has become more serous or the collection is seen to have resolved on the appropriate imaging modality.

Pearls

- Always aspirate as much pus as possible at time of insertion of catheter. Using a three-way tap aspirate into a 50 ml syringe and then inject straight into the drainage bag.

- Locules may be broken down with a guidewire or with the pigtail of the catheter to aid drainage.
- Multiple drainage catheters may be required for optimal drainage.
- Consider fistulous connection if there is prolonged drainage or high output after the initial aspiration (contrast injection can often demonstrate this).

Suggested reading

Jaffe TA, Nelson RC, DeLong DM *et al.* Practice patterns in percutaneous image-guided intraabdominal abscess drainage: survey of academic and private practice centers. *Radiology* 2004;**233**:755–756.

7.3 Nephrostomy

Nephrostomy is one of the commonest interventional procedures performed as an emergency outside of normal working hours. See Fig. 7.3.

Indications

Indications for emergency nephrostomy:
Pyonephrosis.
Hydronephrosis of single functioning kidney.

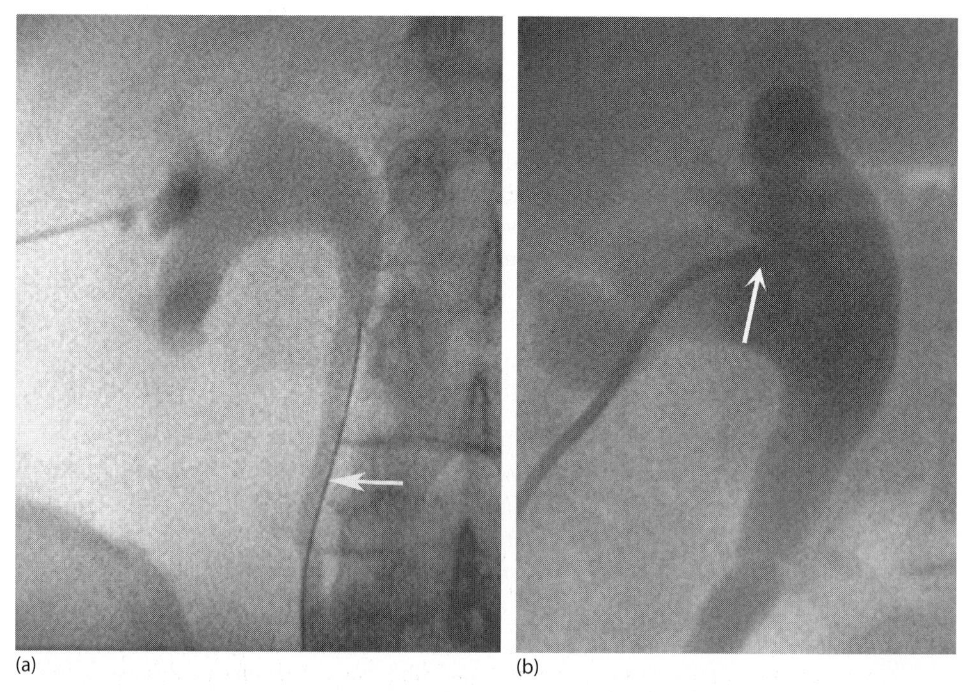

Fig. 7.3. (a, b) Hydronephrosis and nephrostomy. Renal ultrasound in a septic patient showed mild to moderate hydronephrosis secondary to calculus disease. (a) Fluoroscopic image shows guidewire (arrow) in collecting system and ureter. (b) Fluoroscopic image shows successful insertion of an 8 French locking pigtail drain (arrow).

Relative contraindications

Coagulopathy.
Severe uremia (high serum potassium) and bilateral hydronephrosis. (Nephrostomy can be performed post-dialysis when the patient becomes stable.)

Investigations

Ultrasound/intravenous urogram.

Equipment

18 G needle for direct puncture or micropuncture (AccuStick set).
Guidewire.
Drainage catheter (generally 8-Fr locking pigtail).
Vascular/fascial dilators.
Sedation (midazolam occasionally required).

Procedure

1. Intravenous antibiotics administered according to hospital guidelines.
2. Patient positioned prone/prone oblique on table.
3. Ultrasound-guided puncture of mid to lower pole calyx; posterior to mid-posterior approach best.
4. A guidewire is passed into the collecting system over which a suitable draining catheter may be placed (contrast may be used to outline the system prior to placement of the guidewire).
5. Secure the drain to the patient and leave system on free external drainage.

Complications

1. Hematuria: common, generally settles within 24/48 hours and rarely requires embolization.
2. Pneumothorax: Rare in mid to lower pole punctures.
3. Visceral injury (e.g. colon) rare but caution in more anterior approaches.
4. Urosepsis: Bacteremia sometimes seen but septic shock is rare.

Pearls

- Choose a suitable ultrasound window to target the dilated calyx. Reposition the patient if necessary.
- The 22 G needle may be passed down through a larger needle (e.g. spinal needle) which is placed to renal capsule level only. This can stabilize the smaller needle for more accurate placement.
- If the drainage catheter is resistant in passing over the guidewire, ensure there is no kink in the system and predilate the track with vascular/fascial dilators if necessary. Use a stiffer guidewire if needed.
- Minimize the volume and force of contrast injection to decrease risk of bacteremia and rupture of the collecting system. Formal nephrostograms can be obtained electively at a later stage.
- A ruptured system will usually heal following 7–10 days of external drainage.

Post-procedure

Routine observations plus alert staff about the potential for diuresis.
Arrange follow-up studies/procedures e.g. antegrade stenting.

Suggested reading

Lang EK, Price ET. Redefinition of indications for percutaneous nephrostomy. *Radiology* 1983;**147**:419–426.

Millward SF. Percutaneous nephrostomy: a practical approach. *J Vasc Interv Radiol* 2000;**11**:955–964.

7.4 Angiography

Perfemoral access is the mainstay of angiography and once access has been obtained angiography of peripheries, viscera, thorax and head and neck can be performed and treatment instituted by an appropriately trained radiologist. See Fig. 7.4.

Equipment

1. Fluoroscopic equipment with digital subtraction angiographic facility plus power injector for contrast.
2. Angiographic set to include following:
   Antiseptic solution, local anesthetic, N-Saline etc.
   Needles for instillation of local anesthetic (25/21-gauge) and arterial puncture (generally 18-gauge will accommodate 0.035 inch guidewire).
3. Selection of syringes e.g. 20, 10 and 5 ml.
4. Blade for skin nick.
5. Vascular sheaths (5 Fr initially).
6. Selection of catheters non-selective and selective (4/5 Fr pigtail for diagnostic peripheral angiogram).
7. Three-way taps, high-pressure connecting tubing for injector.

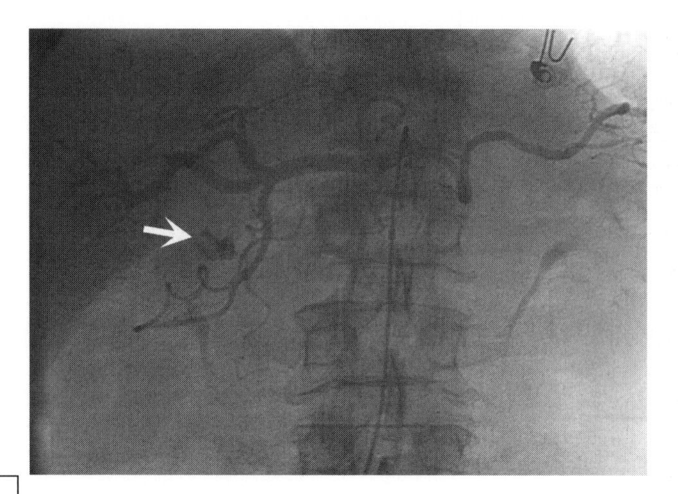

Fig. 7.4. Bleeding duodenal ulcer. Celiac angiogram shows active extravasation (arrow) from a branch of gastroduodenal artery which was subsequently embolized.

Procedure

1. Assess pulses and decide best access route.
2. Infiltrate local anesthetic into groin over artery.
3. Retrograde puncture common femoral artery (usually over midpoint of femoral head), a combination of landmark, fluoroscopic and ultrasound-guided techniques may be necessary in difficult cases.
4. A guidewire is passed into the abdominal aorta.
5. Sheaths, selective and non-selective catheters can be passed/manipulated over the guidewires to perform angiography.

Lower limb angiography

Generally, a non-selective catheter such as 4/5 Fr pigtail is placed in distal aorta and DSA runs carried out of iliac, femoral, popliteal and run-off vessels. A small volume of contrast is injected, e.g. 18–20 ml at 6–8 ml/second (rates vary according to individual patient and institution). Additional oblique views may be necessary to outline the internal iliac or profunda femoris origins.

Visceral/mesenteric angiography

Generally, selective catheters such as Cobra or reverse curve Sidewinder are used to access the vessels. The curve of catheter chosen depends on gender of patient and aortic size, with males requiring catheters with a larger curve than females, and also increases with aortic size i.e. Cobra 1–3 and Sidewinder 1–3. Hydrophilic wires and hydrophilic versions of these catheters can allow further superselection of vessels, alternatively microcatheters are used in this scenario. Obliqued or angled views may be necessary to ideally profile vessels. It is usual to commence angiography with the vessel most likely to demonstrate the suspected pathology. For instance, if the patient has hematemesis and a known duodenal ulcer then commence with celiac axis run which will demonstrate gastro-duodenal artery. With large vessels an injector pump is used, e.g. celiac/SMA use 25 ml at 5–6 ml/s with frame rate 2/s initially decreasing to 1/s for venous phase. For smaller vessels, e.g. GDA and IMA hand injections are performed.

Arch angiography

May be required in trauma patients to evaluate aortic transection or as a prelude to bronchial, cerebral or upper limb angiography. Generally a 5 Fr pigtail catheter is used with an injection of 40 ml at 15–20 ml/s at a frame rate of 2–4 per second. Obliqued views at 30 degrees LAO to show arch and great vessel origins in profile and additional more steep LAO views may be helpful. Selective catheters such as Headhunter, Berenstein and Cobra may be used to catheterize the great vessels for cerebral and upper limb angiography.

Pearls

- If the patient is hypotensive use ultrasound to puncture the vessel.
- Ensure that your assistant knows where all the relevant catheters, wires etc. are located.
- Use the pump injector where possible to minimize radiation dose to operator.

- Patients with gastrointestinal bleeding can also have peripheral vascular disease, hence take care when accessing the iliac system.
- If unable to access a small or branch vessel, change something (i.e. catheter, wire or consider a microcatheter).
- If patient has difficulty with breath holding for subtraction use cine runs at a high frame rate.
- Always assess runs on subtracted and non-subtracted views to allow discrimination between bowel movement and bleeding.
- Consider antegrade approach to femoral artery as indicated.

Suggested reading

Refer to Section 7.1.

7.5 Embolization

Emergency embolization is generally performed in patients with life-threatening hemorrhage. The aim is to occlude the arterial supply to the site of hemorrhage as selectively as possible thus minimizing the risk of ischemia. The procedure should only be performed by an experienced interventionalist. See Fig. 7.5.

Indications

1. Gastrointestinal bleeding.
2. Hepatic and splenic traumatic vascular injuries.
3. Urinary tract hemorrhage.
4. Otolaryngologic e.g. severe epistaxis, post-tonsillectomy or tumor resection, traumatic vascular injuries.

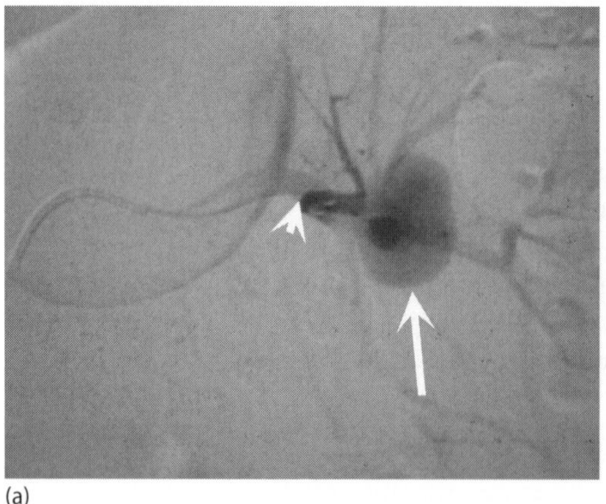

(a)

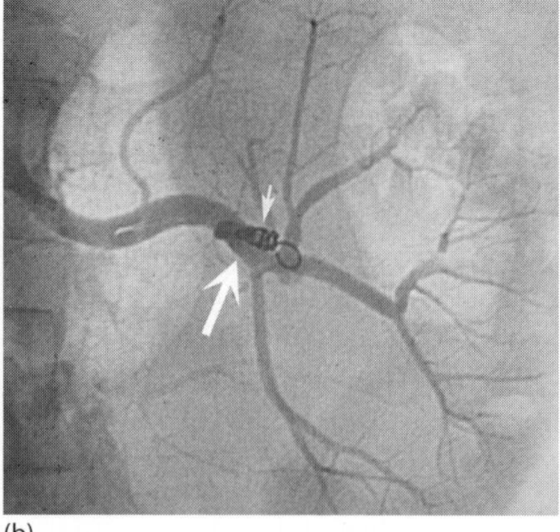

(b)

Fig. 7.5. (a, b) Renal artery embolization. (a) Selective angiogram of left renal artery shows a large pseudoaneurysm (long arrow) secondary to previous renal biopsy. (b) Left renal angiogram following successful embolization shows complete exclusion of the pseudoaneurysm (large arrow) with preservation of the majority of renal blood supply.

5. Respiratory, e.g. bronchial artery bleeding from mycetoma or vascular malformation, intercostal artery hemorrhage post-trauma.
6. Pelvis, e.g. post-partum hemorrhage or pelvic trauma.

Contraindications

Unstable patient.

The surgical team should be on stand-by (non-selective balloon occlusion may allow temporary stabilization in selected cases).

Embolization agents

The agents that offer the potential for temporary occlusion of the vessel are gelatin, sponge pledgets or autologous blood clot. Mechanical agents such as coils and detachable balloons as well as sclerosants (pure alcohol/poly vinyl alcohol (PVA) particles and sodium tetradecyl sulphate) and adhesives lead to permanent vessel occlusion. The size of coil, balloon and particles used will vary with the vessel which needs to be occluded. The commonest agents used are coils, PVA particles and Gelfoam pledgets. Coils are made of platinum or stainless steel and have fibers which help promote thrombosis. The chosen coil must be compatible with the inner lumen of the catheter through which it is delivered and be of suitable size and length for the target vessel. The commonest sizes are 2–10 mm coiled diameter. PVA particles come in a range of particle size from 150 μm to 1000 μm, with the size chosen dependent on the target vessel (300–500 μm commonest). Gelfoam pledgets are cut to size at the time of procedure, generally 1–2 mm. PVA and gelfoam pledgets are mixed with iodinated contrast to visualize the material during embolization.

Equipment

Vascular angiography set (see above).

Selection of end hole-only selective catheters, e.g. Cobra, Sidewinder, Headhunter and microcatheters, e.g. Progreat or Tracker systems.

Relevant embolization agents.

Procedure

1. Ensure patient has received appropriate replacement blood products and is actively having any coagulopathy corrected.
2. Perform angiogram to outline bleeding point.
3. Ensure that endhole catheter is placed as selectively as possible (may require microcatheter system) and that its position is stable.
4. Choose a suitable embolic agent.
5. Deliver agent in a controlled manner under constant fluoroscopic guidance.
6. Perform angiogram post-procedure to ensure there is no additional supply feeding the bleeder (in many cases this "back door" needs to be closed first).

Post-procedure

1. Ensure patient gets appropriate level of monitoring for stability, ischemic complications and pain relief.

2. Ensure patient has appropriate follow-up imaging/investigation where necessary to exclude underlying sinister pathology which may be primary source of the bleed, e.g. large bowel tumor in lower GI hemorrhage.

Pearls

- Have a second trolley and syringes for all particulate/sclerosant agents.
- Always second check every agent that is being injected.
- Always fluoroscope when passing embolic agent into vessel.
- Allow sufficient time for embolization agent to work.
- If patient is too unstable and will require urgent surgery, temporary non-selective balloon occlusion may help stabilize situation for transfer to operating room.

Suggested reading

Refer to Section 7.1.

7.6 Catheter-directed thrombolyis/thrombectomy

Lysis

Catheter-directed thrombolysis is used intra-arterially for acute limb ischemia, thrombosed grafts and arteriovenous fistulae and less commonly for deep venous thrombus, pulmonary embolism and thrombotic cerebrovascular events. The most frequent use is for acute lower limb ischemia. Here the commonest underlying pathology is longstanding stenotic disease with an acute superimposed thrombotic episode. If lysis is successful then the underlying stenosis is also treated. Embolic episodes, e.g. relating to atrial fibrillation or myocardial infarction are less commonly the underlying cause. See Fig. 7.6.

Indications

Acute limb ischemia due to native vessel/graft thrombosis or embolic event.
Iatrogenic thrombosis/embolism during interventional procedures.

Contraindications

Absolute: Recent stroke within 2 months, recent bleeding/surgery/major trauma within 14 days, intracranial neoplasm, potential source of bleeding, e.g. active peptic ulcer, bleeding diathesis/coagulopathy, and irreversible limb ischemia.
Relative: Diabetic retinopathy, age greater than 80 years, emboli from cardiac source, vein graft thrombosis >48 hours, neoplasia with increased risk of hemorrhage, pregnancy, uncontrolled hypertension.

Thrombolytic agents and administration

The three commonest agents which have been used are streptokinase, urokinase and recombinant tissue-plasminogen activator (r-tPA). The commonest agent used in the UK and North America is currently r-tPA.

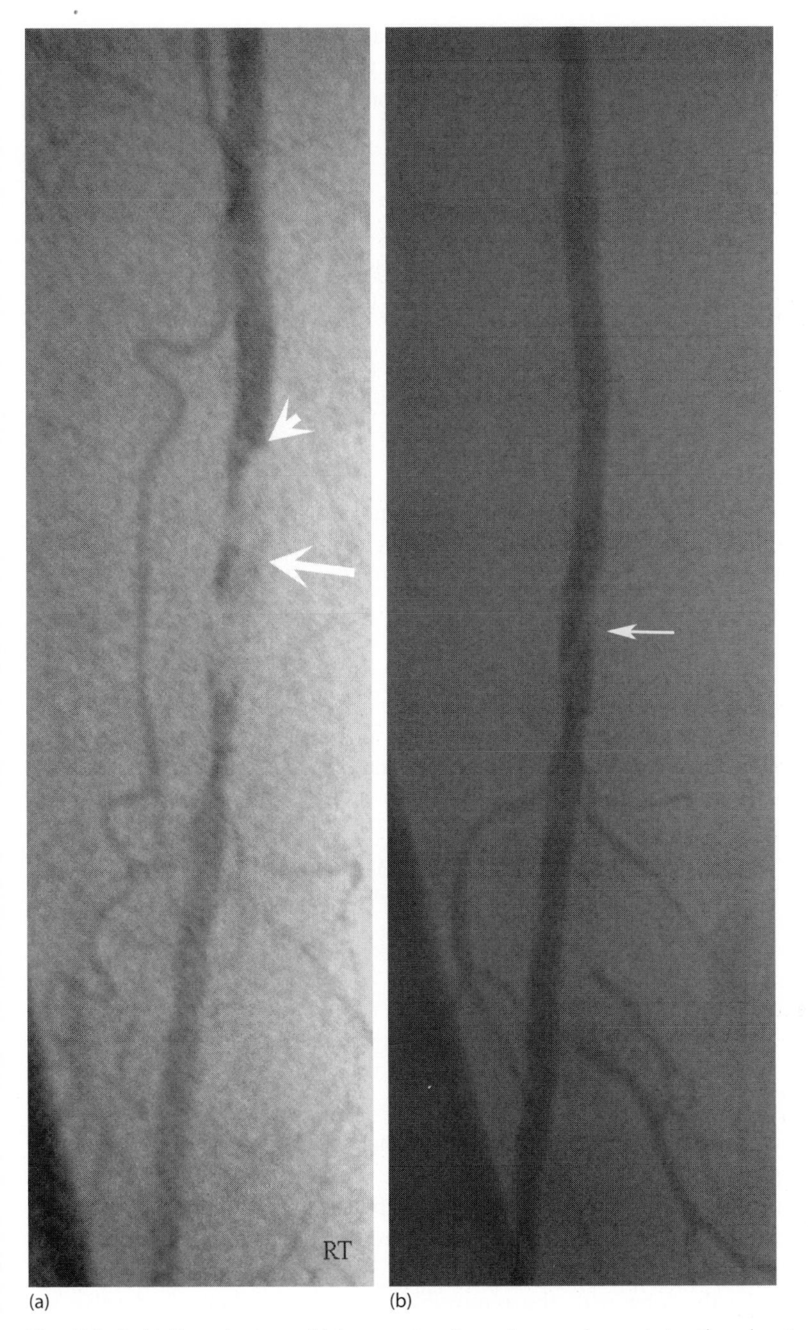

Fig. 7.6. (a, b) Thrombectomy. (a) Lower-extremity angiogram demonstrates thrombus in the right superficial femoral artery (arrow) above the adductor canal. "Mensical sign" (arrowhead) indicates acute thrombosis. (b) Angiogram post-thrombectomy with Angiojet thrombectomy device and 5 mm angioplasty.

Generally thrombolysis is administered via a pump as a continuous low-dose infusion (0.5–1 mg r-tPA/hour) with the catheter tip embedded in the thrombus. Check angiography is carried out at 4–6 hours and at 12/24 hours after commencement (only rarely is lysis extended beyond 24 hours).

Equipment

Vascular angiography set (see above).
Infusion catheters and pumps.
Angioplasty balloons, stents and thrombectomy catheters/devices for adjuvant procedures.

Procedure

1. Perform baseline angiogram.
2. Commence appropriate lysis regime.
3. Re-image/treat as per hospital protocol bearing in mind endpoints such as sufficient clot lysis, deteriorating or static thrombus/clot burden, deteriorating clinical condition or bleeding complications.
4. Perform any adjunctive procedures.

Peri-procedure

Ensure patient is monitored in a high-dependency area.
Observe and treat complications (bleeding can be fatal).

Pearls

- Be wary of hemorrhagic complications; always ensure availability of a high-dependency bed.
- Choosing appropriate access route is a key step.
- Successful endovascular treatment often includes a combination of lysis, thrombectomy and angioplasty/stenting.

Thrombectomy

Thrombosuction/thrombectomy are used both as primary endovascular techniques and also as adjunctive procedures to lysis.

In thrombosuction a large-bore catheter e.g. 6/7 Fr is passed over a guidewire (through a vascular sheath with a removable valve) to the site of thrombus. The guidewire is removed and suction is applied with a 50 ml syringe, then the catheter is slowly withdrawn and removed from the sheath along with the removable valve. The catheter and valve are flushed to remove the thrombus and the valve replaced on the sheath. This procedure is repeated to remove as much thrombus as possible. With mechanical thrombectomy, special catheters and devices, designed for percutaneous use, are used to fragment the thrombus and either remove it from the circulatory system or macerate it into particles small enough to pass through the more distal circulation. There are numerous devices on the market (e.g. Amplatz, Angiojet, Hydrolyser, Oasis, Rotarex and Thrombex PMT).

Suggested reading

Gould D, Wyatt MG, Watkinson AF. Mechanical thrombectomy: is it worthwhile? In Wyatt MG, Watkinson AF, eds. *Endovascular Intervention – Current Controversies*, pp. 199–204. tfm Publishing Limited, 2004.

Working Party on Thrombolysis in the Management of Limb Ischemia. Thrombolysis in the management of lower limb peripheral arterial occlusion, a consensus document. *J Vasc Interv Radiol* 2003;**14**(9 pt 2):S337–S349.

7.7 Transjugular intrahepatic porto-systemic shunt (TIPSS)

A TIPSS procedure is a percutaneous method of forming a channel between the hepatic venous and portal venous systems thus shunting blood away from the liver and reducing pressure in portal venous hypertension. It is generally performed as an emergency procedure for variceal bleeding resistant to medical management and endoscopic techniques such as banding. It may be carried out semi-electively for refractory ascites. In our unit it is performed under general anesthetic but some units use conscious sedation. See Fig. 7.7.

Indications

Acute/subacute uncontrollable bleeding from esophageal varices.
Bleeding due to portal gastropathy.
Budd–Chiari syndrome.

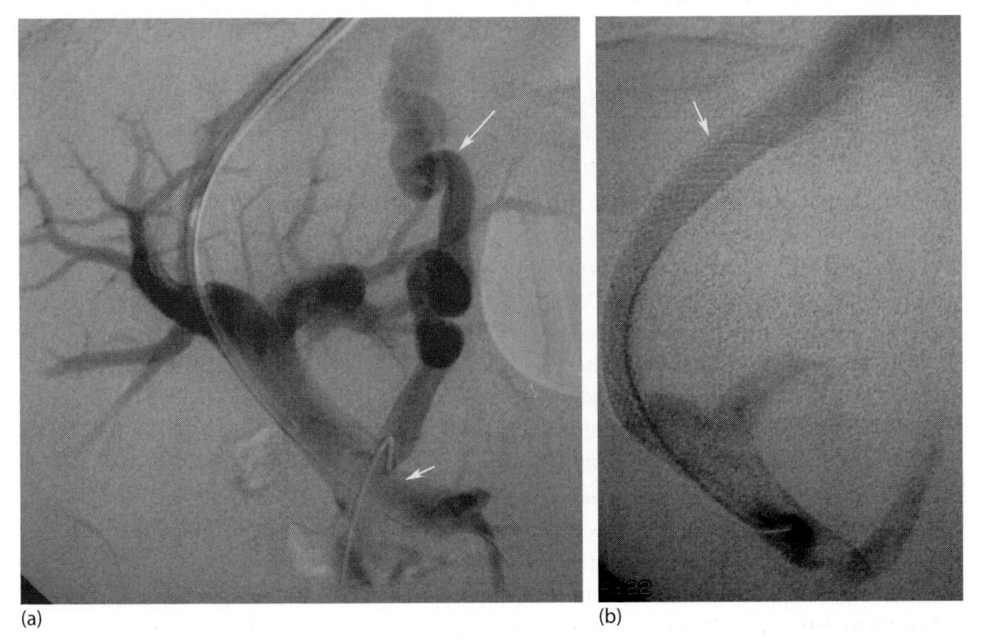

Fig. 7.7. (a, b) TIPSS. (a) Portal venography prior to TIPSS procedure demonstrating a large gastro-esophageal varix (arrow) arising from the main portal vein (small arrow). (b) Portogram post-insertion of Viator TIPPS stent shows prompt flow through the shunt (arrow) into the right hepatic vein and IVC. The gradient dropped from 25 mmHg to 8 mmHg post-TIPSS procedure, with cessation of variceal bleeding.

Contraindications

Severe congestive heart failure.
Severe encephalopathy.
Occluded portal vein.

Equipment

Ultrasound for vascular puncture.
Pressure transducer for measuring portal pressures/porto-systemic pressure gradient.
Vascular angiography set (see above).
TIPSS set e.g. Cook set; generally includes:
10 Fr sheath 40 cm, curved guide catheter with metal inner stiffener and a 60 cm needle with outer sheath which will take 0.035 wire when the needle is removed.
Additional selective catheters e.g. Cobra, multipurpose, Sidewinder and 4 Fr straight hydrophilic 65 cm.
Guidewires generally 0.035, soft, stiff and hydrophilic varieties of varying lengths.

Procedure

1. Obtain access to common femoral artery and right internal jugular vein (ultrasound guided).
2. Pass the 10 Fr TIPSS sheath into the SVC or right atrium.
3. Manipulate a guidewire into the right hepatic vein (RHV) using a selective catheter e.g. Cobra or multipurpose.
4. Confirm position of wire in RHV by screening laterally (should pass posteriorly in liver) or ultrasound.
5. Exchange for stiff wire such as Amplatz.
6. Portal vein outlined by selectively catheterizing SMA from groin and viewing venous phase of SMA angiogram (alternatively some centers use CO_2 wedged hepatic venography).
7. Pass TIPSS sheath and curved stiff guide catheter into RHV over stiff wire.
8. Withdraw sheath, slowly remove stiff wire and angle guide catheter towards right portal vein branch which lies anteriorly.
9. Puncture right branch of portal vein with sheathed needle, remove needle and introduce 180 cm terumo wire into portal venous system.
10. If the sheath of the puncture needle will not pass sufficiently far into portal system for safe exchange with a stiff wire then a 4 Fr slippy 65 cm catheter will pass through the guide catheter over the terumo allowing extra length.
11. Pass the guide catheter and sheath into the portal vein (the tract may have to be balloon dilated prior to this with e.g. 8 mm balloon).
12. Most operators perform portal venography to outline varices and portal pressures may be taken.
13. The shunt tract is now stented. Calibrated catheters or balloons may be used to estimate lengths of stent required. The stent is placed from the RHV to the right branch of portal vein ideally.
14. Balloon dilate shunt to 8 mm and check pressure gradient (general endpoint is gradient of 12 mmHg or less). Additional balloon dilatation to 10 mm may be required. Perform post-procedural portal venography.

Post-procedure

Patient should be monitored in ITU or HDU setting.
Duplex ultrasound follow-up of shunt with venography and re-intervention as necessary.

Pearls

- Puncturing the right portal vein branch 1–1.5 cm from the bifurcation should ensure that the tract is intrahepatic throughout its course.
- In gastric fundal varices ensure the splenic vein is patent.
- TIPSS will not help if the varices drain into the renal or other veins.
- If patient continues to bleed, embolize the main varix through the shunt (which will require large coils).

Suggested reading

Luca A, D'Amico G, La Galla R *et al.* TIPS for prevention of recurrent bleeding in patients with cirrhosis: meta-analysis of randomized clinical trials. *Radiology* 1999;**212**:411–421.

Saravanan R, Nayar M, Gilmore IT *et al.* Transjugular intrahepatic portosystemic shunt: 11 years' experience at a regional referral centre. *Eur J Gastroenterol Hepatol* 2005; 17(11):1165–1171.

7.8 Inferior vena-caval filters

Inferior vena-caval filters are devices which are placed in the vena cava to prevent large venous emboli reaching the pulmonary circulation. The filters placed are either permanent or temporary/recoverable, and there are several of each type commercially available. The early retrievable filters were only recommended for removal in the first couple of weeks post-implantation. However, some of the newer recoverable filters have been removed after much longer time periods. See Fig. 7.8.

The majority of filters can be placed via the internal jugular veins or the femoral veins. Filter types include Greenfield, Birds Nest, Gunther Tulip, Recovery and ALN.

Indications

Emergency

Recurrent pulmonary embolus (PE), despite adequate anticoagulation.
Pulmonary embolus or large thrombus load, e.g. iliofemoral DVT with contraindication to anticoagulation.
Pulmonary embolectomy with residual thrombus in the leg veins.

Semi-emergent

Patients requiring surgery who are at high risk of PE.
Immobile patients e.g. post severe trauma.
Patients with known PE/DVT and severely limited cardiorespiratory reserve.
Progression of DVT or free-floating iliofemoral/IVC thrombus despite anticoagulation.
DVT/PE in pregnancy.

Contraindications

Thrombosis of entire IVC.

Equipment

Angiographic suite.
Duplex ultrasound.
Vascular angiography set.
Selection of guidewires/catheters.
Suitable filter and its information leaflet/brochure.

Procedure

1. Ultrasound jugular/femoral veins to help choose the appropriate device and access site.
2. Obtain venous access and advance a catheter to just above the iliac veins.
3. Perform venography to demonstrate caval/iliac vein anatomy, size of cava, position of renal veins and extent of thrombus.
4. If the renal vein positions are not clear from the venogram then selective catheterization will be necessary to outline their location. Following the filter information leaflet guidelines, position the filter in a suitable location and deploy. Perform a venogram post-implantation to document correct deployment. Generally, the filter is placed below the level of the renal veins and above the iliac bifurcation or caval thrombus. Occasionally, a decision is made to place the filter in a supra-renal position due to the extent of thrombus. This can predispose to renal vein thrombus, but occasionally renal vein thrombus may also be the indication.

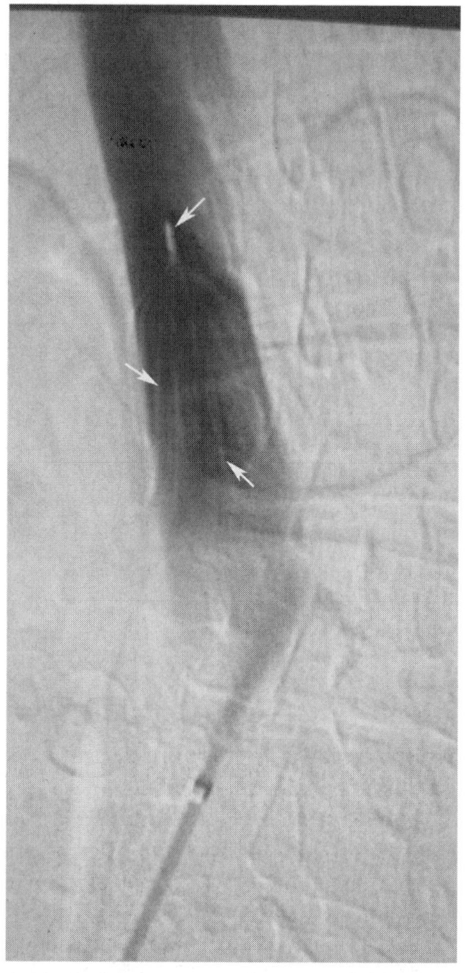

Fig. 7.8. Inferior vena-caval filter. Filter (arrows) is placed below renal veins after confirming infra-renal position by inserting it in left renal vein to outline junction with IVC. Note flow void from unenhanced blood entering cava from the left renal vein.

Follow-up

Observe for complications (e.g. access site thrombosis now rare, caval thrombosis (5–10%), filter migration, strut perforation of caval wall and strut fractures).

Make arrangements for removal if deploying a temporary filter.

Pearls

- Ultrasound the femoral/iliac veins to assess location of thrombus.

- Assess vena caval size (usually less than 3 cm diameter) at venography or on CT if already carried out (occasionally the cava may be large which may alter the choice of filter used).
- Beware of variant venous anatomy e.g. left-sided IVC and duplication of the IVC with the left iliac vein draining to left renal.
- Anticoagulation should be continued post-insertion unless there is a contraindication.
- Clearly state in the patient's chart what the plan is for the filter; if it is intended to be retrieved then have a system in place as a reminder.

Suggested reading

Becker D, Philbrick J, Selby J. Inferior vena cava filters: indications, safety, effectiveness. *Arch Intern Med* 1992;**152**:1985–1994.

Binkert CA, Sasadeusz K, Stavropoulos SW. Retrievability of the recovery vena caval filter after dwell times longer than 180 days. *J Vasc Interv Radiol* 2006;**17**:299–302.

7.9 Emergency aortic stent-grafting

Stent-grafting may also be used in the emergency treatment of complicated acute type B thoracic dissections, aortic intramural hematomas and traumatic aortic pseudoaneurysms. See Fig. 7.9.

The stent-graft is a device which is placed via an endovascular route. It comprises a metal stent (stainless steel or nitinol) with a fabric covering made with either

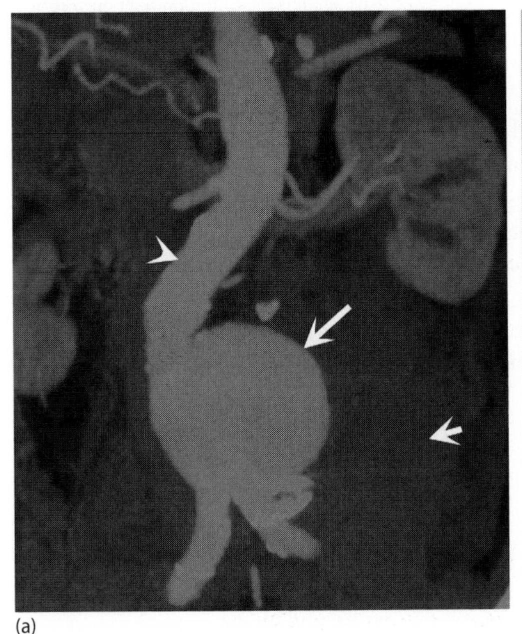

(a)

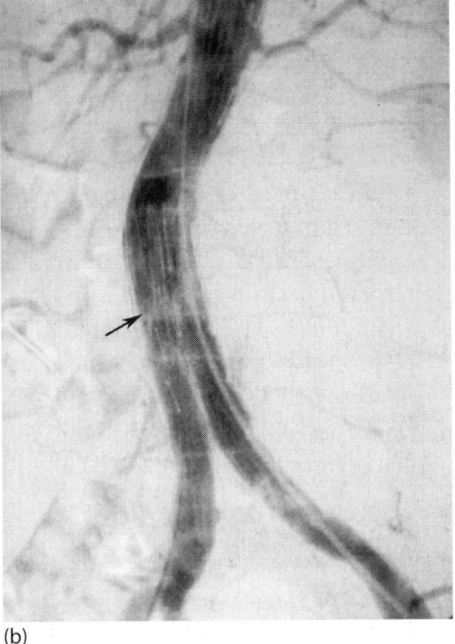

(b)

Fig. 7.9. (a, b) Endovascular aortic stent graft. (a) Coronal reformat image of CTA shows infra-renal abdominal aortic aneurysm (arrow) with large left retroperitoneal hematoma (small arrow). Note there is an adequate neck (proximal sealing zone) of the aneurysm (arrowhead). (b) DSA image following successful exclusion of the leaking abdominal aneurysm shows placement of endovascular stent graft (arrow) without an endoleak into the residual aneurysm sac.

polytetrafluoroethylene or polyester. The concept is to place the stent-graft across the aneurysm or tear to exclude it from the circulation, the radial force of the stent keeping the device in situ. The device can be placed from the femoral arteries following the surgical exposure of the vessels (occasionally an entirely percutaneous procedure is carried out). The devices essentially come in three varieties: tube stent-grafts (used in the thoracic aorta), aorto-uniiliac and modular bifurcated devices (used for abdominal ruptures).

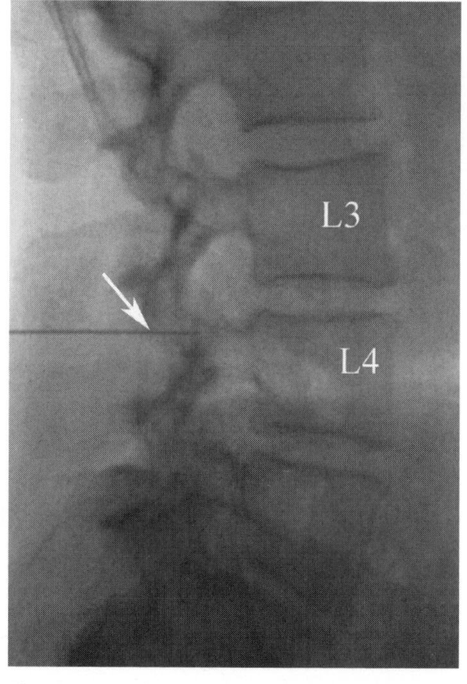

Fig. 7.10. Lumbar puncture. Fluoroscopic image of lateral view of lumbar spine demonstrates positioning of the coaxial needle (arrow) for lumbar puncture.

Equipment

Facilities for conversion to open repair.
Multidisciplinary team.
Angiographic set.
Long guidewires (ordinary plus stiff).
Vascular access sheaths 5 Fr to 16 Fr.
Occlusion balloon for emergency control.
Suitable stent-graft.
Moulding balloons.

Procedure

1. Groin dissection/percutaneous femoral access obtained (under local anesthetic).
2. Guidewires passed into the thoracic aorta.
3. Catheter placed to obtain angiogram.
4. An occlusion balloon may be placed above the level of an abdominal rupture in unstable cases to obtain hemostatic control. The graft can be placed below this and the balloon retrieved post-deployment.
5. Stent-graft is passed to the approximate position of deployment and arteriogram performed to mark final position. Deployment is carried out under continuous fluoroscopy.
6. Check angiography is carried out post-procedure in order to assess exclusion and patency of vital arteries.

Pearls

- In some cases a subclavian artery bypass procedure may be required for chronic upper limb ischemia – acute limb ischemia is rare.
- In bifurcated abdominal aortic device, the contralateral iliac stump must be cannulated and limbs extended into the iliac arteries to seal the aneurysm.

Follow-up

Patients who undergo endovascular repair of an aortic rupture or transection should be entered on a suitable surveillance program to detect late complications.

Suggested reading

Murphy M, McWilliams RG, eds. *A Companion to Specialist Surgical Practice. Vascular and Endovascular Surgery, 3rd edition*. Elsevier, 2006.

7.10 Lumbar puncture

Indications

Suspected meningitis or encephalitis.
Suspected subarachnoid hemorrhage.
Prior to intrathecal chemotherapy or contrast injection.

Contraindications

Suspicion of mass lesion or raised intracranial pressure, local infection at site of puncture.
Coagulation/clotting abnormalities.

Equipment

Fluoroscopy C arm/angiography suite.
Lumbar puncture set/needle.
CSF pressure measurement equipment.
Sterile drapes/antiseptic solution.
Towel/sponge holder or long forceps.

Procedure

1. Position patient in left lateral-fetal position (knees and chin tucked as close as possible together).
2. Screen in frontal and lateral positions to locate optimal LP level, usually L3–4 interspace.
3. Slowly advance LP needle (typically 22 gauge) in the midline with a mild cranial tilt (bevel facing lateral – parallel to nerve roots – to minimize nerve root injury).
4. Intermittent screening is usually sufficient.
5. Forceps or sponge holder may be used if continual screening.
6. Withdraw stylette when needle felt to penetrate dura mater.
7. Take pressure measurements and samples as appropriate.

Post-procedure

Ensure samples are labeled and sent appropriately.
Chart patient for appropriate analgesia and administer neurological observations.

Pearls

- In adults 4–5 cm is typical distance to thecal sac.
- Have a member of oncology team to inject any intrathecal chemotherapy agents.
- CT brain prior to LP is essential in suspected intracranial mass lesion or raised intracranial pressure.
- In double-needle technique for difficult cases, an 18-gauge needle is passed towards the duramater for more stability and then pass the 22-gauge needle through this to pierce the dura.

Suggested reading

Slipman CW. *Interventional Spine – An Algorithmic Approach*. Saunders Elsevier, 2008.

Pediatrics

Shivarama Avula and Nick Barnes

8.1 General principles

Although medical imaging of children is in many ways similar to that of adults, some special consideration should be given to the way an examination is carried out. See Fig. 8.1.

Clinical assessment

Ensure that the child is in a stable condition for imaging. A full clinical assessment is important to guide appropriate radiological investigation and aid in interpretation of images.

Selection of imaging technique

Radiographs, ultrasound, fluoroscopy and computed tomography are commonly used.

In most emergency situations magnetic resonance imaging is inappropriate and unnecessary; it plays a role in further investigation of abnormalities once a patient has undergone initial evaluation and management.

Nuclear medicine plays no real role in acute imaging but can be used as a planned procedure for follow-up investigation in some conditions.

Interventional techniques in children are specialized procedures that should only be carried out in pediatric centers.

Selection of an imaging technique depends very much on the clinical assessment. Basic indicators such as the child's age and knowledge of the type of illness are important guides to possible causes of a problem.

Radiation protection

Children are more "sensitive" to the effects of radiation because of increased cellular division during growth and the overall relative life expectancy compared with adults. The risks and benefits of a technique involving ionizing radiation should be weighed before resorting to imaging. Pulse fluoroscopy and image capture should almost always be used rather than continuous fluoroscopy.

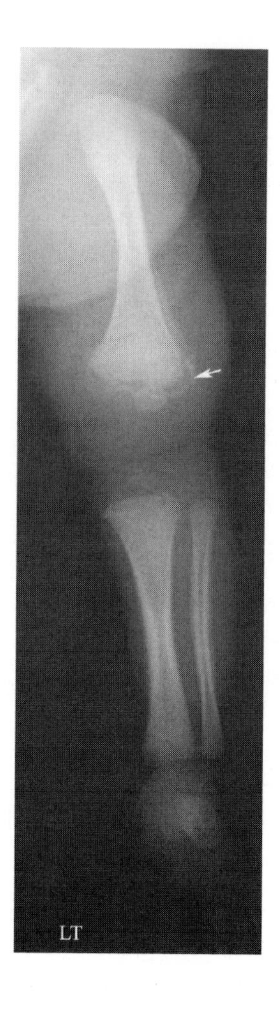

Fig. 8.1. Non-accidental injury. Anteroposterior radiograph of the left lower extremity in an infant with suspected NAI showing a typical bucket handle metaphyseal fracture of the distal femur (arrow) and metaphyseal corner fractures also involving the proximal and distal tibia. Subperiosteal new bone formation noted along the lateral femoral and fibular diaphyses. (Photo courtesy of Dr. Susie Muir, UCLA.)

Environment

Maintain an environment conducive to keeping the child as relaxed as possible. Allow the parent to interact with the child during any imaging and permit distractions such as toys. Sedation should be used with caution and only with appropriate support staff present.

The radiographer should be skilled and patient to achieve the required images without repetition. Effective immobilization is important to avoid repeat radiography and hence increase in radiation exposure.

Sedation should be used with caution and only with appropriate support staff present. A general anesthetic may rarely be needed in the emergency situation.

An imaging room used for infants and children should be kept warm to prevent loss of body heat and hypothermia.

Non-accidental injury (NAI)

A lack of correlation between history and injuries seen on imaging can sometimes be the first indication of NAI; it is always the radiologist's responsibility to raise the possibility of NAI when appropriate. However, it should be remembered that the investigation of NAI is a multidisciplinary effort and radiological imaging is only a small facet in the overall analysis of such cases.

Selection of contrast agent

When examining the gastrointestinal system in the acute situation use a water-soluble contrast medium with a strength of around 150 mg I/ml to limit any potential osmotic effect that the contrast may have on fluid balance between the blood and intestinal lumen, particularly important in sick neonates. If water-soluble contrast of a 150 mg I/ml is not available then dilute 300 mg I/ml contrast 50:50 with water. Warming the contrast prevents lowering the patient's core body temperature.

Suggested reading

Kuhn JP, Slovis TL, Haller JO. *Caffey's Pediatric Diagnostic Imaging, 10th edition*, pp. 1657–1662. Mosby, 2004.

Stringer DA, Babyn PS, eds. *Pediatric Gastrointestinal Imaging and Intervention, 2nd edition*, pp. 486–491. BC Decker, 2000.

8.2 Bowel atresia

Duodenal atresia and stenosis

Congenital abnormality comprising narrowing or complete obliteration of the duodenal lumen. See Fig. 8.2.

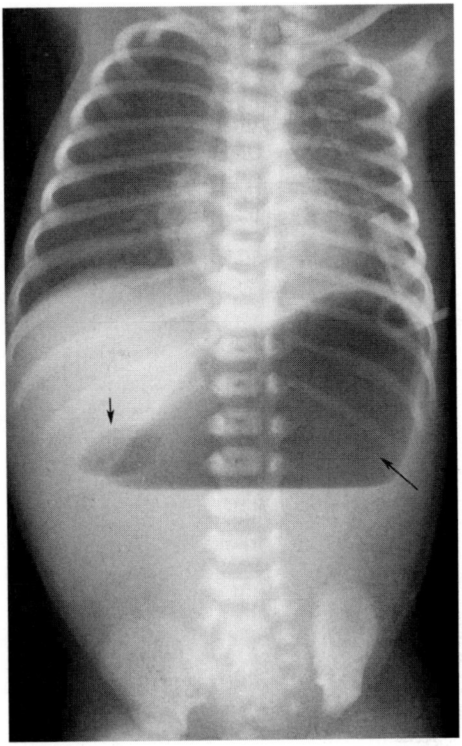

Fig. 8.2. Duodenal atresia. A chest and abdominal radiograph of a neonate shows markedly distended gas-filled stomach (long arrow) and a small gas-filled duodenal cap (short arrow) with paucity of gas in the rest of the abdomen, consistent with "double-bubble" sign of duodenal atresia.

Clinical

Presents in the first few hours or days of life as vomiting, abdominal distension with duodenal atresia.

Vomiting is usually bilious except in rare cases when the obstruction is above the ampulla of Vater. The neonate can rapidly deteriorate due to fluid loss and electrolyte imbalance.

Technique

Plain abdominal radiograph.

Upper GI contrast with dilute water-soluble contrast under fluoroscopy may confirm the diagnosis. An NG tube should always be in situ by the time a neonate with possible duodenal atresia attends for an upper GI study. After checking the NG tube position it can be used to introduce contrast into the stomach. If necessary the NG tube can be positioned in the duodenum. This technique is only required if there is suspicion of partial obstruction on plain radiograph without a "double-bubble" sign.

Findings

1. "Double-bubble" sign seen as gaseous distension or air–fluid levels within the stomach and duodenum.
2. Paucity of gas within the remaining small and large bowels.
3. Duodenal narrowing or stenosis on upper GI contrast study.

Pearls

- Aspiration of fluid from the stomach with a nasogastric tube and injection of 20–30 ml of air may demonstrate the double-bubble sign on radiograph.
- When associated with esophageal atresia the plain radiograph shows an opaque upper abdominal mass, which on ultrasound is seen as a fluid-filled sonolucent stomach and duodenum.
- Look for associated anomaly such as an anorectal malformation, or an abnormality of the cardiac or genitourinary systems (VATER).
- Duodenal atresia/stenosis is seen more frequently in trisomy 21 and is also associated with other gastrointestinal, biliary and renal abnormalities. Vertebral and rib anomalies can be identified on the plain radiograph.
- Antenatal ultrasound may show polyhydramnios and double-bubble sign.
- Duodenal obstruction can also be extrinsic to the bowel – due to Ladd's bands, small bowel malrotation or an annular pancreas.

Suggested reading

Fonkalsrud EW, deLorimier AA, Hays MD. Congenital atresia and stenosis of the duodenum: a review compiled from the member of the surgical section of the American Academy of Pediatrics. *Pediatrics* 1969;**43**:79–83.

Traubici J. The double bubble sign. *Radiology* 2001;**220**:463–464.

Jejuno-ileal atresia

Congenital obliteration or stenosis of the jejunal/ileal lumen. Thought to be secondary to an ischemic insult to the developing gut in utero.

Clinical

Complete obstruction presents as bilious vomiting usually within hours of birth, commonly after the first feed.

The abdomen can be scaphoid, normal or distended depending on how distal the lesion is. Stenosis can be more difficult to diagnose and can present later in life.

Technique

Plain abdominal radiograph as an initial investigation.

Water-soluble contrast enema to exclude other causes of lower GI obstruction involving the colon (see Sections 8.4, 8.5, 8.7).

Findings

1. Abdominal radiograph: Multiple loops of gas-filled bowel. The "higher" the obstruction the smaller the number of dilated loops. The "triple-bubble" sign has been described in cases of proximal jejunal obstruction. The bowel distal to a complete obstruction will be gasless.
2. Water-soluble contrast enema: Demonstrates a varying degree of microcolon. The higher the small bowel obstruction the less the degree of microcolon.

Pearls

- The key use of the water-soluble contrast enema is to distinguish colonic causes of obstruction from ileal obstruction. There may be a role for a water-soluble contrast upper GI study in demonstrating a proximal ileal obstruction or stenosis.
- Apple peel syndrome: Autosomal recessive inheritance, proximal jejunal atresia, shortened small bowel distal to atresia spiraling around its vascular supply consisting of left branch of ileocolic artery "the apple peel."
- Very proximal obstruction (jejunal) is not associated with microcolon but distal small bowel obstruction from ileal atresia is commonly associated with microcolon.

Suggested reading

Berrocal T *et al.* Congenital anomalies of the small intestine, colon, and rectum. *RadioGraphics* 1999;**19**:1219–1236.

Leonidas JC *et al.* Duodenojejunal atresia with "apple peel" small bowel. A distinct form of intestinal atresia. *Radiology* 1976;**118**(3):661–665.

8.3 Small bowel malrotation and volvulus

Abnormal position of the small bowel due to failure, incomplete or reversed rotation of the gut during fetal development. This results in a narrow mesenteric attachment that can predispose to mid-gut volvulus which can compromise blood circulation in the affected bowel. See Fig. 8.3.

Clinical

Most cases present in first month of life, typically with bilious vomiting. Older children present with recurrent attacks of abdominal pain, distension and vomiting.

If the volvulus is not recognized early, the child can rapidly deteriorate due to bowel infarction and this may be fatal.

Technique

Plain abdominal radiograph as an initial investigation.

Upper gastrointestinal contrast study is the most accurate (although not perfect) way of demonstrating malrotation. In the acute situation, low osmolar contrast is best injected down an NG tube into the stomach. If contrast is slow to leave the stomach the NG tube can be placed through the pylorus into the duodenum. In older children in the non-acute situation barium is the preferred contrast of choice.

Findings

Plain abdominal radiograph

1. Normal or show slight distension of the stomach and proximal duodenum.

Upper GI contrast study

2. On the AP view, the duodeno-jejunal (DJ) junction lies to the right of the spine and inferior to the level of the pylorus in malrotation, but this can be extremely variable (in a normal patient it lies to the left of the left vertebral pedicle and at the level of the pylorus).

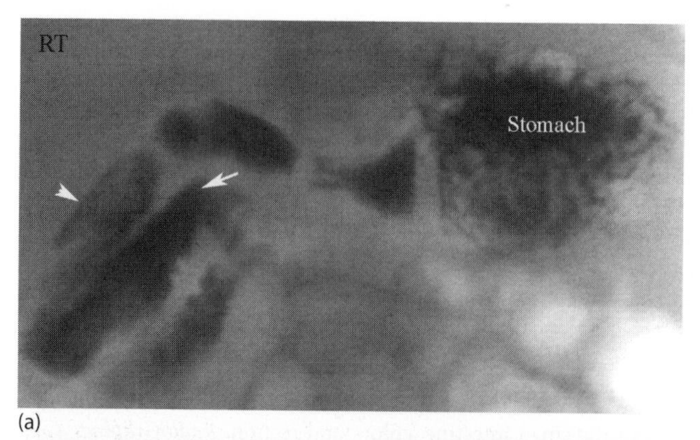

(a)

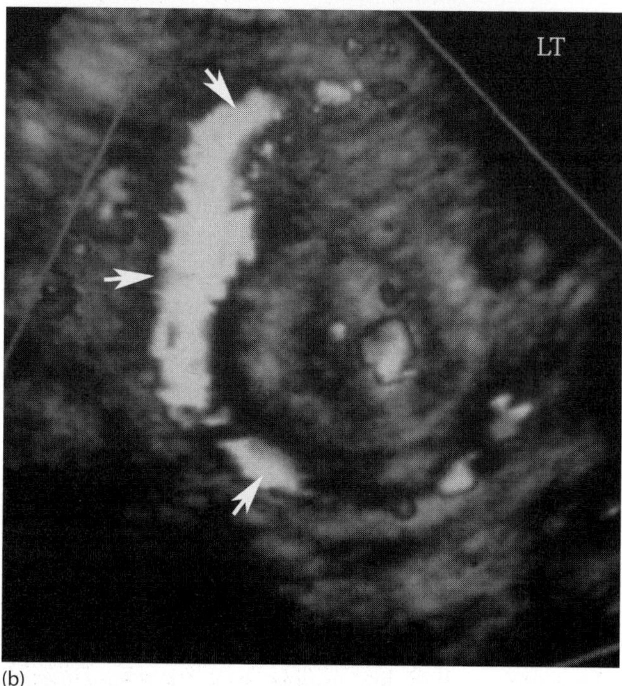

(b)

Fig. 8.3. (a) Malrotation. Upper GI contrast shows the duodenal loop (arrowhead) and duodenal-jejunal flexure (arrow) lie to the right of the spine and below the pylorus due to malrotation. (b) Malrotation and volvulus. A Doppler ultrasound image taken at the level of the super mesenteric artery in an infant shows an abnormal spiral pattern (arrows) to the vessels due to the small bowel rotation around a small mesenteric attachment. Although the "spiral" is counter-clockwise this child had a proven malrotation.

3. On the lateral view the junction of the 2nd and 3rd parts of the duodenum (are normally retroperitoneal) sharply turn anteriorly in malrotation.
4. A cork-screw appearance of the duodenum and jejunum is highly suggestive of a concurrent volvulus.
5. With volvulus and complete obstruction, the proximal duodenum is distended with tapering of the 3rd part giving a beaked appearance.

Pearls

- Delayed films showing the ileocecal junction may show the cecal pole to be higher and more towards the left of the abdomen. Normal position of the cecum does not exclude malrotation.

- Malrotation is also associated with peritoneal (Ladd) bands that can cause duodenal obstruction causing a double-bubble appearance on the plain radiograph.
- The relation of the superior mesenteric vein (SMV) to that of the superior mesenteric artery is altered in 2/3 of children with the SMV lying to the left of the artery. Ultrasound is however only complementary to fluoroscopy as this sign is neither sensitive nor specific.
- Color Doppler imaging can also demonstrate the "whirlpool" sign of the SMV spiraling around the SMA in children with volvulus. A counterclockwise spiral has been reported as a normal variant, however, so this sign should be treated with caution.
- If there is marked bowel distension the appearances should be interpreted with caution as the true position of the DJ flexure can be distorted producing false positive and negative results.
- In babies < 4 years of age normal DJ junction may be mobile. The enlarging spleen, an indwelling nasogastric tube or manual palpation can alter the DJ position in normal babies.
- Diagnosis of malrotation using an upper GI study can be difficult because of the confounding factors mentioned above. Reference to the suggested reading below may help in difficult cases.
- Acute mid-gut volvulus is an emergency and needs immediate surgical attention.

Suggested reading

Refer to Section 8.1.

Long FR *et al*. Intestinal malrotation in children: tutorial on radiographic diagnosis in difficult cases. *Radiology* 1996;**198**(3):775–780.

8.4 Meconium ileus

Distal small bowel obstruction in neonates due to impaction of meconium. See Fig. 8.4.

Clinical

More than 90% of cases of meconium ileus are associated with cystic fibrosis (CF) and this is the earliest clinical manifestation of CF. Neonates present with vomiting, abdominal distension and failure to pass meconium. Complications include volvulus, ischemia, necrosis and meconium peritonitis.

Technique

Plain radiographs of the abdomen.

Contrast enema using water-soluble contrast agent is the gold standard technique. Once the diagnosis is established half strength gastrografin can be used as a therapeutic agent with extreme caution in conjunction with the surgical team and adequate fluid resuscitation.

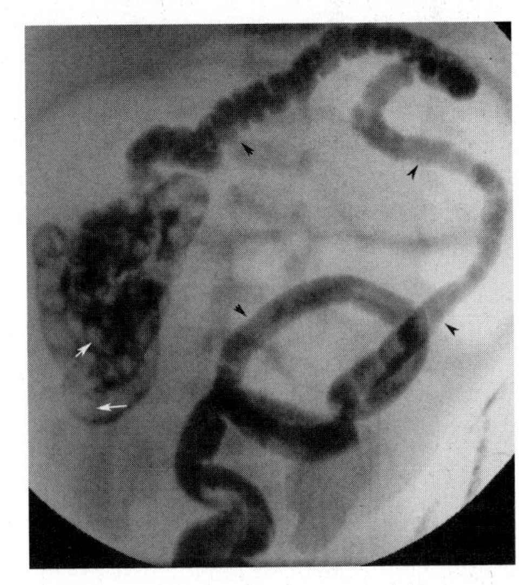

Fig. 8.4. Meconium ileus. A water-soluble contrast enema shows a microcolon (arrowheads) and meconium plugs (arrows) within the terminal ileum in a neonate with meconium ileus and cystic fibrosis.

Findings

1. Multiple dilated bowel loops with a soap bubble appearance in the right iliac fossa caused by a mixture of meconium and gas on radiograph.
2. Contrast enema shows typically a small caliber colon (microcolon). This is non-specific and can be seen in ileal atresia and stenosis.
3. Contrast when refluxed into the distal ileum outlines multiple pellets of meconium and may then pass into dilated small bowel.
4. Meconium ileus can be complicated by volvulus which can lead to ischemic necrosis and perforation of bowel. The spilled meconium can either form a psuedocyst or give rise to meconium peritonitis or meconium hydrocele.
5. Meconium peritonitis can appear as intraperitoneal free fluid separating the bowel loops associated with multiple calcified psuedocysts.
6. Scrotal calcifications can also be seen due to passage of intraperitoneal meconium into the scrotum through a patent tunica vaginalis.

Pearls

- Filling of the terminal ileum must be attempted in every case to demonstrate the inspissated meconium pellets.
- Gastrografin, being hypertonic, helps to soften the meconium by drawing water into the lumen, thus acting as a therapeutic agent. The infant should be well hydrated with intravenous fluid to prevent shock and electrolyte imbalance as a result of the procedure. Repeated studies can be performed to dissolve the thick meconium. If no improvement, surgery is indicated.
- The procedure carries a 5% risk of intestinal perforation.
- Additional laboratory tests for CF will contribute to the diagnostic process.
- Calcification within the abdomen indicates the presence of meconium peritonitis secondary to in utero perforation.

Suggested reading

Refer to Section 8.1.

Kao SC *et al.* Non-operative treatment of simple meconium ileus: a survey of the Society for Pediatric Radiology. *Pediatr Radiol* 1995;25:97–100.

8.5 Meconium plug syndrome

Meconium plug syndrome (MPS) is a transient form of colonic obstruction caused by inspissation of meconium in a functionally immature colon. See Fig. 8.5.

Clinical

Most infants present within the first 24–36 hours with abdominal distension, failure to pass meconium and vomiting. It is common with infants born to mothers who are diabetic or who have received magnesium sulphate, and sometimes occurs in infants with cystic fibrosis.

Technique

Plain radiograph of the abdomen shows non-specific features of distal bowel obstruction.

Water-soluble contrast enema to confirm the diagnosis.

Findings

1. Contrast enema results in a characteristic "double-contrast effect" with contrast between the meconium and the bowel wall.
2. In some infants, especially those associated with maternal diabetes, a small contracted descending colon is seen. This has led to the term Small left colon syndrome. The segment of colon proximal to the transition zone is moderately distended with inspissated meconium.

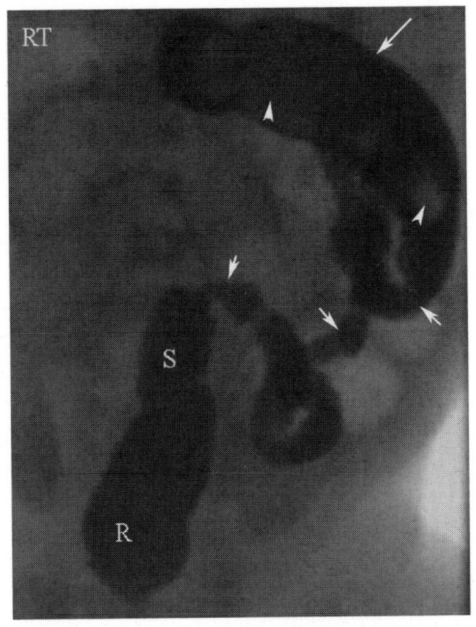

Fig. 8.5. Meconium plug syndrome. A water-soluble contrast enema shows the descending colon has a small caliber (short arrows) with a transition point in the region of the splenic flexure to dilated colon (long arrow) containing a filling defect that is the meconium plug (arrowheads). Note the rectum is still larger than the sigmoid colon.

Pearls

- Hirschsprung's disease is an important differential which must be excluded before considering the diagnosis of MPS.
- Plain radiographs can show a bubbly appearance mimicking necrotizing enterocolitis (NEC). NEC usually presents 48–72 hours after birth, unlike MPS which presents earlier, but clinical findings play an important role in distinguishing the two.
- The contrast enema is therapeutic with resolution of intestinal dilatation once the meconium is passed.

Suggested reading

Berdon WE *et al.* Neonatal small left colon syndrome: its relationship to aganglionosis and meconium plug syndrome. *Radiology* 1977;**125**:457–462.

Swischuk LE. *Imaging of the Newborn, Infant, and Young Child, 4th edition*, pp. 460–463. Philadelphia, Lippincott, Williams & Wilkins, 1997.

8.6 Necrotizing enterocolitis

Necrotizing enterocolitis (NEC) is an inflammatory/ischemic bowel pathology of unknown etiology presenting in the neonatal period, most commonly in premature neonates. See Fig. 8.6.

Clinical

Necrotizing enterocolitis commonly affects the preterm neonate. It can also affect term infants with bowel obstruction as in Hirschsprung's disease, polycythemia, dehydration and cyanotic congenital heart disease. Initial symptoms are non-specific, simulating neonatal sepsis. These include lethargy, hypoglycemia, feed intolerance and temperature instability. Late signs include vomiting, diarrhea, abdominal distension with discoloration and shock. The mortality rate is approximately 30%.

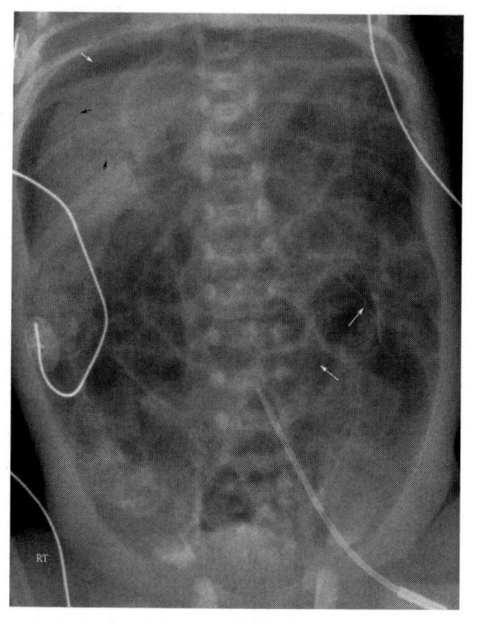

Fig. 8.6. Necrotizing enterocolitis. A plain abdominal radiograph demonstrating free intraperitoneal air in the abdomen (short white arrow) of a neonate with NEC. Rigler's sign (gas on both sides of the bowel wall) (long white arrows) and portal venous gas (black arrows) are noted.

Technique

Plain radiograph (supine AP as standard and cross-table, lateral and decubitus plain abdominal X-rays when looking for small amounts of free gas).

Ultrasound is complementary in diagnosis and monitoring.

Findings

1. Dilatation of large and small bowel or isolated gastric dilatation. A bowel loop that is wider than the coronal width of L1 is considered dilated. Serial radiographs demonstrate persistent dilatation of some loops.
2. Bowel wall appears thickened or contains air (pneumatosis intestinalis) which gives a bubbly appearance when submucosal and curvilinear "tram track" when subserosal.
3. Air in the portal venous system, seen as a peripheral branching leucency on plain radiograph and bubbles in the portal venous system on US.
4. Pneumoperitoneum, free intra-abdominal fluid or focal fluid collection suggest perforation, which is an indication for surgery.

Pearls

- Though pneumatosis is a specific sign, it is not seen in all neonates and mere dilatation of the bowel in an acutely unwell neonate should raise suspicion of NEC, particularly if dilatation is persistent.
- Serial radiographs every 6–12 hours may be required to monitor NEC and the development of bowel perforation – free intraperitoneal air.
- Signs of perforation: In supine radiograph a small amount of air outlining the bowel from both sides – "Rigler sign." Large intraperitoneal air can outline peritoneal cavity, undersurface of diaphragm and falciform ligament – "football sign."

- Ultrasound is more sensitive than plain radiographs in detecting fluid collection, ascites, and portal venous gas; the latter appears as flowing echogenic particles within the portal vein and multiple echogenicities within the peripheral liver parenchyma. Pneumatosis intestinalis and bowel wall thickening (inflammation) or thinning < 1 mm (ischemia) can also be well appreciated on US.
- Bowel dilatation alone can be present in premature infants who do not tolerate feeding, infants receiving continuous positive pressure ventilation, infants with ileus or following resuscitation. So the imaging findings must be correlated with the clinical history.

Suggested reading

Daneman A *et al.* The radiology of neonatal necrotizing enterocolitis. A review of 47 cases and the literature. *Pediatr Radiol* 1978;7:70–77.

Silva CT *et al.* Correlation of sonographic findings and outcome in necrotizing enterocolitis. *Pediatr Radiol* 2007;**37**(3):274–282.

8.7 Hirschprung's disease

Functional low-bowel obstruction secondary to absence of parasympathetic ganglia in bowel extending from the anus to variable lengths of proximal colon. See Fig. 8.7.

Clinical

The extent of disease can range from involvement of the anus alone (ultra-short segment disease) to total colonic aganglionosis (5%). The most common (80%) form is the short-segment disease where the aganglionic segment extends to the recto-sigmoid region. Neonates present with failure to pass meconium in the first 48 hours, abdominal distension and vomiting. Older children present with chronic constipation sometimes associated with intermittent paradoxical diarrhea. Complications include enterocolitis (up to 30%), volvulus and perforation.

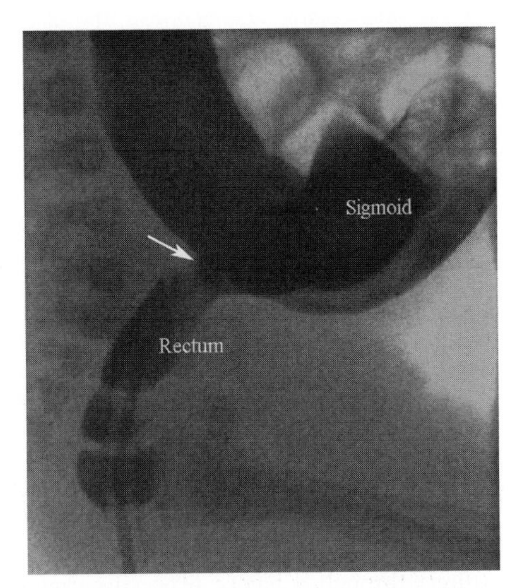

Fig. 8.7. Hirschprung's disease. An image from a water-soluble contrast enema in a baby with Hirschprung's disease shows that despite good distension the rectum remains of smaller caliber than the sigmoid colon, which contains meconium. A transition zone of caliber change (arrow) is seen at the recto-sigmoid junction.

Technique

Plain radiographs show signs of distal bowel obstruction. There is absence of gas in the rectum but this is a non-specific finding.

Contrast enema using water-soluble agent is the investigation of choice. A soft catheter should be used and inserted just into the rectum. The balloon should not be inflated. Rectal examination and bowel preparation prior to examination is best avoided as this will change the appearance of imaging. Contrast is best injected into the catheter using a 20 ml syringe. Commence the study with child in left lateral position, document the rectosigmoid region in lateral and AP. Establish the presence of transition zone level. Once it is demonstrated, stop the procedure.

Findings

1. Transition zone noted between the narrow aganglionic segment of bowel and the distended innervated segment that appears as an inverted cone. The transition zone may not be easily identified in some cases, especially in neonates.
2. Abnormal contractions and irregular peristalsis is sometimes seen in the aganglionic segment.
3. The ratio of the transverse diameters of the rectum and sigmoid (recto-sigmoid index) which is normally > 1 is reversed in short segment disease.
4. Mucosal edema and ulceration is seen when the disease is complicated by colitis.

Pearls

- Definitive diagnosis is made by biopsy and analysis. A contrast enema can be safely performed 24 hours after a suction biopsy and 4 days after a full thickness biopsy using a water-soluble agent.
- In total colonic aganglionosis, the plain radiographs show signs of distal small bowel obstruction. The contrast enema may demonstrate a normal colon, a microcolon or a short colon. Abnormal contractions can be noted throughout the colon.

Suggested reading

Refer to Section 8.1.

8.8 Obstructed hernia

Intestinal obstruction secondary to extraperitoneal or rarely intraperitoneal (mesenteric) herniation of a segment of bowel. See Fig. 8.8.

Clinical

Inguinal hernia is the common form of bowel herniation in children. It is almost always indirect through a patent processus vaginalis. A majority of hernias are asymptomatic, presenting as a groin swelling. An incarcerated hernia presents with clinical features of intestinal obstruction depending on the segment of bowel involved. A small proportion can develop strangulation of the bowel.

Umbilical hernia is also commonly seen in children – it usually disappears spontaneously.

Technique

Plain abdominal radiograph and ultrasound.

Findings

1. Plain radiograph will reveal multiple distended bowel loops and a gas-filled loop may be seen in the region of the inguinal canal or scrotum.
2. In an incarcerated hernia where the bowel loop is fluid-filled, the hernia may appear as thickening of the inguino-scrotal fold on the affected side.
3. Ultrasonography can be used to visualize the inguinal structures which may contain fluid or air-filled bowel and omentum. In female children the ovary and fallopian tube can also herniate through the canal of Nuck causing a prominent labial fold.

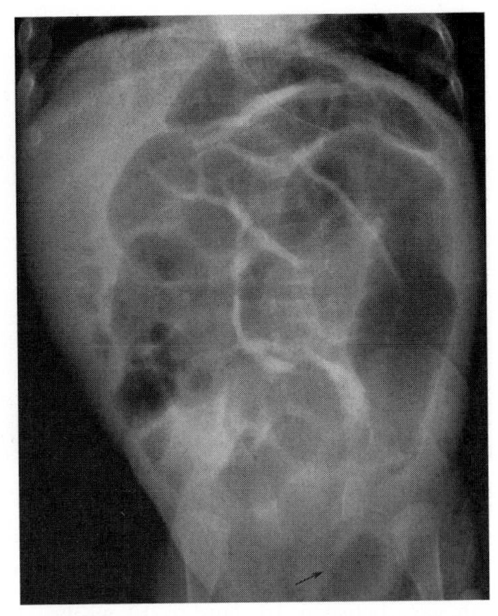

Fig. 8.8. Incarcerated inguinal hernia. A plain abdominal radiograph in a young child with an obstructed inguinal hernia shows multiple loops of distended gas-filled bowel and gas within the left scrotum (arrow).

Lack of peristaltic activity in the dilated bowel loop in the hernial sac is highly suggestive of strangulation.

Pearls

- In a child with bowel obstruction, always look at the inguinal/scrotal region for bowel gas that may indicate a hernia as the cause of obstruction.

Suggested reading

Carty HML. Paediatric emergencies: non-traumatic abdominal emergencies. *Eur Radiol* 2002; 12:2835–2848.

Irish MS *et al.* The approach to common abdominal diagnosis in infants and children. *Pediatr Clin N Am* 1998;45(4):729–772.

8.9 Pyloric stenosis

Hypertrophy and hyperplasia of the pyloric musculature leading to partial gastric outlet obstruction. See Fig. 8.9.

Clinical

Infants usually typically present at between 3–5 weeks with non-bilious projectile vomiting which may lead to dehydration, hypochloremic alkalosis and weight loss. The age of onset

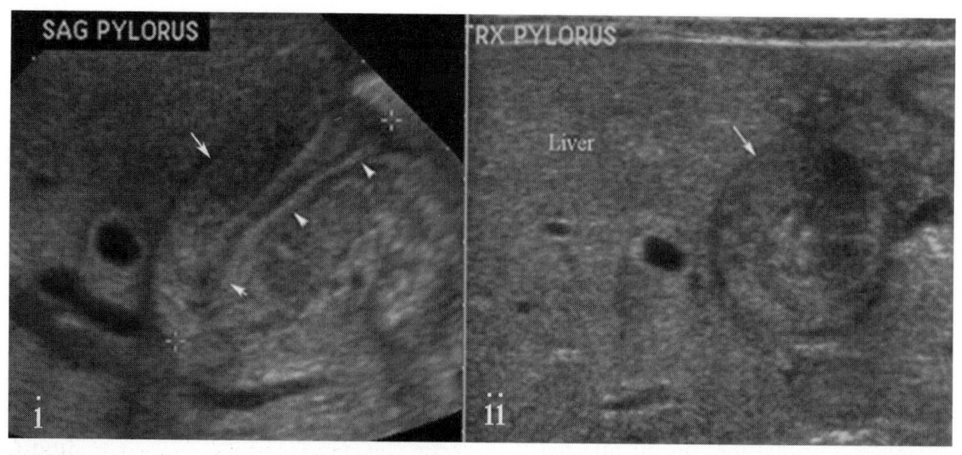

Fig. 8.9. Pyloric stenosis. Ultrasound images of a patient with history of non-bilious vomiting shows an enlarged pylorus (arrow) with increased pyloric wall thickness and increased pyloric length (arrowheads) due to pyloric stenosis.

can vary between 10 days to 12 weeks. An olive-shaped mass may be palpable in the epigastric region.

Technique

Ultrasound examination of the pylorus. Linear high frequency probe. Study is done with patient in right lateral decubitus. Fluid is usually present within the distended stomach.

Findings

1. Gastric distension in a vomiting infant.
2. The hypertrophied pylorus appears a target sign on transverse section with a hypoechoic ring of muscle surrounding a central echogenic mucosal layer.
3. A single wall muscle thickness of ≥ 3 mm or a pyloric canal length ≥ 17 mm is diagnostic of pyloric stenosis.
4. Failure of opening of the pyloric canal during gastric peristalsis – this is not a reliable sign on its own.
5. Upper GI contrast study (which is rarely performed) may be useful if the ultrasound study is not conclusive. Contrast meal shows a "double-track" sign of contrast within the pyloric canal separated by redundant intervening mucosa. A "string" sign of a streak of contrast through the pyloric canal. "Antral beak" sign with pyloric impression on the antrum with a streak of barium pointing to the pyloric canal.
6. Fluoroscopy may show vigorous peristalsis called a "caterpillar" sign stopping abruptly at the pyloric antrum. Thickened pyloric muscles give extrinsic impression on the barium column, named the "Shoulder" sign.

Pearls

- Feeding the infant during the scan with appropriate fluid is useful to appreciate gastric peristalsis and to check for fluid transit via the pylorus.

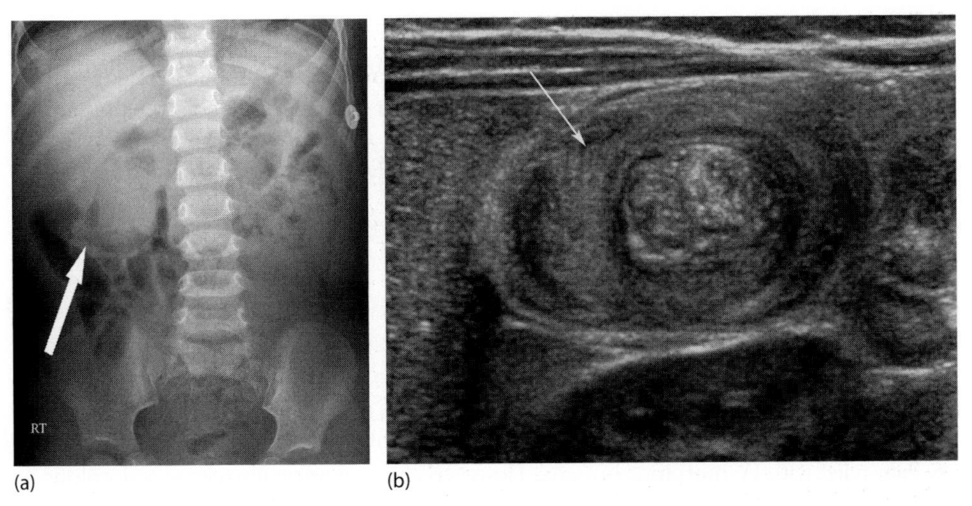

Fig. 8.10. (a) Intussusception. A plain radiograph in a young child demonstrating a soft tissue mass in the right upper quadrant (arrow) due to an intussusception mass. (b) Intussusception. Ultrasound of a transverse section of an intussusception producing the classical target appearance (arrow).

- Pyloric muscle thickness of 2 mm and canal length of 14 mm are considered normal. In infants with equivocal imaging findings i.e. pyloric muscle thickness of 2–3 mm and canal length between 14–17 mm a repeat scan after 24 hours may be useful. In spasm, the pyloric wall thickness is less than 3 mm.
- Upper GI contrast studies may also exclude other causes of upper GI obstruction such as malrotation or duodenal stenosis.

Suggested reading

Aspelund G, Langer JC. Current management of hypertrophic pyloric stenosis. *Semin Pediatr Surg* 2007;**16**:27–33.

Hernanz-Shulman M. Infantile hypertrophic pyloric stenosis. *Radiology* 2003;**227**(2):319–331.

8.10 Intussusception

Intussusception is the invagination of bowel into more distal bowel. See Fig. 8.10.

Clinical

It typically presents between 6 months and 2 years with sudden onset of crampy abdominal pain, vomiting, lethargy and bloody diarrhea ("redcurrant jelly"). Peritonitis and hypovolemic shock are late signs. If untreated it can lead to bowel infarction. The most common form is ileo-colic intussusception.

The abdominal radiograph frequently is not helpful; it may reveal a meniscus of soft tissue mass in an air-filled colon, frequently in the right lower quadrant (or in the region of transverse colon) and signs of small bowel obstruction.

Technique

Ultrasound, linear high frequency probe. A full abdominal scan should be performed. Start in right lower quadrant and scan the whole abdomen. If normal, it excludes the presence of intussusception.

Fluoroscopic intussusception reduction – should only be attempted by a radiologist with appropriate training and experience.

1. Patient must be fully hydrated with IV access.
2. Contraindications – peritonitis and/or shock.
3. Informed consent is necessary.
4. Surgeons and anesthetists with pediatric experience should be aware of the procedure and be on site. Preferably the surgeon should be present at the time of the reduction.
5. Personnel competent in pediatric resuscitation should be present.
6. Pain relief with IV morphine is useful. However, children normally release endorphins.
7. Pneumatic reduction is favorable using a specifically designed device that can measure pressure. Hydrostatic reduction can be used by experienced personnel.
8. The starting pressure should be 80 mmHg. Three sustained attempts at reduction of 3 minutes long are recommended with a maximum pressure of 120 mmHg.
9. Successful reduction is indicated by seeing air filling the terminal ileum but this can sometimes be difficult to see. Careful comparison between a control (pre-inflation image) and post-reduction image can be helpful.
10. A second attempt at reduction can be helpful 2–8 hours later but this is controversial.
11. Bowel perforation leads to a pneumoperitoneum and the procedure should be stopped immediately. If the pneumoperitoneum causes respiratory compromise then a needle puncture of the abdomen can relieve the pressure.

Findings

1. Transverse scan through the mass demonstrates concentric rings of alternating hyper- and hypoechoic layers (target/doughnut sign).
2. Longitudinal scans show hypoechogenicity on either side of an echogenic mesentery (pseudo kidney).
3. The lesion is often found in the right upper quadrant except in cases where the intussusception has progressed more distally into the transverse colon.
4. Absence of blood flow on color Doppler may indicate bowel necrosis but is not a contraindication for air reduction in itself.
5. Free fluid can be seen within the abdomen but does not mean air reduction will be unsuccessful.
6. Pneumoperitoneum indicates a perforation and is a contraindication for air reduction and an indication for surgery.

Pearls

- The entire abdomen must be scanned as the intussusception mass can lie anywhere between the cecum and the sigmoid colon.

- Children >3 years are likely to have a pathological lead point (Meckel's diverticulum, lymphoma, Henoch–Schonlein purpura, bowel duplication cyst).
- Peritonitis, pneumoperitoneum and recurrent intussusception are contraindications to pneumatic reduction.

Suggested reading

British Society of Paediatric Radiology draft guidelines for intussusception reduction. Dr. K. McHugh. http://www.bspr.org.uk/intuss.htm.

Carty H, Brunelle F, eds. *Imaging Children, 2nd edition*, pp. 1498–1501. Edinburgh: Elsevier Churchill Livingstone, 2005.

Daneman A, Navarro O. Intussusception. Part 2: An update on the evolution of management. *Pediatr Radiol* 2004;34(2):97–108.

8.11 Acute appendicitis

Infection and inflammation of the appendix most often due to obstruction of the appendiceal lumen. See Fig. 8.11.

Clinical

Appendicitis presents as fever, nausea, vomiting, diarrhea and right lower quadrant pain. It most commonly affects individuals in the 2nd and 3rd decade. Non-specific presentations are more common in younger children. Complications include perforation and peritonitis.

Technique

Ultrasound imaging with linear probe using a graded compression technique.

CT has a greater accuracy in diagnosing appendicitis and is increasingly used, especially in patients with a strong clinical suspicion and equivocal findings on ultrasound.

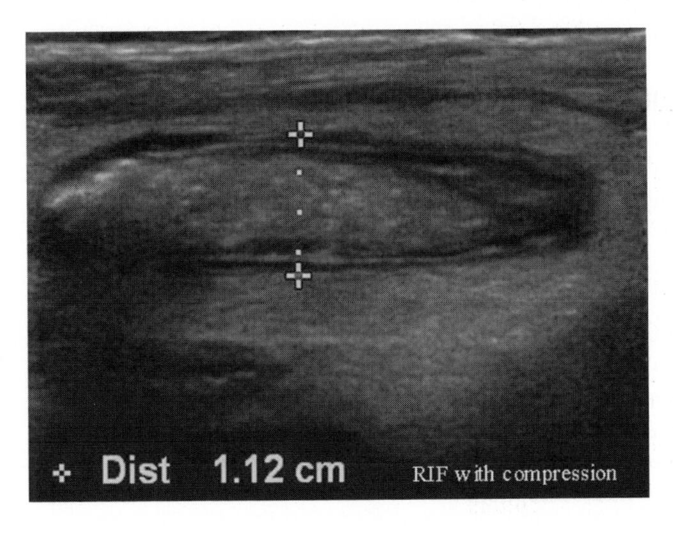

Fig. 8.11. Appendicitis. Ultrasound of the right iliac fossa demonstrating a non-compressible tubular structure (between the calipers) representing an inflamed appendix. (Photo courtesy of Dr. Gurdeep Mann, Alder Hey Children's NHS Foundation Trust.)

Findings

1. Plain radiographs may reveal an appendicolith (7–15%), abrupt cessation of transverse colon gas at the hepatic flexure and distortion of the right psoas margin. In perforation there may be evidence of small bowel obstruction with displacement of bowel loops from the right iliac fossa.
2. On ultrasound swollen, tubular, fluid-filled, blind-ending structure which is non-compressible and measures $\geq$ 6 mm in diameter on cross-section.
3. Diffuse hypoechogenicity with poorly defined mucosal layer in the right iliac fossa is indicative of appendicitis/appendix mass even if the appendix is not itself visualized.
4. Fecolith can sometimes be seen (6%).
5. Enlarged reactive lymph nodes are commonly noted.
6. Perforated appendix appears as an intraperitoneal fluid collection.
7. On CT there is circumferential thickening of the appendix with periappendiceal fat stranding and soft tissue mass indicative of inflammation. Appendicolith is noted in 25%. Focal thickening of the cecal apex is often seen.

Pearls

- Complete ultrasound scan of the abdomen and pelvis should be performed to exclude other causes of acute abdomen.
- False negative ultrasound scans are due to a retrocecal position of the appendix, if the appendix is gas filled, resolving appendicitis or if the inflammation is restricted to the tip of the appendix.

Suggested reading

Levine CD *et al.* Pitfalls in the CT diagnosis of appendicitis. *Br J Radiol* 2004;77:792–799.

Stephen AE *et al.* The diagnosis of acute appendicitis in a pediatric population: to CT or Not to CT. *J Pediatr Surg* 2003;**38**(3):367–371.

8.12 Complicated ovarian cyst

Fluid-filled cysts in the ovaries are most often functional cysts developing from the ovarian follicle. They may occasionally enlarge and undergo complications such as rupture, hemorrhage or cause ovarian torsion. See Fig. 8.12.

Clinical

Hemorrhagic ovarian cysts (HOC) present with sudden, severe and transient lower abdominal pain. Ovarian torsion also presents as acute lower abdominal pain and is sometimes associated with nausea, vomiting or constipation.

Some patients have recurrent pelvic pain suggesting bouts of torsion and de-torsion. The non-specific nature of the symptoms may mislead physicians into diagnoses such as appendicitis, gastroenteritis and intussusception.

Technique

Transabdominal ultrasound scan of the pelvis and entire abdomen. Use Doppler to evaluate for possible torsion.

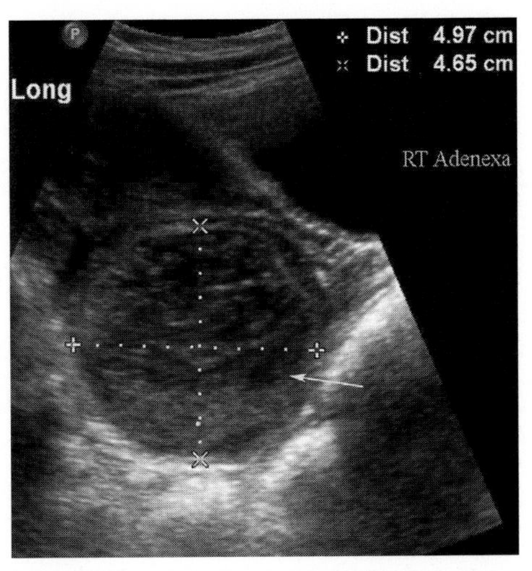

Fig. 8.12. Complex right ovarian cyst. Ultrasound of the right ovary of a teenage girl with acute right iliac fossa pain demonstrates a 5 cm complex cyst in the right adnexum (arrow).

Findings

Hemorrhagic ovarian cyst

1. HOCs are usually heterogeneous with hypo- or hyperechoic areas separated by thin or thick linear echoes (reticular pattern). The cysts are sometimes hypoechoic with a round echogenicity of varying size which represents the retracted clot.
2. The echogenicity changes with time appearing bright in the early stages and progressively decreasing in echogenicity as the blood products resolve.

Ovarian torsion

1. The appearance of the ovary is variable depending on the presence of hemorrhage, edema or infarction. It is usually markedly enlarged (volume > 10 ml) with a central hyperechogenic area and multiple peripheral cysts measuring 8–15 mm (secondary to transudation).
2. Fluid debris levels may be noted within the peripheral cysts.
3. Absence of flow on color Doppler is indicative of torsion but presence of flow does not exclude it.
4. Free fluid in the cul-de-sac is sometimes seen but is non-specific.

Pearls

- Conditions such as tubo-ovarian abscess, ectopic pregnancy, benign cystic teratomas and an appendix abscess are important differential diagnoses to consider and clinical correlation is vital in the management.

Suggested reading

Hayes-Jordan A. Surgical management of the incidentally identified ovarian mass. *Semin Pediatr Surg* 2005;**14**(2):106–110.

Pfeifer SM, Gosman GG. Evaluation of adenexal masses in adolescents. *Pediatr Clin N Am* 1999; **46**(3):573–592.

8.13 Testicular torsion

Twisting of the spermatic cord resulting in compromise of blood flow to the testis and epididymis. See Fig. 8.13.

Clinical

Testicular torsion is common in peripubertal boys, presenting as sudden severe scrotal pain, sometimes radiating to the groin and abdomen. It may be associated with nausea and vomiting. Low-grade fever and leukocytosis are sometimes present but urine analysis usually shows negative results. Testicular atrophy is a complication if surgical detorsion is delayed. Testicular salvage rate is 80% in the first 6 hours decreasing to 20% if surgery is delayed for 24 hours.

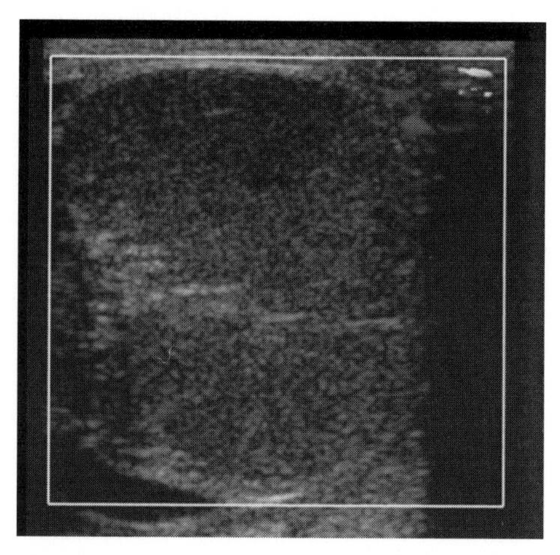

Fig. 8.13. Proven testicular torsion. The testis is hypoechoic and demonstrates no flow due to torsion.

Technique

Gray scale and Doppler ultrasound scan of the testes using a high frequency linear transducer.

Findings

1. Testicular and epididymal enlargement with hypoechogenicity and a secondary hydrocele (10%). The testis may be of normal echogenicity and size within the first 6 hours.
2. Enlarged twisted spermatic cord.
3. Change in the axis of testis (compare with the contralateral testis).
4. If there is a delay in diagnosis the testis may appear heterogeneous due to hemorrhage or necrosis.
5. There can be absence or decreased vascularity on color Doppler imaging.

Pearls

- Ultrasound diagnosis of torsion can be difficult and the clinical history and examination are paramount.
- The demonstration of normal blood flow does not exclude torsion due to spontaneous detorsion in some cases. If the torsion is less than 360° the vascularity may be present but diminished and comparison to the normal side is helpful.
- Differential diagnoses include torsion of the appendix testis/epididymis, epididymo-orchitis and cellulitis where the testicular vascularity is normal or increased.
- Advancement in ultrasound technology has decreased the use of nuclear scintigraphy with Tc 99 m pertechnetate in testicular torsion. If present, torsion manifests as decreased perfusion with a halo of increased activity.

Suggested reading

Gatti JM, Murphy PM. Current management of the acute scrotum. *Semin Pediatr Surg* 2007;**16**:58–63.

Kass EJ Lundak B. The acute scrotum. *Pediatr Clin N Am* 1997;**44**(5):668–679.

8.14 The painful hip

A painful hip is a common complaint in pediatric practice and can be a result of a number of conditions. See Fig. 8.14.

Clinical

Pathology of the pediatric hip can present in a number of ways depending on the age of the child and cause of the pathology. The baby and infant may simply present with irritability and fever which on closer inspection is associated with reduced movement of a leg. A toddler may stop walking and an older child may complain specifically of pain in the hip. Pain can be referred to the thigh or knee. A number of pathologies are common in the hip in children and the type of pathology is often age related.

Irritable hip or *transient synovitis* is usually a post-viral phenomenon seen in 3- to 8-year-olds. Symptoms overlap with those of septic arthritis and osteomyelitis but the child is usually well but with pain in the hip and limited movement. Irritable hip must be a diagnosis of exclusion.

Perthes disease or *avascular necrosis* of the femoral head occur most commonly from ages 4–8 years. The child is afebrile and has restricted hip movements; the classical risk factors for avascular necrosis of the hip are usually absent. 20% of children will have bilateral disease.

Slipped capital femoral epiphysis (SCFE) occurs in late childhood and adolescence affecting boys more than girls and is often associated with a weight > 90th centile. Bilateral disease is found in up to 36% of cases.

Osteomyelitis and *septic arthritis* will usually present in a child who is systemically unwell.

A full blood count and ESR may help to distinguish between infective conditions and other causes of painful hip but infection must always be excluded when investigating a painful hip.

Juvenile idiopathic arthritis (JIA) can also cause inflammation of the hip and should always be considered as a cause of pain and reduced movement in the hip.

Technique

Plain films and ultrasound together are the emergency imaging of choice. Nuclear medicine and MRI are second-line investigations that can be used in difficult cases.
Plain films: Anterioposterior and frog-leg views of the pelvis.
Ultrasound: Of the anterior hip using a linear high-frequency probe.

Findings

1. Plain film.

    Can be normal in all the above conditions except slipped capital femoral epiphysis.

    Irritable hip: Appearances should be normal. Look for joint effusion.

    Perthes disease: Initially normal progressing from subarticular lucency to sclerosis and fragmentation.

    SCFE has diagnostic appearances of widening of the epiphyseal plate and varying degrees of displacement of the upper femoral epiphysis medially and posteriorly. A line

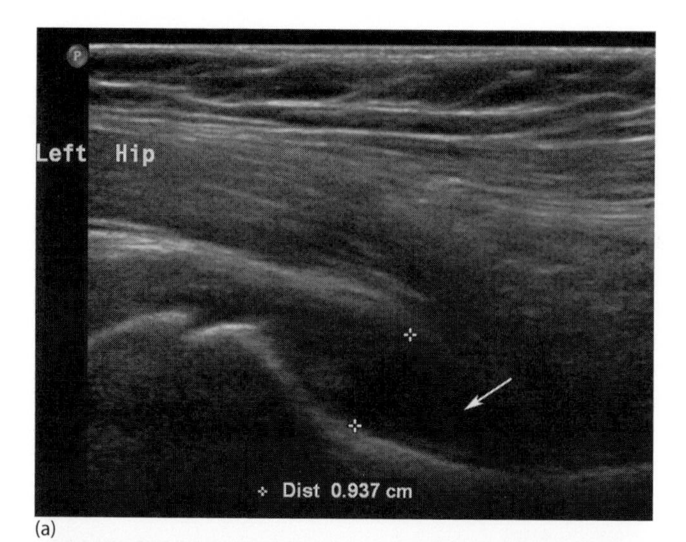

(a)

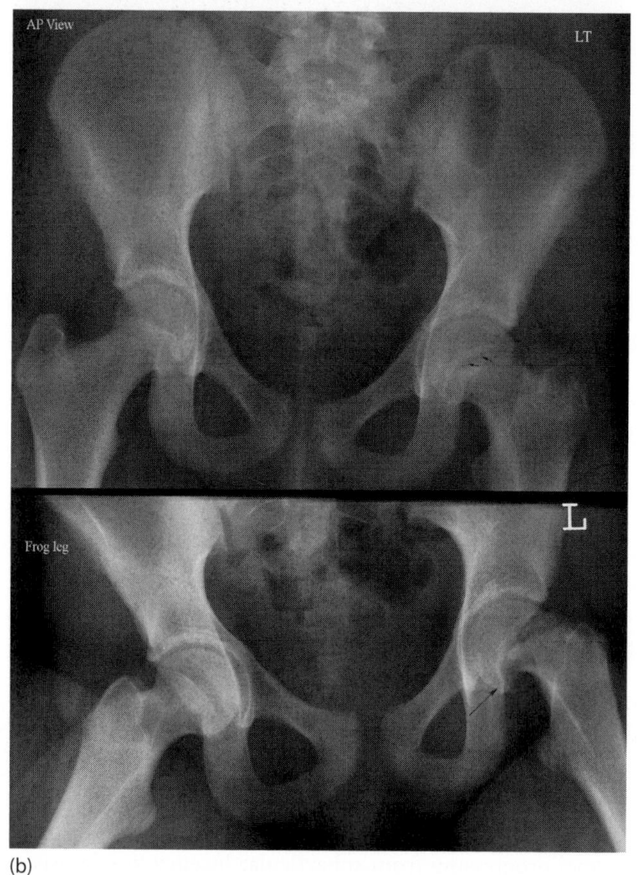

(b)

Fig. 8.14. (a) Left hip effusion. Ultrasound of the left hip demonstrating anechoic collection suggestive of hip effusion (arrow). (b) Slipped capital femoral epiphysis. AP and frog-leg views on a child with a left slipped upper femoral epiphysis shows the growth plate on the left is enlarged (short arrows) compared with the right side. The slip is much more apparent on the frog-leg view (long arrow).

drawn along the upper border of the femoral neck line of Klein should intersect the upper capital epiphysis. If the line passes lateral and above the epiphysis this is strongly suggestive of SCFE. The frog-leg view will demonstrate more subtle degrees of slip and is important in determining whether a slip is present on the contralateral side.

Osteomyelitis and septic arthritis: Most often normal.

Juvenile idiopathic arthritis: Initially normal progressing from periarticular lucency to loss of joint space and joint erosions.

2. Ultrasound.

All of the above conditions (except perhaps commonly SCFE) can present with fluid in the hip joint seen as a lifting of the joint capsule from the anterior neck of the femur. Fluid can be hypoechoic to echogenic.

Thickening of the synovium of the hip can also be identified but is a non-specific finding.

In osteomyelitis, lifting of the periosteum also at the femoral neck and diaphysis may be seen.

Pearls

- Septic arthritis in the neonate and infant should be treated as an emergency if damage to the hip joint is to be prevented. If there is strong clinical suspicion then immediate drainage of the joint without the need for imaging is appropriate.
- The absence of fluid in the joint on US does not exclude septic arthritis as a cause for hip pain.
- On US of the hip the echogenicity of the joint fluid does not indicate the presence or absence of septic arthritis.
- Clinical correlation with imaging and laboratory findings is essential to make a correct distinction between causes of a painful hip.
- MRI scanning in the non-emergency situation is often an essential further investigation.

Suggested reading

Koop S, Quanbeck D. Three common causes of childhood hip pain. *Pediatr Clin N Am* 1996; 43(5):1053–1065.

8.15 Miscellaneous

Congenital diaphragmatic hernia

Congenital diaphragmatic hernia is one of the more common congenital anomalies seen in the newborn. Almost 90% of congenital diaphragmatic hernias are through the foramen of Bockdalek on the left side and can contain bowel, and solid abdominal organs. It has a significant morbidity and mortality. See Fig. 8.15.

Clinical

Most large congenital diaphragmatic herniae should be detected on antenatal ultrasound. The newborn baby with a diaphragmatic hernia presents with respiratory distress, cyanosis and scaphoid abdomen.

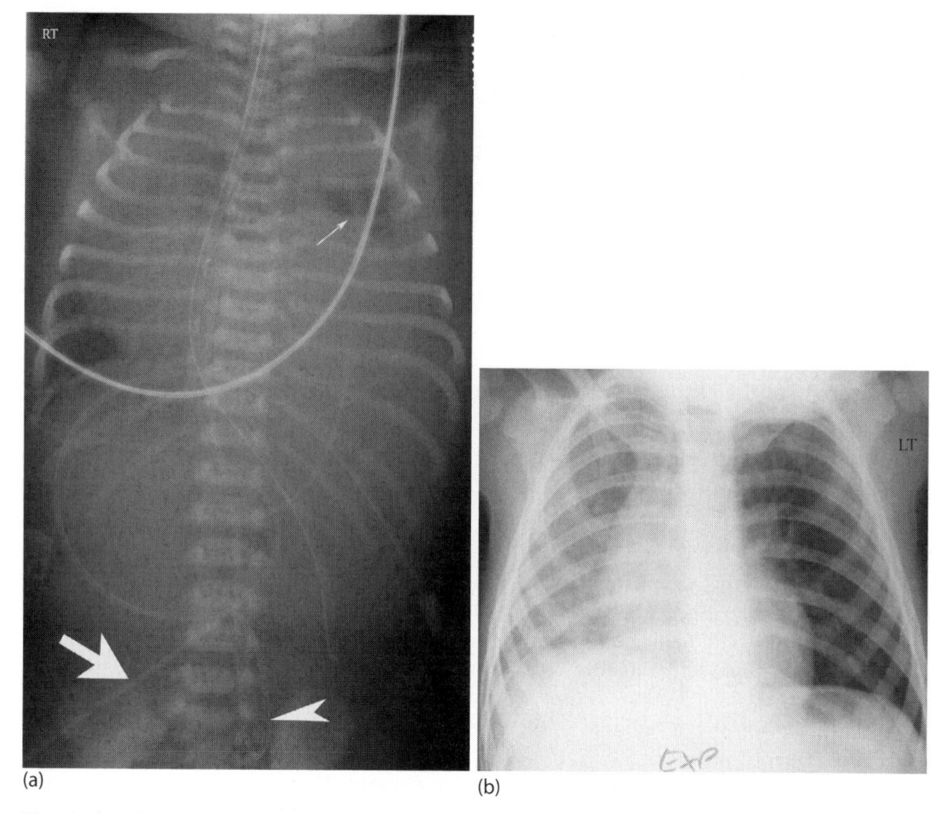

(a) (b)

Fig. 8.15. (a) Congenital diaphragmatic hernia. A chest and abdomen radiograph shows almost complete opacification of the left chest with marked mediastinal shift to the right. Note the NG tube and umbilical arterial line (arrowhead) are shifted to the right within the chest. The umbilical venous line (arrow) takes a very unusual course suggesting the liver is contained in the herniation. The lucencies in the upper left chest represent gas-filled loops of bowel (thin white arrow). (b) Inhaled foreign body. Frontal radiograph of the chest in expiration demonstrating relative hyperlucency of the left hemithorax to the right in a child with history of foreign body aspiration. This is secondary to a ball-valve effect causing air trapping within the affected lung.

Findings

1. Chest radiograph: Early films may simply show an opaque hemithorax with minimal midline shift. As air fills the bowel, multiple cystic structures are seen with shift of mediastinum to the contralateral side.
2. Both lungs are hypoplastic so that even after corrective surgery midline shift persists and the ipsilateral hemithorax fills to some degree with fluid depending on the degree of hypoplasia of the lungs.
3. Abdominal radiograph: Scaphoid gasless abdomen.
4. Ultrasound showing diaphragmatic defect with bowel loops in the thorax showing peristalsis.

Pearls

- CT/MR shows defect in the posterolateral part of the diaphragm and bowel loops in continuity in the thorax and abdomen and is confirmatory.

- Prenatal sonography may show hydramnios, intrathoracic mass comprising liver, stomach or bowel showing peristalsis in the thorax.
- The heart and renal tract should also be examined with US to exclude common associated anomalies.
- An upper GI contrast study is not recommended in a suspected congenital diaphragmatic hernia as this can distend the bowel in the chest and lead to further respiratory compromise.
- Despite advances in surgical techniques, pulmonary hypoplasia and hypertension are major survival factors.

Suggested reading

Guibaud L Filiatrault D, Garel L *et al.* Fetal congenital diaphragmatic hernia: accuracy of sonography in the diagnosis and prediction of the outcome after birth. *Am J Roentgenol* 1996;**166**:1195–1202.

Inhaled foreign body

Young children are most at risk from aspiration of a foreign body into the airway. Food is the most common foreign body but anything small enough to fit in the airway of a child can be aspirated.

Clinical

Most small foreign bodies will lodge in the right main bronchus.
Acute onset of respiratory symptoms: Choking, coughing and wheezing. If the upper airways are obstructed severe respiratory distress, cyanosis and collapse.
Chronic onset: Often with no specific history of aspiration but presenting with cough and wheeze or even recurrent pneumonia and bronchiectasis. A high degree of clinical suspicion is required to spot and diagnose these patients.

Technique

Plain radiograph: Unless a foreign body is radio-opaque only the secondary signs it creates will be seen on a radiograph.
Chest radiograph: AP – inspiratory and expiratory.
Neck: Lateral.

Findings

1. Normal chest radiograph in 80% of cases.
2. Classically obstructive hyperinflation of the affected lung/lung segment: Ball valve effect.
3. Contralateral mediastinal shift and ipsilateral paradoxical or restricted hemidiaphragm movement during breathing.
4. Focal collapse and consolidation.
5. Chronic changes: Bronchiectasis.

Pearls

- A decubitus film can be used in children who cannot perform an expiratory film. Air trapping and static lung volumes on affected side are suggestive of obstruction in right or left decubitus radiograph.
- Where there is a clinical suspicion of aspiration then bronchoscopy is the investigation of choice even if plain radiography is normal. A CT scan may be helpful in detailed investigation before or after bronchoscopy.
- CT scan is useful in detection of radiodense as well as radiolucent foreign bodies. Apart from detection of an opaque or non-opaque foreign body, it can also demonstrate obstructive and reactive changes in distal airways and lung parenchyma.

Suggested reading

Donnelly LF *et al.* The multiple presentations of foreign bodies in children. *Am J Roentgenol* 1998;**170**:471–477.

Yedururi S *et al.* Multimodality imaging of tracheobronchial disorders in children. *RadioGraphics* 2008;**10**.1148/r.e29.

Chapter 9

Skeletal trauma

John Curtis and Mayil S. Krishnam

9.1 General principles

Spinal trauma may cause both soft tissue and skeletal injury. Occasionally there is significant soft tissue and cord injury without bony injury. Therefore, absence of radiographic and CT signs of trauma does not exclude ligamentous or cord injury. It is important to know the basic anatomy of the normal cervical spine to understand the mechanism and to detect radiological signs of spinal injury. See Figs 9.1 and 9.2.

The vertebrae are aligned in an arc which is smooth, gently lordotic and without steps. The vertebrae are stabilized by strong ligaments (summarized in Fig. 9.1). In the entire spine, the anterior and posterior longitudinal ligaments (ALL and PLL) run along the length of the anterior and posterior vertebral bodies respectively. The nucleus pulposus (NP) lies between an annular structure called the annulus fibrosus. Fibers of the annulus fibrosus (AF) merge with the ALL anteriorly and the PLL posteriorly. Together the AF and NP comprise the intervertebral disc, which acts like a shock absorber for the spine. The bony spinal canal is a cylindrical space containing the spinal cord, nerve roots, thecal sac and cerebrospinal fluid. Its anterior boundary comprises the posterior vertebral body which is supported by the posterior longitudinal ligament. Laterally its boundary is composed on each side of the neural arch: pedicles (or lateral masses) and laminae. Its posterior boundary comprises the junction of the laminae and the spinous process at the so-called spinolaminar line. The posterior ligamentous complex comprises the facet joint capsules, ligamenta flava, interspinous and supraspinous ligaments.

Computerized tomography and MR have greatly improved detection of subtle injuries not visible on plain films. MR is useful to detect subtle cord injury.

The categorization of injuries can be by:

Mechanism of injury.
Stability or instability.
Anatomical location.

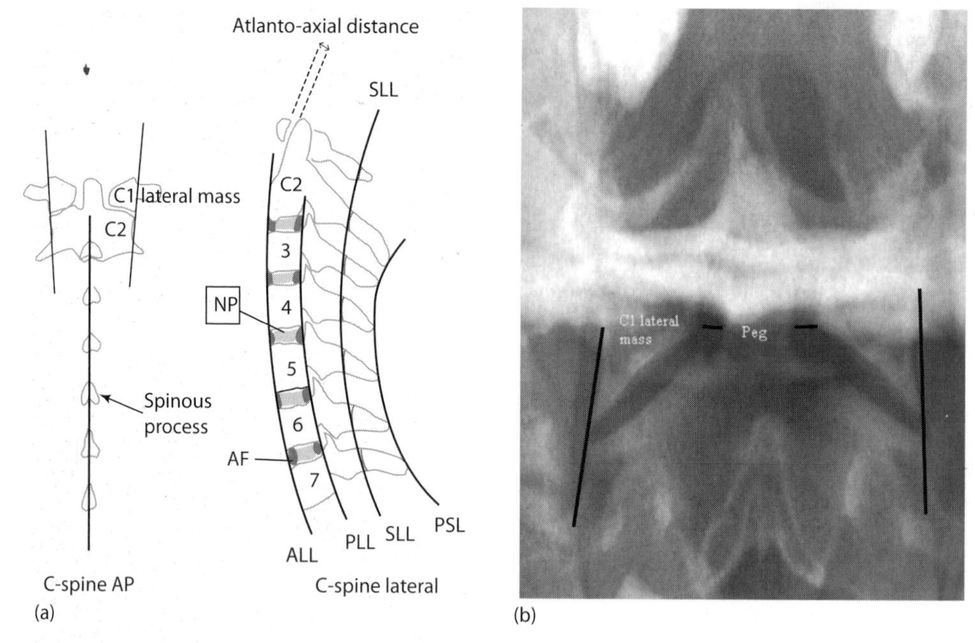

Fig. 9.1. (a) C-spine lines. ALL, anterior longitudinal ligament; PLL, posterior longitudinal ligament; SLL, spinolaminar line; PSL, posterior spinal line; NP, nucleus pulposus; AF, annulus fibrosus. (b) Normal peg. Open mouth view of the cranio-cervical junction shows C2 body, odontoid peg and normal alignment of lateral masses. There is symmetrical distance between the lateral border of the Peg and medial margin of lateral masses.

The majority of spinal injuries will occur at three sites – upper cervical (C1–2), lower cervical (C5–7) and thoracolumbar areas. Multiple sites of trauma occur in about 10% of cases, which has led to the policy of performing CT of the whole cervical spine in cases of significant trauma.

Anatomical consideration

Compressive forces on the spine (cervical and thoracolumbar) tend to cause significant bony injury without significant intervertebral disc or ligament injury. This is because discs and ligaments are able to withstand large compressive forces, rather like spinal "shock absorbers." The intervertebral disc and spinal ligaments are weak when subjected to rotation or horizontal shear forces.

The bony end plates are disrupted during axial loading forces because the disc and ligaments are resistant to compression. This results in end-plate fracture with herniation of the nucleus pulposus into the bone marrow.

During rotation or shear forces the ligaments will disrupt before bony injury occurs and this leads to dislocation/subluxation with or without bony injury.

Stability of injury

Injuries involving the spinal ligaments are considered unstable, especially those ligaments forming the posterior complex.

The spine is divided into three columns as follows:

Anterior column: Anterior longitudinal ligament (ALL), anterior annulus fibrosus (AF). Anterior 2/3 of vertebral body.

Middle column: Posterior longitudinal ligament (PLL), posterior annulus fibrosus (AF). Posterior 1/3 of vertebral body.

Posterior column: Posterior bony arch (pedicles, laminae and spinous process).

Posterior ligament complex: Capsular ligaments, ligamentum flavum (LF).

Interspinous ligaments (ISL).

Supraspinous ligaments (SSL).

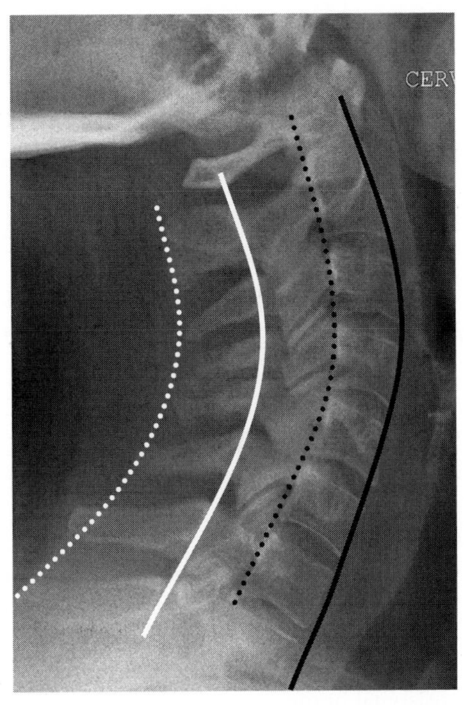

Fig. 9.2. Normal cervical spine. Normal lateral cervical spine radiograph showing course of various spinal lines. Black line, ALL; black dotted line, PLL; white line, SLL; white dotted line, PSL.

Minor injuries

Isolated fractures of the posterior elements without disruption of the interspinous ligament constitute minor stable injury.

Major injuries

These involve more than one column or disruption of any of the interspinous ligaments. The middle column is the most important in determining stability and if disrupted, instability exists.

Signs of instability in the middle column

Vertebral displacement greater than 2 mm implying ligament disruption.

Widening of the interpedicular distance, interlaminar space and facet joints.

Disruption of the posterior margin of the vertebral body.

Classification of injury by mechanism

Hyperflexion, rotation-flexion, rotation-extension, compression, hyperextension.

Pearls

- Axial loading forces cause bony injury.
- Rotatory/shearing forces cause subluxation/dislocation.

Suggested reading

Blackmore CC *et al.* Helical CT in the primary trauma evaluation of the cervical spine: an evidence-based approach. *Skeletal Radiol* 2000;**29**:632–639.

Hanson JA *et al.* Cervical spine injury: a clinical decision rule to identify high-risk patients for helical CT screening. *Am J Roentgenol* 2000;**174**:713–717.

Imhof H, Fuchsjäger M. Traumatic injuries: imaging of spinal injuries. *Eur Radiol* 2002;**12**:1262–1272.

Lee JS *et al.* The significance of prevertebral soft tissue swelling in extension teardrop fracture of the cervical spine. *Emerg Radiol* 1997;**4**(3):132–139.

Perry JR *et al.* Lateral radiography of the cervical spine in the trauma patient: looking beyond the spine. *Am J Roentgenol* 2001;**176**:381–386.

Rao SK *et al.* Spectrum of imaging findings in hyperextension injuries of the neck. *RadioGraphics* 2005;**25**:1239–1254.

Timothy J *et al.* Cervical spine injuries. *Curr Orthopaed* 2004;**18**:1–16.

Tins BJ, Cassar-Pullicino VN. Imaging of acute cervical spine injuries: review and outlook. *Clin Radiol* 2004;**59**:865–880.

9.2 Cervical spine injury

Technique

Cervical spine radiograph

Good quality AP and lateral radiographs with open-mouth views.

Always check that the top of T1 is seen on the lateral radiograph. Pulling the shoulders down or a swimmer's view may be necessary.

Most injuries are best demonstrated on the lateral film which is centered at C4 with a horizontal beam.

Cervical spine CT

Helical CT direct may be the preferred option for those patients with the following:

High risk for injury, e.g. high-velocity road traffic accidents (RTA) or falls greater than 10 feet. Pelvic fractures are a marker for severe trauma in patients with neck injury.

Patients who are difficult to clinically assess, i.e. unconscious or intoxicated patients or patients with severe degenerative disease.

Associated head injury.

Focal neurological signs and symptoms.

Inability to see C7/T1 on the lateral film.

Inability to do a swimmer's view in upper limb trauma.

Detection of injury on the cervical spine radiographs.

Findings

1. Soft tissue swelling.
2. Inspect the soft tissues looking for prevertebral soft tissue swelling. Follow the lines of the ALL, PLL, spinolaminar and interspinous lines looking for any "step" in alignment. This process should be carried out from top to bottom and repeated from bottom to top searching for any "steps."
3. On the lateral film look for superimposition of the lateral masses of the vertebrae. Any loss of superimposition may be due to rotation which can be positional or traumatic. Examine the AP view. The spinous processes should be in alignment (see Fig. 9.1).

4. Look for individual bony injury.
5. Look at the cranio-cervical junction for signs of fracture, dislocation and distraction and the skull and the sphenoid sinus for an air–fluid level.

Pearls

- Absence of prevertebral soft tissue swelling is not a reliable indicator for excluding spinal injury.
- The presence of prevertebral soft tissue swelling is seen with anterior bony and ligamentous injury.
- Significant posterior ligamentous injury may not result in radiographically visible soft tissue swelling.
- Indirect indicators of cervical spine injury: retropharyngeal soft tissue swelling prevertebral fat stripe displacement (difficult and unreliable sign), and laryngeal/tracheal disruption.
- A normal cervical spine series does not exclude injury.
- The prevertebral soft tissue varies with lateral neck movements, phonation and distress. The presence of endotracheal or nasogastric tubes may also alter the prevertebral soft tissue appearance.
- Normal atlantoaxial interval (atlantodental distance) should not be greater than 3 mm in adults and 5 mm in children.
- Between C1–C4 the prevertebral soft tissue width should not exceed 7 mm or 33% of the AP width of the vertebral body. Below C4 the soft tissue should not exceed 22 mm or the AP width of the vertebral body.

9.3 The cranio-cervical junction

The distance between the basion and the posterior arch of C-1 is equal to the distance between the anterior arch of C-1 and opisthion (the posterior margin of the foramen magnum). See Fig. 9.3.

Normal individuals: Powers ratio $BC/OA = <1$.

>1 is suggestive of anterior atlanto-occipital dislocation. It is best calculated on sagittal CT with flexion extension views.

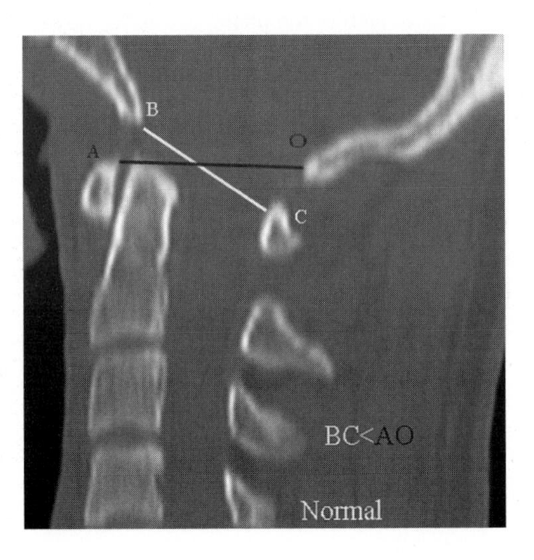

Fig. 9.3. Normal cranio-cervical junction. Sagittal CT of cervical spine showing the distance (white line) between the basion (B) and the posterior arch of C-1 (C), is equal to the distance (black line) between the anterior arch of C-1 (A) and opisthion (O). Also note normal atlanto-axial interval.

In atlanto-occipital dislocation the atlas and axis move posteriorly with respect to the cranium: BC/OA > 1.15.

Powers ratio is best calculated on the sagittal CT reconstruction image which removes the overlapping shadows seen on the lateral film.

Distraction injuries displace the atlas from the occipital condyles > 5 mm. This is best appreciated on the parasagittal CT reconstructed image.

9.4 Fractures of C1 (atlas)

Mechanism

Posterior arch fractures are due to hyperextension-compression injury. The Jefferson fracture is due to axial loading force which drives the lateral masses of C1 apart as they are compressed between the occiput and articular facets of C2. See Fig. 9.4.

Findings

1. Posterior arch fractures: Hyperextension resulting in compression of the C1 posterior arch between the occiput and the posterior arch of C2.
2. Jefferson fracture (burst fracture).
   Fractures of anterior and posterior arches of C1.
   Lateral displacement of the articular masses of C1 (disruption of transverse ligament).
   Marked prevertebral edema and swelling.
   Widening of the atlanto-axial distance (> 3 mm).
3. Anterior arch fractures.
   Lateral mass fractures (very rare).
   Transverse process fracture (very rare).

Pearls

- C1 fractures are not usually associated with neurological problems because of the wide spinal canal relative to the cord diameter at this level.
- CT is very useful to assess the integrity of the anterior arch of the atlas.
- Jefferson fracture is an unstable injury.

9.5 Fractures of C2 (axis)

Odontoid peg fractures

May be difficult to see on plain film if undisplaced. See Fig. 9.5.
55% of C2 fractures are odontoid peg fractures.
Mechanism complex but implies major force.

Findings

Type 1: Tip fractures (avulsion of alar ligament) – rare.
Type 2: Junction of dens and body of C2. 65% of dens fractures.
Displacement of > 4 mm = instability.

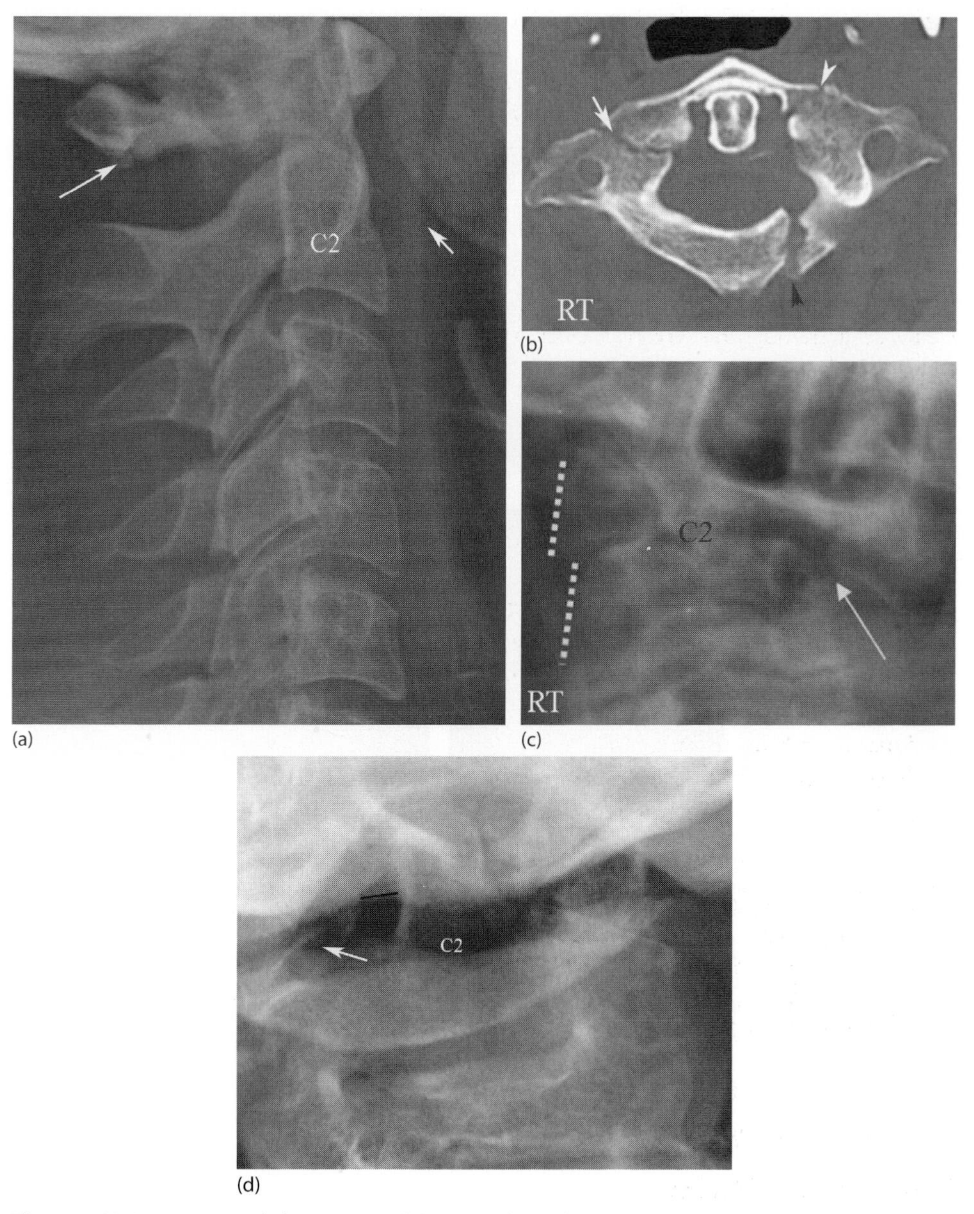

Fig. 9.4. (a) C1 posterior arch fracture. Lateral C-spine radiograph in a trauma patient shows C1 posterior arch fracture (long arrow). Note the lack of soft tissue swelling (short arrow). (b) Jefferson fracture. Axial CT at C1 vertebra shows fractures of the right lateral mass (arrow), left anterior (white arrowhead) and posterior arches (black arrowhead) of C1 with mild lateral displacement of the left lateral mass. (c) Jefferson fracture. Peg view shows marked lateral displacement of the left lateral mass of C1 (arrow) and incongruous lines of the right lateral mass of C1 and C2 (dotted line). The distance between the dens and left lateral mass is >4 mm indicating atlanto-axial rotational fixation injury. (d) C1/2 subluxation. Peg view of C1/2 vertebra shows C1/2 subluxation on right side with oblique pillar fracture of C1 (arrow). Note the asymmetry between the right (black line) and left C1/2 facet joints.

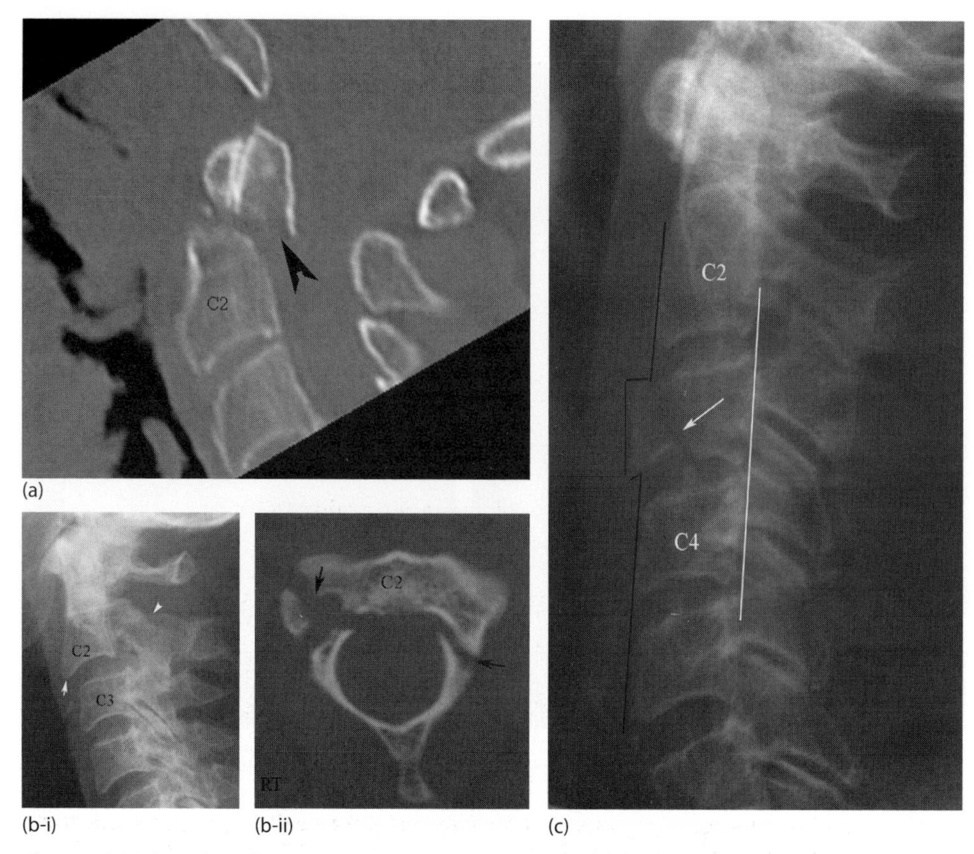

Fig. 9.5. (a) Odontoid peg fracture. Sagittal CT of C-spine shows a peg fracture and separation and displacement of fracture fragments (arrowhead), consistent with type 2 displaced fracture (unstable) of the body of the odontoid peg. (b) Hangman's fracture. (i) Lateral C-spine radiograph shows fractures through both pedicles (arrowhead) and anterior displacement of C2 (arrow) on C3. No retrolisthesis of the posterior elements. (ii) Axial CT at C2 vertebra shows fractures through both pedicles (arrows) with extension of the fracture to the right vertebral foramen. (c) Extension tear-drop fracture C3. Lateral C-spine radiograph shows the posterior longitudinal line (white line) is intact (unlike in flexion tear-drop fracture). Note soft tissue swelling and that the vertical height of the fracture exceeds the width.

Type 3: Horizontal/oblique fractures adjacent to the base of the dens and through into the vertebral body of C2.

Hangman fracture

Unstable fracture of the body and posterior arch of the axis. Mechanisms of injury:

Hyperextension.

RTA, rapid deceleration of head on the windscreen followed by forward flexion.

Falls.

Hanging.

Findings

1. Fractures through both pedicles of C2 with anterior subluxation of C2 on C3.
2. May involve the posterior vertebral body in 20% of cases.

3. Odontoid peg intact.
4. Rarely cord injury – look for bony fragments in the spinal canal.
5. Rarely retrolisthesis of the posterior elements of C2 relative to C3.

Extension tear-drop fracture

Unstable fracture.
Tends to occur in pre-existing osteoporotic bone.
Extension injury.

Findings

1. Avulsion of the antero-inferior portion of the vertebral body (usually C2 or upper cervical vertebrae) with disruption of the anterior longitudinal ligament complex.
2. The bony fragment is less than 25% AP width of vertebral body. The vertical height of fragment exceeds the AP width.

   No vertebral body displacement, unlike flexion tear-drop fracture.
4. Check for any intraspinal canal fragment.

Pearls

- Axial CT may overlook the fracture if it has the same orientation. Reformatted images are essential.
- Type 2 fractures are associated with high rate of non-union (up to 36%) due to osteonecrosis. Disruption of the sclerotic ring of Harris indicates an unstable type 3 fracture or hangman's fracture. This sclerotic "ring" is formed by the superimposition of the cortical bone along the margin of the neurocentral synchondrosis seen on the lateral radiograph.
- CT is useful in the detection of undisplaced fractures of the pedicles. CT will demonstrate bony fragments in the spinal canal.
- Cord injury rare with the above mechanisms due to the relatively large diameter of the spinal canal at C2.
- Distraction cord injury with hanging.
- Acute central cord syndrome may or may not be seen in extension tear-drop injury.

9.6 Lower cervical spinal injuries

Extension tear-drop fracture

Mechanism

Hyperextension results from severe deceleration, forced hyperextension with often rebound forward flexion, typically seen in RTAs. See Fig. 9.6.
Extension tear-drop fracture can occur anywhere but commonest at C2.
Hyperextension dislocation commonly at C5–6 with disruption of the ALL and anterior disc.
The force is greatest at C5–6, a natural site of maximal flexion.

Findings

1. Prevertebral swelling.
2. Mild forward slip of the vertebra below the injury.

3. Subtle avulsion fractures of the inferior end plate.
4. Retrolisthesis of the upper VB on lower VB.
5. Hyperextension dislocation with disruption of the ALL and anterior disc (see Fig. 9.5c).

Flexion tear-drop fractures

Mechanism

Hyperflexion results from a strong force from behind causing the chin to hit the chest. It can result as a "rebound" to hyperextension injuries.
Disruption of ligaments in all three columns.
Usually at C5–6.

Findings

1. The bony fragment, which is between a third and a half of the AP diameter of the vertebral body, occurs in an antero-inferior position and is aligned with the vertebral body below.
2. In 80% of cases the larger fragment is displaced posteriorly which results in a step in the posterior longitudinal line. This feature is usually absent in extension tear-drop fractures (see Fig. 9.6b and c).
3. Anterior cord injury resulting from posterior vertebral body displacement.
4. Often associated with posterior arch and sagittal vertebral body fractures.

Bilateral facet lock

Mechanism

Unstable injury, severe flexion with complete disruption of the ligamentous complex of the posterior, middle and anterior columns.

Findings

1. The facet joints become locked. The posterior part of the facet of the upper vertebra becomes locked anterior to the facet of the vertebra below (see Fig. 9.6d).
2. Severe narrowing of the spinal canal and neural foramina with consequent severe neurological damage.
3. Anterior VB displacement; is typically greater than 50% of the AP diameter of the VB below.
4. Typically associated with absence of fracture.
5. CT: Naked facet sign bilaterally (see Fig. 9.6d-ii).

Clay-shoveller's fracture

Mechanism

Forced hyperflexion.
Stable avulsion injury.

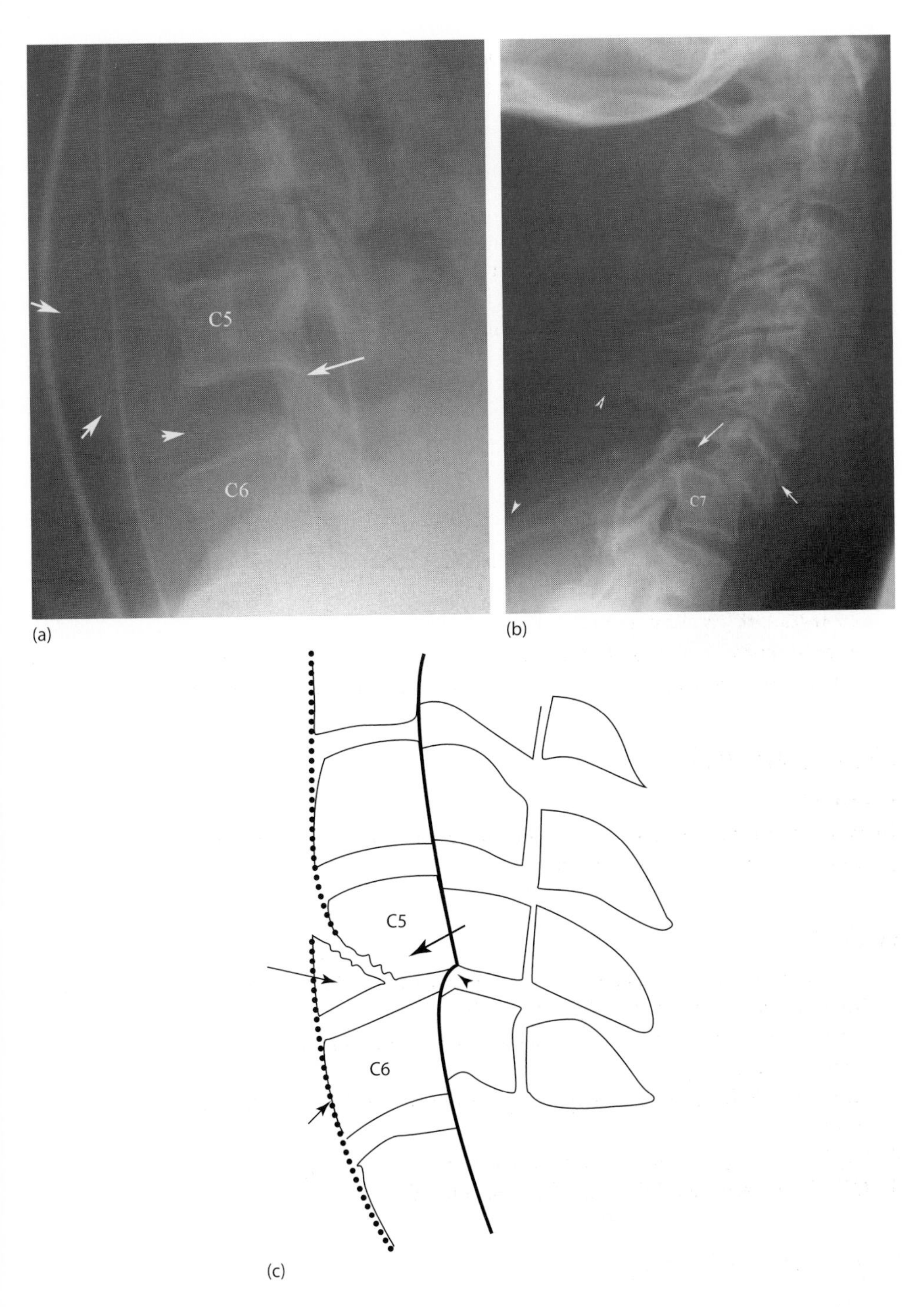

Fig. 9.6.

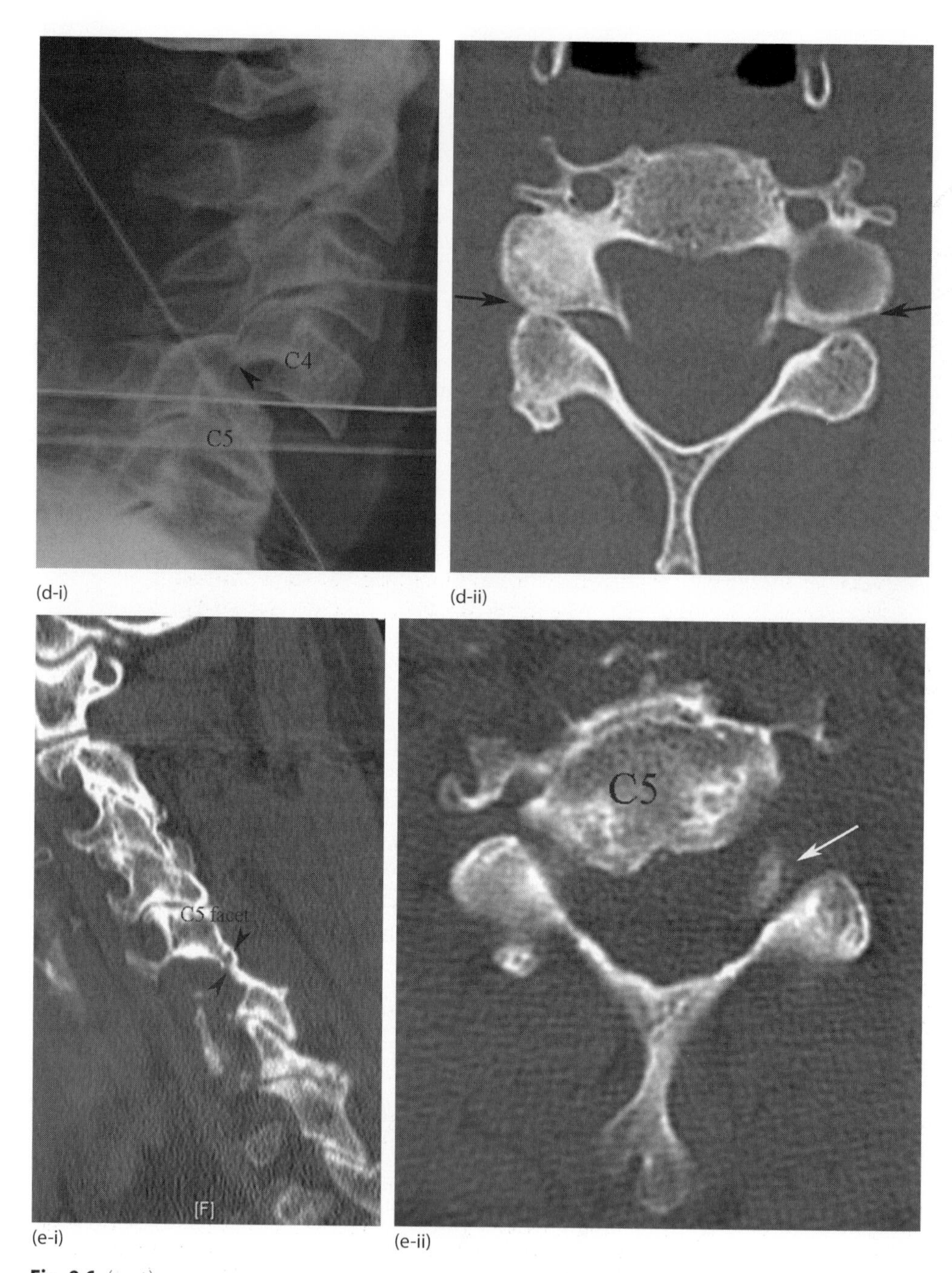

(d-i) (d-ii)

(e-i) (e-ii)

Fig. 9.6. *(cont.)*

Findings

1. Oblique fracture of the spinous process, typically of C7.
2. The interspinous ligament remains intact.
3. Break in the posterior part of the spinous process.

Unilateral facet lock injury

Mechanism

Flexion-rotation injury.
It is unstable and occurs most frequently at C4–5 and C5–6.
It is associated with cord and neural impingment.
Disruption of the interspinous ligament, the posterior longitudinal ligament and the facet capsule.

Findings

1. The ipsilateral inferior facet rotates to lie within the neural foramen which is anterior to the superior facet of the VB below it.
2. The upper VB is anteriorly displaced by no more than 50% of its AP width.
3. Loss of normal superimposition (roofing) of the facets on the lateral view.

Burst fractures

Mechanism

Combination of flexion and axial loading.
Commonest sites atlanto-occipital junction, cervico-thoracic junction and lower cervical spine.
Mechanically "stable" as they are rarely associated with ligamentous injury. Retropulsed fragments may cause neurological compromise.

Findings

1. Crushed vertebral body.
2. Retropulsed fragments of the posterosuperior VB into the spinal canal.
3. Spinal cord injury causing neurological deficit.

Caption for Fig. 9.6 (a) Hyperextension facet-lock injury. There is retropulsion of C5 on C6. Locking (long arrow) occurs at the anterior inferior vertebral body and the superior articular process of the facet joint below. There is widening of the disc space at C5–C6 (arrowhead) and prevertebral soft tissue swelling (short arrows). (b) Hyperflexion lower C-spine injury. There is anterior displacement (small arrow) of C6 on C7 with anterior wedging of C6. Note the widened interspinous distance (arrowheads) and widening of the facet joint of C6/7 (long arrow), due to a combination of unstable bony and ligamentous injury. (c) Flexion tear-drop fracture of C5. Schematic diagram of lower cervical vertebrae shows the antero-inferior triangular fragment (thin arrow) keeps its alignment with vertebral body below (C6). The larger fragment (thick arrow) moves posteriorly, causing a step in the posterior longitudinal line (arrowhead). Note a step in the anterior longitudinal line (short arrow) at upper C5. (d) Bilateral facet-lock injury. (i) Lateral C-spine radiograph shows anterior subluxation, of C4 on C5, spinal canal narrowing at this level and the forward locking of the lateral mass of C4 (arrowhead) on C5. (ii) Axial CT at C4 vertebra shows bilateral "naked facet" sign (arrows). The inferior articular facets of C4 lie anterior to the superior articular facets of C5. (e) Unifacetal subluxation of C5 on C6. (i) Sagittal CT C-spine in a trauma patient shows "perching" of the inferior facet of C5 (arrowheads) on the superior facet of C6. (ii) Axial CT shows C5 vertebral body rotated anticlockwise exposing its naked inferior facet (arrow).

Pearls

- Radiographs may be normal or may show small wedge-like anterior VB compression fractures.
- Flexion tear-drop fractures: *Highly unstable injury.*
- Hyperflexion sprain: Ligamentous injury. *Unstable* injury due to disrupted ligaments in the posterior column and in severe cases disruption of the middle column (posterior longitudinal ligaments and posterior disc).
- Hyperflexion bony injury: These *stable* injuries tend to spare the posterior ligamentous complex but with bony injury to the anterior vertebral column. They are associated with loss of anterior vertebral height (wedging) and soft tissue swelling.
- Extension tear-drop: The only radiographic abnormality may be prevertebral swelling or mild forward slip of the vertebra below the injury. Plain XR may be normal even in unstable injury.
- Posterior slip of the upper vertebral body into the spinal canal at the time of injury can result in severe cord injury. MRI should be performed.

9.7 Thoracic/lumbar spine trauma

90% of thoracolumbar injuries occur between T11 and L4.
60% occur between T12 (mostly T4/5 in children) and L2.
Only 30% of traumatic fractures occur above T10.
Falls, direct trauma or RTAs with all types and direction of force: axial loading, hyperflexion, hyperextension, rotation and distraction forces. See Fig. 9.7.

Technique

AP and lateral spine radiograph. Sensitivity about 60%.
CT of the thoracolumbar spine in cases of trauma and a radiographic abnormality or when there is a high clinical suspicion and negative radiographs.
Thin sections with overlap and orthogonal reconstructions.

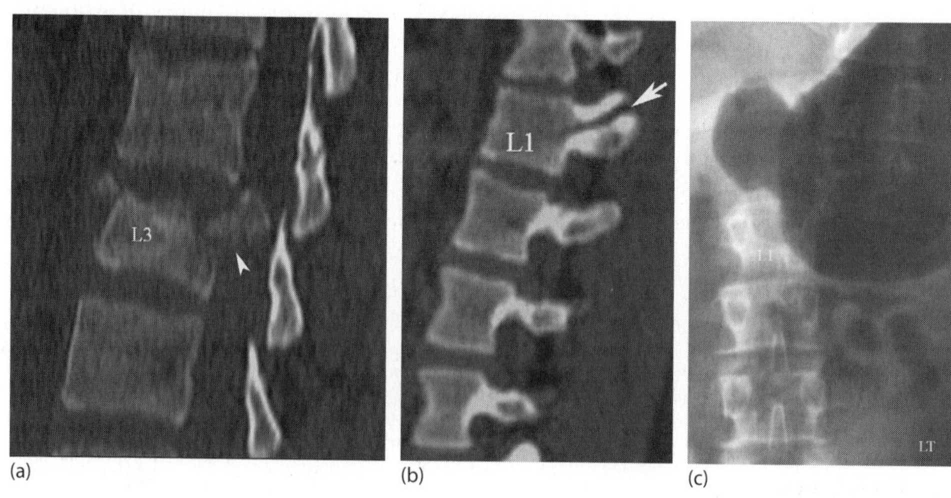

(a) (b) (c)

Fig. 9.7. (a) Burst fracture of L3. Sagittal lumbar spine CT shows burst fracture of L3 and the extent of retropulsion into the spinal canal (arrowhead). (b) L1 chance fracture. Sagittal lumbosacral spine CT shows the horizontal orientation of the fracture through the L1 pedicle (arrow) (photo courtesy of Dr. T. Muthukumar, Stanmore). (c) T12/L1 fracture dislocation. AP radiograph of dorsolumbar spine shows the thoracic spine is rotated and dislocated from the lumbar spine which results in "double vertebrae sign" on axial CT (not shown) (photo courtesy of Dr. D. Parker, Wrexham).

Compression fractures

Compression fractures comprise 50% of all thoracolumbar injuries, the commonest site being the thoracolumbar region. L1 and L2 regions commonly involved. T12 > T7 > L3.

Mechanism

Compressive force in the anterior column but not in the middle and posterior columns. Common in osteoporosis.

Findings

1. Anterior wedging.
2. Preservation of the height of the posterior vertebral body is usual.
3. Occasionally the anterior force is severe enough to cause distraction posteriorly, causing ligamentous disruption.
4. Usually no loss of disc height (discs withstand compressive forces).
5. Kyphosis.

Burst fractures

Burst fractures are unstable injuries. T12, L1 and L2 are the commonest sites. Neurological deficit is common.

Mechanism

Compression with flexion of the anterior and middle columns of vertebral bodies. The compressive force causes disruption radiating outwards from the center of the vertebral body. Usually no force on the posterior column but posterior element injury may be seen in over half of cases.

Findings

1. Increased AP diameter and interpedicular distance.
2. Anterior wedging similar to compression fractures. In addition, the middle column is involved.
3. Loss of congruity of the posterior vertebral line on the lateral film.
4. Retropulsion of bony fragment, narrowing the spinal canal.
5. Associated posterior element fractures, involving the laminae and spinous processes, are very common and more likely seen on CT.
6. CT may better demonstrate a bony fragment emanating from the superior corner of fractured VB. This feature is often obscured by the pedicles on the lateral view of the spine.

Seat-belt fractures

Mechanism

Anterior abdominal wall/seat belt interface acts as the fulcrum. Hyperflexion injury leads to compression of the anterior column and distraction of the middle and posterior columns.

Findings

1. Compression fractures commonly seen at T/L junction L1/2 level.
2. Often associated with abdominal injuries – pancreatic and duodenal trauma.
3. Osseous/ligamentous injury.
4. Posterior element fractures, e.g. horizontal Chance fracture.

Pearls

- Mediastinal hematoma often accompanies severe thoracic trauma.
- Sternal fracture: Suspect thoracic spine trauma and vice versa.
- The upper four thoracic vertebrae are often difficult to visualize on the radiograph – CT is preferred.
- Fracture-dislocation: Rotational shear injury involving all three columns. The middle and posterior columns are distracted and the anterior column suffers compression.
- The same principles of C-spine stability apply to the thoracic spine.
- MRI imaging if suspecting cord injury, ligamentous disruption and epidural hematoma. Ligamentous tears are of high signal on STIR and T2.

9.8 Pelvic trauma

The bony pelvis protects internal organs and high impact injury to this bony region often results in visceral injury. See Fig. 9.8.

Mechanism

The mechanism of injury of pelvic fractures can be broadly categorized into three types:

1. AP loading force.
2. Lateral force.
3. Vertical shear force.

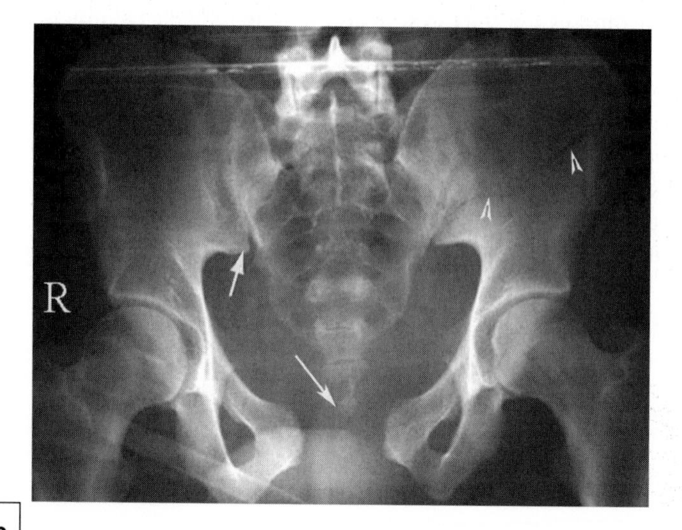

Fig. 9.8. "Sprung" pelvis. AP radiograph of pelvis showing pubic diastasis (long arrow) – "open book" type injury with associated left iliac blade fracture (arrowheads) and widening of the right sacroiliac joint (short arrow).

Acetabular fractures often result from so-called "dashboard" injuries when the knee strikes the dashboard resulting in a force on the posterior acetabulum. They may also result from lateral compression forces.

Pelvic fractures are associated with visceral or vascular injuries of the following types:

I: No disruption of bony pelvic ring.
II: Single fracture through pelvic ring.
III: Two or more fractures through pelvic ring (straddle, and Malgaigne's fractures).
IV: Acetabular fractures.

Technique

Plain film: AP view. In practice further views are usually not carried out. Further imaging usually involves CT.

If there are any signs of internal injury, a contrast-enhanced CT of the pelvis is indicated even if the plain film reveals no fractures. CT often reveals more subtle injuries that may be overlooked on plain films. If vascular injury suspected, a CT angiogram should be performed. Oral and/or rectal contrast required if gastrointestinal injury is suspected.

Findings

1. Pelvic ring fractures.
2. Acetabular fractures.
3. Pelvic hematoma.
4. Thickening of obturator internus.
5. Arterial injury and hemorrhage-contrast extravasation, pseudoaneurysm, focal narrowing due to spasm, or dissection.
6. Bladder injury: Urinoma.

Pearls

- Urethral and bladder injury associated with diastasis of the symphysis, pubic rami fractures. Refer to Section 3.7.
- Nerve injuries more common in sacral fracture.
- Pubic diastasis of >15 mm or overlapping pubic bones suggests severe injury with posterior bony ring disruption. Diastasis can increase the volume of the pelvis for further accumulation of blood. Angiography and embolization may be necessary.
- Straddle injury causes disruption of the anterior bony ring in two places.
- Malgaigne's fracture involves the anterior and posterior pelvic ring.
- CT may be primarily indicated if the patient is unconscious or hemodynamically compromised due to bleeding; associated visceral/vascular injury; history suggestive of disruption of the sacro-iliac joints or other unstable injury; blood is present at urethral meatus (associated bladder or urethral injury); neurological injury.

Suggested reading

Kane WJ. Fractures of the pelvis. In Rockwood CA, Green DP, eds, *Fractures in Adults, 2nd edition*, p. 112. JB Lippincott, 1984.

9.9 Facial trauma – general principles

The facial skeleton comprises buttresses oriented in horizontal and vertical directions which form the framework for the face. A buttress is a supporting pillar of increased bone thickness which connects the facial structures to the skull base and cranium (see Fig. 9.9). There are four transverse buttresses and four paired vertical buttresses.

1. The upper transverse midface buttress runs from naso-frontal suture medially to the squamous part of the temporal bone laterally via the zygomatic arch. Posteriorly this buttress runs horizontally backwards as the relatively thin orbital floor.
2. The lower transverse maxillary buttress is the maxillary alveolar ridge running posteriorly as the hard palate. A palatal fracture in association with a Le Fort injury widens the maxillary arch.
3. The paired lateral vertical midface buttresses are the columns of bone from the upper back molars via the zygomaticomaxillary suture and zygoma body up along the lateral orbital wall across the zygomatico-frontal suture to the frontal bone. It extends backwards as the lateral orbital and maxillary antral walls.
4. The paired medial vertical buttresses of the maxilla are bony columns from the anterior nasal spine extending up via the naso-frontal suture to the frontal bone. Each buttress extends backwards as the medial orbital wall and anteriorly as the lateral nasal wall. The paired posterior maxillary buttresses are bony columns at the pterygomaxillary junction.

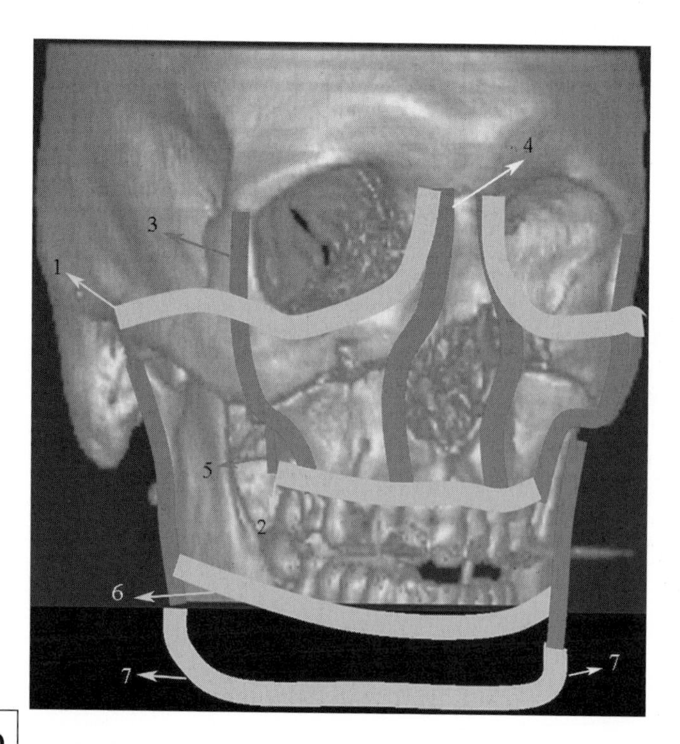

Fig. 9.9. Facial buttresses. 1, the upper transverse midface buttress. 2, the lower transverse maxillary buttress. 3, the paired lateral vertical midface buttresses. 4, the paired medial vertical buttresses of the maxilla – site of naso-orbito-ethmoid fractures. 5, the paired posterior maxillary buttresses. 6, upper transverse mandibular buttress. 7, lower transverse mandibular buttress.

Naso-orbitoethmoid (NOE) fractures

Traumatic disruption of the junction of the medial maxillary buttresses and upper transverse buttress and along the medial orbital wall and floor. Fractures involve the ethmoid sinuses and when bilateral also involve the nasolacrimal duct. Posterior disruption of medial canthus, ethmoids and medial orbital walls distinguishes NOE from simple nasal fracture.

Zygomaticomaxillary fractures

Fractures of the ZMC complex occur across the three buttress-related sutures – tripod fracture. The zygomatico-sphenoid suture may also be disrupted leading to a change in orbital volume – quadripod fracture. A fracture at the temporo-zygomatic junction can often be overlooked and failure to recognize this injury will result in facial widening.

Pearls

- Facial fractures are common following assault and RTAs.
- CT is used for complex fractures.
- CT determines which patients need surgical fixation.
- CT can assess the facial buttress integrity which determines the correct surgical procedure. It is to these buttresses that screws are applied during fixation.
- Any displacement of a buttress is treated with open reduction and internal fixation (ORIF).

Suggested reading

Hopper RA *et al.* Diagnosis of midface fractures with CT: what the surgeon needs to know. *RadioGraphics* 2006;**26**:783–793.

9.10 Le Fort fractures

Le Fort fractures are fractures of the mid-face that account for up to 25% of all facial fractures. Le Fort fractures can be unilateral, bilateral and symmetrical, bilateral and asymmetrical or of any type in combination with any other type. See Fig. 9.10.

Mechanism

Essentially the maxilla becomes separated from the base of the skull by disruption of the pterygo-maxillary junction due to a large force. This is due to fracture of either the pterygoid plates or posterior maxillary antral walls, or both.

Technique

Volumetric CT of the face. Axial, sagittal and coronal reformations are important. Fractures of anterolateral nasal fossa (Le Fort I) and inferior orbital rim (Le Fort II) are best appreciated on coronal images but zygomatic arch fracture (Le Fort III) on axial reformats.

Findings

The pterygoid processes are almost always involved in Le Fort fractures.

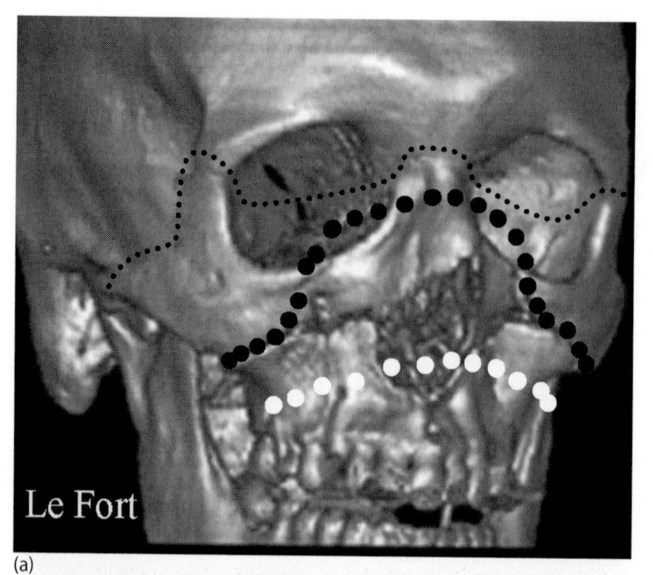

(a)

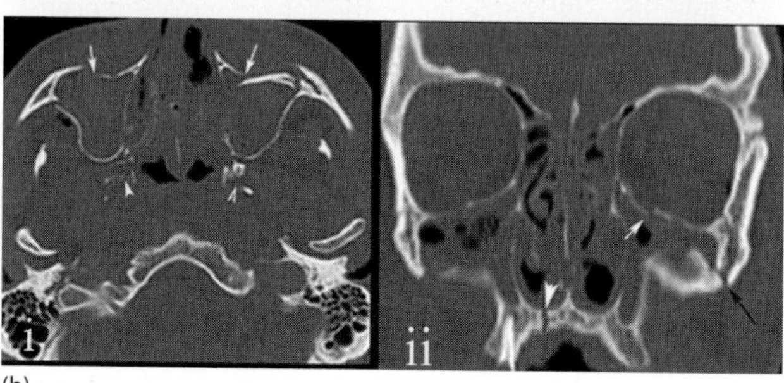

(b)

Fig. 9.10. (a) Le Fort fractures. Volume rendered image of CT face showing type I (white dotted line), type II (black dotted line), and type III (thin dotted line) Le Forte fractures. (b) Le Fort II fracture. (i) Axial facial CT shows bilateral fractures of the pterygoids (arrowheads) confirming a Le Fort fracture and fractures of the anterior walls of both maxillary antra (long arrows). Fractures of nasal bones were present but not shown. (ii) Coronal image shows a fracture through the left zygomatico-maxillary suture (black arrow), the left orbital floor (white arrow), and through the right hard palate (arrowhead).

Le Fort I

1. Fracture involves the inferior vertical buttresses, i.e. the inferior portion of the lateral and medial maxillary antral walls.
2. A fracture through the anterolateral nasal fossa is unique.

Le Fort II

3. Fracture involves the inferior lateral vertical buttress and the superior medial maxillary buttresses, i.e. the superior portion of the lateral maxillary antral wall and fronto-maxillary suture.
4. A fracture through the inferior orbital rim is unique.

Le Fort III

5. Fracture involves the superior transverse maxillary buttress and the superior lateral and medial maxillary buttresses.
6. A fracture through the zygomatic arch is unique.

Pearls

- If a fracture of the pterygoid process is established, a Le Fort fracture is highly likely. When examining the CT of facial trauma, the first task is to establish the presence or not of a pterygoid fracture.
- Clinical: Le Fort I - maxillary arch to move away from the nose and face; Le Fort II - maxillary arch and nose to move away from the remainder of the face; and Le Fort III - the whole face to move away from the base of the skull.
- Fractures of the hard palate allow coronal separation and subsequent widening of the maxillary arch. The hard palate is a posterior part of the lower transverse maxillary buttress.
- In any type of facial trauma always look for associated fractures of the skull vault, base of skull, mandible and upper cervical spine.

Suggested reading

Hopper RA *et al.* Diagnosis of midface fractures with CT: what the surgeon needs to know. *RadioGraphics* 2006;**26**:783–793.

Rhea JT, Novelline RA. How to simplify the CT diagnosis of Le Fort fractures. *Am J Roentgenol* 2005;**184**:1700–1705.

9.11 Orbital fractures

Fractures of the orbit may occur as solitary injuries or as part of injury to the zygomatico-maxillary complex and Le Fort type II injuries. Orbital fractures may occur in up to 16% of all cases of major trauma and 55% of cases of facial trauma. See Fig. 9.11.

Mechanism of blow-out fracture

Following trauma by direct force there is a sudden increase in orbital pressure resulting in disruption of the orbital floor or medial wall (lamina papyracea) with herniation of orbital contents outside the orbit.

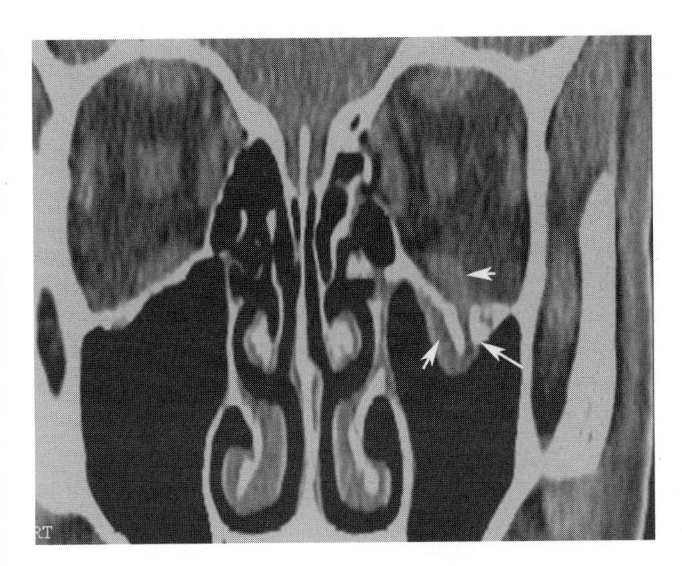

Fig. 9.11. Orbital blow-out fracture. Coronal CT face shows the left inferior rectus muscle (short arrows) trapped between the fracture fragments (long arrow) and slightly swollen compared with the contralateral side.

Findings

1. Orbital emphysema due to fractures of the orbital walls bordering a sinus.
2. Fractures of the orbital floor or medial wall (lamina papyracea).
3. Herniation of orbital contents (fat and/or muscle) outside the orbit.
4. Extra-ocular muscle entrapment – inferior rectus and medial rectus for the orbital floor and medial wall fractures respectively.
5. Cross-sectional shape of the trapped inferior rectus – if it remains flat, then there is no disruption of the fascial sling of the muscle, but if it is rounded and displaced down towards the site of the fracture, there is a strong likelihood that the fascial sling will be disrupted.
6. Associated ZMC fracture.
7. Fractures of the apex of the orbit are rare but may lead to damage to the optic nerve, even if subtle.
8. Look for intra-ocular injuries such as displacement of the lens, vitreous or aqueous hematoma, retrobulbar hemorrhage and any intra-ocular bony fragments or foreign bodies.
9. Look for abnormalities of the orbital vasculature in cases of carotico-cavernous fistulae.

Pearls

- In children the orbital floor is more elastic and following inferior rectus muscle herniation, the floor may spring back into position with permanent entrapment of the muscle. This is called the trap-door effect. Radiologists should be vigilant for this injury and alert the surgeon. This represents a true emergency to reduce the fracture.
- Blow-out fracture may lead to diplopia (herniation of inferior rectus), orbital bruising and swelling.
- Fractures of the apex of the orbit may result in optic nerve injury – a surgical emergency.
- ZMC fracture resulting in increased orbital volume following disruption of the zygomatico-sphenoid suture. This results in less displacement of the orbital floor fracture making it less conspicuous.

Suggested reading

Refer to Section 9.10.

9.12 Miscellaneous: Orbital cellulitis

Infections of the orbit are common. It usually occurs from associated sinus infection via vascular spread. Anatomical location of infection in relation to the orbital septum is important as this will define the type of treatment on offer to the patient. See Fig. 9.12.

Findings

Pre-septal cellulitis

1. Pre-septal soft tissue swelling and fat stranding.
2. Fluid collection.
3. Usually orbital bones are intact.

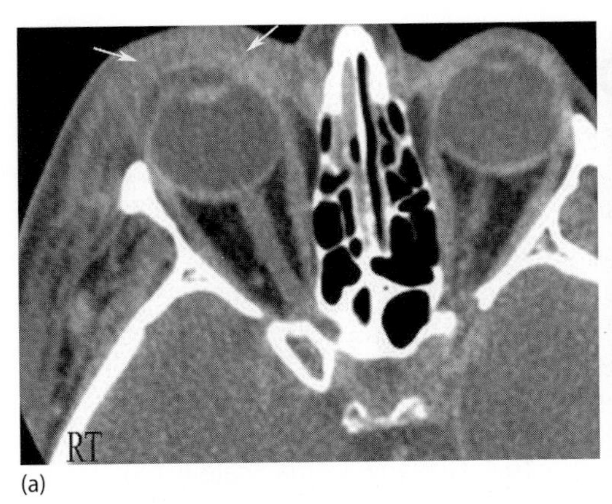

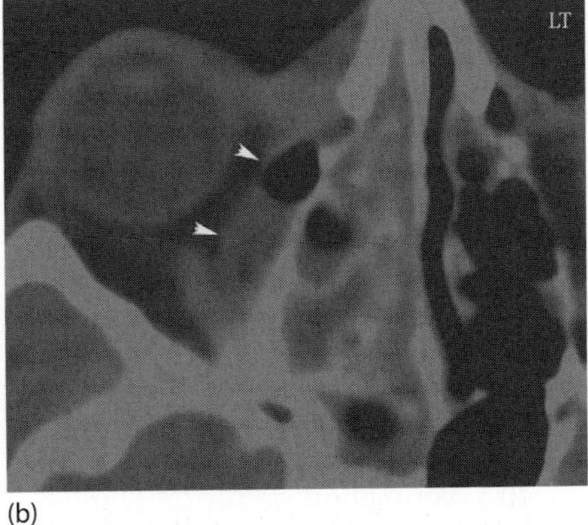

(a) (b)

Fig. 9.12. (a) Pre-septal cellulitis. Axial CT shows marked soft tissue swelling (arrows) anterior to septum. No abscess formation. (b) Intra-orbital cellulitis. Axial CT orbit shows right ethmoidal sinusitis and right intra-orbital abscess (arrowheads).

Post-septal cellulitis

4. Focal peripherally enhancing fluid collection or abscess within the orbit along the post-septal region.
5. May be associated with bony destruction.
6. Soft tissue stranding.
7. Both types are associated with sinus infection.

Pearls

- Pre-septal or periorbital infection is treated with antibiotics.
- Post-septal (subperiosteal collection) or orbital infection is treated with intravenous antibiotics and by surgery if abscess formation occurs.
- Proptosis is greater in orbital than periorbital cellulitis.
- Complications include cavernous sinus thrombosis, intracranial extension of infection, increased intra-orbital pressure and loss of visual acuity.

Suggested reading

LeBedis CA, Sakai O. Nontraumatic orbital conditions: diagnosis with CT and MR in the emergent setting. *RadioGraphics* 2008;**28**:1741–1753.

Chapter

10 Miscellaneous

Swati P. Deshmane and Mayil S. Krishnam

10.1 Ventilation perfusion scan

Although CT pulmonary angiography (CTPA) has become a new gold standard in the diagnosis of pulmonary embolism (PE), non-invasive ventilation perfusion (V/Q) imaging still plays a role as an initial modality of choice in some institutions. Patients who clinically are thought to have PE but have normal chest radiographs and have no previous history of cardiopulmonary disease are potentially good candidates to undergo this study. In this clinical setting, a normal perfusion scan alone is very useful in excluding PE with approximately 96% accuracy. However, the role of V/Q scan is very limited in ER patients with suspected PE, especially out of hours. See Fig. 10.1.

Technique

Perfusion scan

Before injection ask the patient to cough and take deep breaths.
Inject Tc 99 m labeled microaggregates of albumin (1.5–5 mCi).
Obtain images (300 000 counts) in six views: Anterior, posterior, RAO, LAO, RPO, LPO.

Ventilation scan

Tc 99 m DTPA aerosol by inhalation 6 mCi.
Similar six views as perfusion scan.
or
^{133}Xenon gas 5 mCi–10 mCi.
One view scan, usually posterior.

PIOPED criteria

High probability

Two or more large segmental mismatched perfusion defects.
At least 1 large defect with 2 moderate mismatched perfusion defects.
At least 4 moderate mismatched perfusion defects.

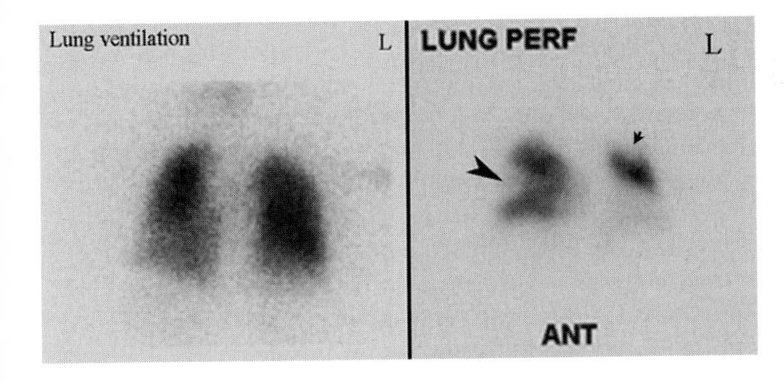

Fig. 10.1. Ventilation and perfusion lung scan. Single anterior view of ventilation scan in a patient with acute onset chest pain and breathlessness shows normal tracer uptake in both lungs. However, corresponding anterior view of the perfusion scan image shows multiple segmental wedge-shaped defects in both lungs as photopenic regions (arrows). These mismatched defects are most consistent with high probability of pulmonary embolism.

Intermediate probability

One moderate to 2 large segmental mismatched perfusion defects.
Single large matched perfusion defects with normal chest radiograph.
Difficult to categorize as low or high.

Low probability

Non-segmental perfusion defects.
Single moderate mismatched segmental perfusion defect with normal chest radiograph.
Any perfusion defect with substantially larger chest radiographic abnormality.
Small segmental perfusion defects with a normal chest radiograph.
Matched perfusion defect involving $< 50\%$ of one lung or $< 75\%$ lung zone.

Normal

Normal perfusion images.

Interpretation

A high probability scan showing mismatched ventilation–perfusion defect confirms the diagnosis of pulmonary embolism while low probability or normal scan, in patients with a low pretest probability, excludes the diagnosis of pulmonary embolism.

If the scan is intermediate or non-diagnostic, further imaging with CTPA or catheter pulmonary angiography is required to reach a diagnosis.

A low-probability scan does not completely rule out PE. If the pretest clinical probability for PE is high, proceed to CTPA.

Pearls

- Causes of V/Q matched defects (abnormal ventilation corresponding to the region of perfusion defect): Chronic obstructive pulmonary disease, pneumonia, emphysema.
- Causes of V/Q mismatched defects (normal ventilation in the region of perfusion defects): Pulmonary embolism (thrombus/air/fat/tumor/sickle cell disease), extrinsic vessel compression – bronchogenic carcinoma, lymphadenopathy, pulmonary artery sarcoma, absent or hypoplastic pulmonary artery, pulmonary stenosis, pulmonary veno-occlusive disease, primary pulmonary hypertension, vasculitis.

- False positive V/Q mismatch can be seen: Any emboli other than thrombus, vasculitis, IV drug abusers.
- False negative V/Q mismatch: Saddle embolus in the pulmonary artery bifurcation. A perfusion defect is not necessarily seen because the central occlusion is only partial, enabling microaggregates to travel into peripheral arteries.
- *In revised PIOPED criteria*, a single, moderate-sized mismatched segmental defect was held inappropriate for low probability. Also, multiple-matched defects are considered to be of low probability if they are the only perfusion defects present. This was further modified by grouping together low and intermediate probability ventilation perfusion scans as "non-diagnostic" category. This group of patients requires further imaging with CTPA to diagnose or rule out pulmonary embolism.
- Doppler ultrasound of leg should be carried out in compliance with the VQ scan to rule out deep venous thrombosis.
- Advantages of CTPA include direct visualization of intra-luminal emboli or thrombi, right heart strain (increased RV/LV ratio), clot burden, pulmonary perfusion abnormality, peripheral infarction, pleural effusion and, if needed, simultaneous CT venogram of the pelvic and lower extremity deep veins at the same sitting. CTPA will also demonstrate alternative pathology.

Suggested reading

Gottschalk A. New criteria for ventilation – perfusion lung scan interpretation: a basis for optimal interaction with helical CT angiography. *RadioGraphics* 2000;**20**:1206–1210.

Gottschalk A *et al.* Ventilation perfusion scintigraphy in the PIOPED study. Part II. Evaluation of the scintigraphic criteria and interpretations. *J Nucl Med* 1993;**34**:1109–1118.

10.2 Contrast media reaction

Intravenous iodinated contrast media reaction

Adverse reactions to IV non-ionic water-soluble iodinated contrast media are rare (incidence of severe and very severe reactions is 0.04% and 0.004% respectively) but they do occur idiosyncratically. Most reactions occur within 20 minutes following intravenous administration of contrast. Patients with an increased risk of contrast reactions can be supervised for 30–60 minutes before discharge from the radiology suite. Before administering contrast media the radiologist should be aware of adverse reactions and the first line of treatment. An emergency box should be well-stocked (adrenaline 1:1000, H1 antihistamine IV, atropine, beta-2 agonist, IV fluids such as 0.9% normal saline or Ringer lactate solutions, hydrocortisone IV), ready to hand and maintained regularly. Staff in the Radiology department should be familiar with the location of such equipment (oxygen, crash trolley, sphygmomanometer, nebulizers, suction tubes) and its proper use.

Clinical features and management

Mild reaction

Clinical signs and symptoms: Nausea, vomiting, urticaria, sensation of warmth and flushing.

Treatment: General assurance. Observe, usually no treatment is required. Chlorpheniramine IV and hydrocortisone IV may be considered.

Moderate reaction

Clinical signs and symptoms: Urticaria, vasovagal reaction (hypotension with bradycardia), mild bronchospasm, tachycardia with hypotension.

Treatment: Monitor vital signs. O_2, Trendelenberg position, IV fluids for hypotension, benedryl 50 mg PO/IM/IV or vistanl 25–50 mg PO/IM/IV, β agonist inhalation/nebulizer for bronchospasm, epinephrine (adrenaline) 1:1000 IM 0.1–0.3 ml (if no cardiac contraindications). Monitoring is essential for adrenaline injection.

Severe or generalized anaphylactoid reaction

Clinical signs and symptoms: This is a life-threatening emergency and needs immediate and aggressive treatment. Manifestations include cardiorespiratory distress/collapse, diffuse erythema, profound vasovagal reaction, severe bronchospasm or laryngeal edema, seizures, cardiac arrest, pulmonary edema.

Treatment: Urgent cardiopulmonary resuscitation, advanced life supporting devices, call for cardiac arrest team. O_2 (6–10 L/min), Trendelenberg position, IV fluids, epinephrine (adrenaline) ideally 0.5 mg 1:1000 intramuscular (1 ml 1:10000 IV slowly, this is time consuming and needs close monitoring) and atropine 0.6–1 mg IV slowly up to 2 mg total dose for bradycardia.

Hypertension (severe)

Call medical team. Vitals, Nitroglycerin sublingual 0.4 mg (may repeat up to 3 mg). If no response, labetalol IV.

Vasovagal reaction

Hypotension and bradycardia. Treat with oxygen (6–10 L/m), elevate legs, rapid IV fluids with 0.9% normal saline or Ringers, atropine 0.6–1 mg IV (max 3 mg or 0.04 mg/kg). Ensure clear throat, suction if necessary.

Seizures

Secure airway, O_2, vitals, diazepam 5 mg IV or midazolam 0.5–1 mg IV.

Pulmonary edema

Semi-erect position, O_2, vital signs, call medical team.

Diamorphine 1–3 mg IV slow, frusemide 20–40 mg IV slow.

Delayed reaction

1. Delayed cutaneous reactions: Macular rash, maculopapular rash, pustules. This needs close observation and symptomatic treatment.
2. Contrast-induced nephropathy (CIN): It is more common in patients with pre-existing renal disease or those with associated risk factors.
3. Mumps.
4. Polyarthropathy.

Prophylaxis

Familiarize yourself with local policy for the prophylaxis that has been implemented in your institution/practice.

Prednisolone 50 mg PO at 13 hours, and 7 hours, and 1 hour before contrast media injection plus diphenhydramine (benedryl) 50 mg PO/IM/ IV 1 hour before contrast media injection or methylprednisolone (Medrol)-32 mg PO 12 hours and 2 hours before contrast media injection plus diphenhydramine (benedryl) 50 mg PO/IM/ IV 1 hour before contrast media injection.

If patient is unable to take oral medication, hydrocortisone 200 mg IV at 13 hours, 7 hours, and 1 hour before contrast media injection.

In emergency situations, hydrocortisone 200 mg IV every 4–6 hours plus diphenhydramine (benedryl) 50 mg PO/IM/ IV 1 hour before contrast media injection.

Adverse reactions of gadolinium-based contrast media

Risk factors

1. Chance of developing an adverse reaction is greater and likely to be more severe in patients who have had a reaction at the time of the previous administration.
2. Patients with allergy, atopy, asthma (< 4% chance of developing significant reaction).
3. Patients with previous reaction to iodinated contrast media (6% chance of developing significant reaction).

Clinical and treatment options are similar as for iodinated contrast media adverse drug reactions. Delayed complications include nephrogenic systemic fibrosis (NSF).

Intravenous contrast extravasation

Extravasated contrast media causes an acute inflammatory response in the surrounding soft tissue. Usually there are no sequelae but sometimes tissue necrosis can lead to ulceration and even compartmental syndrome.

Treatment

Elevate the limb above the heart level.
Cold/hot compresses.
Surgical consultation depending upon symptoms and signs.

Iodinated gastrointestinal contrast media

Barium sulphate: Causes inflammation if aspirated.
HOCM: More prone to induce pulmonary edema if aspirated.
LOCM: Reduced risk of pulmonary edema; less mediastinal and peritoneal irritation; less risk of hypovolemia.

Pearls

- Informed consent may be necessary before injection of any intravenous contrast media. Check local policy.
- If the patient has previously developed a contrast allergy it is not an absolute contraindication to administering contrast. However, details of previously administered contrast media and reactions should be known and the treatment should be ready beforehand if such reaction occurs. Also appropriate premedication should be given as a prophylaxis.

- If there is no history of renal impairment in the past and there is no history suggestive of any risk factors for renal damage, recent serum creatinine is not usually necessary.
- In diabetic patients on metformin, there is increased risk of lactic acidosis. Metformin should be stopped at the time of the contrast procedure. The patient should resume metformin after 48 hours. Recent advice from the Royal College of Radiologists (2009) states that in patients with normal serum creatinine and/or eGFR $>$ 60 ml/min there is no requirement to stop metformin if 100 ml or less of contrast medium is administered.
- Contrast media crosses the placental barrier, so avoid contrast administration in pregnancy and in breastfeeding women. In situations where the benefit outweighs the risk and there is no alternative imaging modality to answer the problem, it should be used with caution. Breastfeeding women should express milk via a breast pump before the procedure, and should discard breast milk for 12–24 hours following contrast administration.
- Patients should be warned about the occurrence of delayed contrast reaction although they will most likely be minor ones. Patient should be advised to approach the dermatologist should they occur.
- Pretesting does not predict the occurrence of future reaction and is therefore not recommended.

Suggested reading

American College of Radiology. *Manual on Contrast Media, version 6*, 2008.

Bettmann MA. Frequently asked questions: iodinated contrast agents. *RadioGraphics* 2004;**24**:S3–S10.

Metformin: updated guidance for use in diabetics with renal impairment. June 2009. Ref. no. BFCR (09) 7. www.rcr.ac.uk.

10.3 Nephrogenic systemic fibrosis (NSF)

When gadolinium was introduced as an MRI contrast media it was considered a safe intravenous drug even in patients with renal failure. But there are reports linking high-dose intravenous gadolinium chelate with nephrogenic systemic fibrosis (NSF), especially in patients with severe renal insufficiency (more common with gadodiamide gadopentate dimeglumine).

Nephrogenic systemic fibrosis causes fibrosis of the skin, subcutaneous tissues and many organs such as lung, esophagus, heart, diaphragm, liver, kidneys and skeletal muscles.

Mechanism of NSF induction

Postulated mechanism is that in patients with severe renal insufficiency/renal failure, prolonged excretion of gadolinium causes dissociation of gadolinium ions from the chelate (transmetallation). Free gadolinium forms an insoluble precipitate which accumulates at different sites causing fibrosis. Associated proinflammatory conditions such as infection, major surgery, vascular events or thrombosis increase the risk of NSF.

Recommendations for use of gadolinium

Ask for the relevant history suggestive of renal insufficiency in every patient.

Ask for the estimated GFR before proceeding to gadolinium administration within 6 weeks in patients with renal disease, high-risk patients such as the elderly, diabetics, hypertensive patients, renal transplant patients, patients with severe liver disease.

In high-risk patients:

1. Select alternative imaging modality if possible.
2. Avoid administration of gadolinium. Proceed to the non-contrast MRI study.
3. Use lowest dose possible after taking informed consent if the benefits outweigh the risks (0.1 mmol/kg).
4. Avoid double- or triple-dose study.
5. Avoid gadodiamide and other gadolinium chelates which are most commonly associated with NSF.
6. In patients with end-stage renal disease on renal dialysis, CT with iodinated contrast media may be preferred over MR with contrast.
7. If contrast-enhanced MR is essential, then the study should be done just prior to dialysis (the role of dialysis in prevention of NSF is not proven yet).
8. In cases of renal failure (GFR$<$ 30 ml/min/1.73 m^2) who are not on dialysis *avoid* any intravenous contrast media. If it is essential to administer contrast, the lowest possible dose of gadolinium should be administered after informed consent.

Suggested reading

American College of Radiology. *Manual on Contrast Media, version* 6, 2008.

Sadowski EA *et al.* Nephrogenic systemic fibrosis: risk factors and incidence estimation. *Radiology* 2007;**243**:148.

Royal College of Radiologists. Standards for iodinated intravascular contrast agent administration to adult patients. Ref. no. (05) 7. http://www.rcr.ac.uk

Thomsen HS *et al.* Management of acute adverse reactions to contrast media. *Eur Radiol* 2004;**14**:476–481.

10.4 Glasgow Coma Scale (GCS)

The Glasgow Coma Scale (GCS) is an objective way of describing the level of consciousness of a person.

Three types of responses are checked. Overall score is summation of all three responses from a minimum of 3 to a maximum of 15.

Each category has different grades.

(A) Best motor response: 6, obeying commands; 5, pain localization; 4, withdrawal to pain; 3, flexor response to pain; 2, extensor response to pain; 1, no response to pain.

(B) Best verbal response: 5, orientated to time, place and person; 4, disoriented and confused conversation; 3, inappropriate speech; 2, incomprehensible speech; 1, none.

(C) Eye opening: 4, spontaneous eye opening; 3, eye opening in response to speech; 2, eye opening in response to pain; 1, no eye opening.

Interpretation: Severe injury $</=8$; Moderate injury: 9–12; minor injury: 13–15.

Suggested reading

Teasdale G. Assessment of coma and impaired consciousness: a practical scale. *Lancet* 1974; **304**:81–84.

10.5 Cardiac arrest

The radiologist should be aware of diagnosing as well as treating cardiac arrest at the time of onset. However it is imperative to call for immediate help to get the cardiac arrest team to attend.

Diagnosis

Unconscious and apneic patient with absent carotid pulse.

Management

1. Ask for the cardiac resuscitation team and defibrillator.
2. Precordial thump over the lower third of the sternum and recheck carotid pulse.
3. Start CPR and do not interrupt it except for defibrillation.
4. Maintain the airway by tilting the head and lifting chin. Be sure to clear the mouth.
5. Breathing: Give artificial breathing using bag and mask 2 times, each inflation being for 2 seconds.
6. Chest compression: Chest compressions should be given over lower third of sternum in a ratio of 5:1 and if you are alone 15 compressions to 2 breaths.
7. Try to help the arrest team after it takes over. If appropriate, check the scan when complete for any life-threatening findings such as PE, pneumothorax, significant coronary lesion, etc.

Ventricular fibrillation or tachycardia

8. Defibrillate immediately (shock of at least 300 J initially). Then CPR should be done for 60–90 seconds. If VF/VT is not reversed then additional shocks of maximum 360 J can be given. Adrenaline 1mg IV every 3 min can be given in case of failed defibrillation.
9. If repeated attempts fail to defibrillate, IV amiodarone or lidocaine may need to be given intravenously. Check local policy with arrest team.

Cardiac asystole/electromechanical dissociation

10. External pacing: Atropine 0.6 mg/5 min IV if pacing is unavailable. Adrenaline 1:10 000 1 mg IV every 3 min.
11. IV assess: Should be established at the outset.
12. Intubation.
13. ECG monitoring.
14. Epinephrine (adrenaline) and/or atropine by IV route.
15. If IV not established, intratracheal adrenaline and/or atropine can be given in diluted form (10 ml 0.9% NS) at 3 times the IV dose. Then 5 ventilations to increase the absorption.
16. Acidosis can occur after prolonged resuscitation.
17. Once the patient survives shift the patient to ICU.
18. Remember to regularly check the Crash trolley in the department for emergency drugs.

19. Aware of ABC (Airway, Breathing, and then Circulation) and call for help immediately in cardiac arrest. Try to recognize pre-arrest arrhythmias on ECG.
20. Most common cause of VF or VT is ischemic heart disease. This can proceed to asystole. Common causes of EMD are pneumothorax, PE, hypothermia, drug overdose, etc.

Suggested reading

Longmore M, Wilkinson I, Turmezei T, Cheung CK, eds. *Oxford Handbook of Clinical Medicine.* Oxford University Press, 2007.

http://www.rcr.ac.uk

10.6 Medications

Metformin

Metformin is an oral antidiabetic drug of the biguanide group used to treat non-insulin dependent diabetes mellitus. The most important side effect is the development of lactic acidosis in high-risk patients; 90% of metformin is excreted unchanged from the kidney by glomerular filtration.

Risk factors for lactic acidosis with metformin

Factors decreasing metformin excretion: Renal insufficiency, administration of contrast media in a renal compromised status.

Factors causing increased blood lactate levels by increasing anerobic metabolism: Cardiac failure, cardiac or peripheral muscle ischemia, infection.

Factors depressing metabolism of lactate: Liver dysfunction, alcohol abuse.

Administration of contrast media in patients on metformin

1. If renal function is normal and there are no associated risk factors: There is no need to discontinue metformin prior to administration of contrast media.
2. If renal function is normal but patient has associated risk factors: Discontinue metformin during the procedure and for 48 hours after the procedure is over. Serum creatinine measurement should follow local policy. Reinstitute metformin after 48 hours.
3. Patient with renal compromise: Substitute the procedure with alternative imaging if possible. Weigh up the risk versus benefit of the procedure. Discontinue metformin before contrast media administration. Serum creatinine serially checked by referring physician until it is safe to reinstate metformin.
4. No special precaution is required for MR with gadolinium-containing contrast media.

Suggested reading

American College of Radiology. *Manual on Contrast Media, version 6*, 2008.

Metformin: updated guidance for use in diabetics with renal impairment. June 2009. Ref. no. BFCR (09) 7. www.rcr.ac.uk

Metoprolol

Metoprolol is a beta-adrenergic blocker used to treat angina and hypertension. It is also used to lower the heart rate to < 65 beats per minute (bpm) prior to CT coronary angiography.

Administration

1. If heart rate less than 65 bpm and regular – no need for metoprolol. Proceed to CT.
2. If heart rate is greater than 65 bpm administer metoprolol after ruling out contraindications.
3. Metoprolol 50–100 mg can be given ideally an hour before the cardiac CT scan. If the heart rate is still over 70/min at the time of scan, intravenous metoprolol can be administered just before data acquisition while the patient is on the scanner.
4. Intravenous metoprolol 5 mg every 5 minutes to a maximum dose of 15 mg (some centers advocate up to 40 mg) to reduce the heart rate to less than 65/min on inspiration.
5. Continuous monitoring of pulse, blood pressure until 10 minutes after the scan is recommended.
6. Time to peak after oral administration of metoprolol is 1–2 hours for regular tablet while it is less than 20 min for IV metoprolol.

Contraindications

Asthma on ß-agonist inhalers, heart block, sinus bradycardia (heart rate of less than 60 bpm), severe aortic stenosis (not HOCM), systolic blood pressure of less than 100 mmHg, allergy to the medication or its constituents, cardiac failure, active bronchospasm, pregnant patients, cocaine abuse.

Drug interaction

1. Metoprolol interacts with calcium channel blockers and digoxin that lower both blood pressure and heart rate.
2. Metoprolol can mask signs and symptoms of hypoglycemia in diabetic patients so these patients need to be cautiously watched.

Diazepam

Diazepam belongs to the benzodiazepine group used to treat anxiety, delirium, seizures, tremors.

Administration

1. Usual dose is 2–20 mg IM or IV depending on the indication. Intravenous injections should be given very slowly taking at least 1 min to inject each 5 mg in adults. For pediatric patients >6 months old it should be given in the dose of 0.25 mg/kg IV very slowly over 3 min.
2. Before administering diazepam check for history of kidney disease, liver disease, glaucoma, breathing problems or alcohol intake.

Contraindications

Allergy to benzodiazepine or diazepam, pregnancy (can cause fetal sedation, congenital anomalies), breastfeeding, and narrow angle glaucoma.

Pearls

- Diazepam can cause drowsiness, fatigue and ataxia hence patient should not be allowed to drive or use machinery. Patient's relatives should be informed not to leave the patient alone.
- Antidote is flumazenil.

Chlorpheniramine maleate

Chlorpheniramine maleate is an antihistaminic (H1 antagonist) drug used for prevention and treatment of allergic reaction. Its brand name is chlor-Trimeton.

Contraindications

Hypersensitivity to chlorpheniramine maleate, severe prostatic enlargement, peptic ulcer disease, narrow angle glaucoma, bladder neck obstruction, acute asthma, and newborns (if administered, may possibly cause sudden infant death syndrome).

Drug interaction

Additive effect if used with tricyclic antidepressants, CNS depressants, MAO inhibitors.

Hydrocortisone

Hydrocortisone is a corticosteroid used for the treatment of contrast reaction as well as its prevention in high-risk patients. As systemic oral corticosteroids have onset of action 4–6 hours after administration, they may not be as useful in acute reaction but they help to reduce persistent bronchospasm or hypotension. Intravenous hydrocortisone of 100–200 mg has a potential application in the prevention of contrast reaction in acute setting and in the treatment of patients with acute iodinated contrast reaction.

Index